Biomedical Aspects of Solid Cancers

Rama Krishna Kancha
Editor

Biomedical Aspects of Solid Cancers

Springer

Editor
Rama Krishna Kancha
Centre for Plant Molecular Biology
Osmania University
Hyderabad, India

ISBN 978-981-97-1801-6 ISBN 978-981-97-1802-3 (eBook)
https://doi.org/10.1007/978-981-97-1802-3

This Springer imprint is published by the registered company Springer Nature Singapore Pte Ltd.
The registered company address is: 152 Beach Road, #21-01/04 Gateway East, Singapore 189721, Singapore

This book is dedicated to Padma Shri Late Prof. M. R. S. Rao (1948–2023).

Preface

Cancer is a group of diseases and is the second most leading cause of deaths worldwide next only to the heart disease. The physical, emotional and financial burden imposed by cancer both on individuals and society is immense thus making it an important health challenge. Despite the progress in basic and translational research in the past decades, several gaps still exist in our understanding of the mechanistic basis of cancer. Diagnostic and therapeutic advances in the recent past have improved the patient survival but limited to a few cancers or their sub-types. The introduction of cancer as a subject or a topic in undergraduate and postgraduate courses of biology and medicine testifies the importance of preparing students for a career in cancer research. In most textbooks, biological and medical aspects of cancer were presented separately; therefore, it is also important to present both the aspects in a single textbook to help students and researchers of both biology and medicine streams gain an integrated understanding of the disease. A consortium of biologists and clinicians was thus formed to adequately achieve this objective by authoring 26 chapters each dedicated to a solid cancer. Each chapter of the book details the biomedical aspects of a certain solid cancer including epidemiology, risk factors and diagnosis as part of the introduction section followed by the classification into sub-types based on various criteria, pathophysiology, treatment, conclusion and references. Multiple classifications are presented for each cancer. Under pathophysiology section, the basic anatomy of the organ, cell of origin of that cancer type or sub-type and genetics along with known mechanisms of disease progression are discussed. In treatment section, surgery, radiotherapy, chemotherapy, targeted therapy and immunotherapy are presented. This inter-institutional and cross-disciplinary collaborative work is possible due to constant support and encouragement from Prof. D. Ravinder, the Vice Chancellor of Osmania University. In addition, many professors, scientists, oncologists and students supported this work both directly and indirectly to realise this vision. In summary, all the basic biomedical aspects of each solid cancer are presented in a simple manner for the benefit of readers belonging to both biology and medicine communities.

Hyderabad, India　　　　Rama Krishna Kancha

About the Book

This book offers a comprehensive overview of essential basics of 26 solid cancers and thus serves as a beginner's guide to biomedical students, clinicians and researchers. The evolving landscape of cancer research and treatment requires that the basic scientists understand clinical challenges and oncologists understand the biological basis of cancer. This book serves these objectives by providing a quick, simplified and updated review of various aspects of solid cancers thereby addressing an unmet need for upcoming researchers in the present era of genetic or genomic medicine.

The clinical information presented in the book evokes interest in biological researchers to understand cancer from a medical point of view and helps frame new hypotheses and questions to address the challenges in each solid cancer. On the other hand, the genetic and molecular details provided in the book helps medical students and practitioners understand the biological mechanisms underlying disease pathogenesis and treatment response. Each chapter provides the epidemiology, risk factors, classification, pathophysiology, genetics and treatment of solid cancers in a systematic and easy-to-understand manner, catering to the needs of biological researchers, students and medical practitioners in the era of personalised cancer medicine.

Contents

1 Lung Cancer

Salwa Hareem, Veena Akula, Sandhya Annamaneni,
Krishna Chaitanya Puligundla, and Rama Krishna Kancha

1.1 Introduction

1.1.1 Epidemiology

In 2020, lung cancer ranked second with a global incidence of 22,06,771 diagnoses, accounting for 11.4% of all cancers, and mortality with 17,96,144 deaths, accounting for 18% [1]. The 5-year survival rate for men and women is 17% and 24%, respectively. According to GLOBOCAN, the incidence is highest in Eastern Asia (10,12,021 cases), followed by Central and Eastern Europe (1,51,632 cases), and Western Europe (1,46,460 cases). Similarly, mortality is highest in Eastern Asia (8,41,174 deaths), followed by North America (1,59,641 deaths), and Central and Eastern Europe (1,30,596 deaths). The global incidence is significantly higher in males (14,35,943 cases, cumulative risk of 3.78) than in females (7,70,828 cases, cumulative risk 1.77). Similarly, global mortality rates are also higher in males (11,88,679 deaths, cumulative risk 3.08) than in females (607,465 deaths, cumulative risk 1.34). As per the SEER data in the United States, the median age of diagnosis and death is 71 and 72 years, respectively.

S. Hareem · V. Akula · R. K. Kancha (✉)
Molecular Medicine and Therapeutics Laboratory, CPMB, Osmania University, Hyderabad, India
e-mail: ramakancha@osmania.ac.in

S. Annamaneni
Department of Genetics and Biotechnology, Osmania University, Hyderabad, India

K. C. Puligundla (✉)
Department of Medical Oncology, MNJ Institute of Oncology and Regional Cancer Centre, Hyderabad, India

R. K. Kancha (ed.), *Biomedical Aspects of Solid Cancers*,
https://doi.org/10.1007/978-981-97-1802-3_1

1.1.2 Risk Factors

Among modifiable risk factors, smoking tobacco is the major cause of lung cancer [2]. Cigarette smokers constitute about 90% of all lung cancer cases, and second-hand smokers have a 20–30% increased risk [2, 3]. The frequency of past or present smokers among lung cancer patients is about 80% and 50% among men and women, respectively [4]. There is about a 30-fold increase in the risk of lung cancer in smokers compared to nonsmokers [2]. Drinking three or more alcoholic beverages per day was linked to a 2.5-fold increased risk of squamous cell carcinoma of the lung [5]. Carotenoids in food and physical activity were linked to a decreased risk [3, 6, 7]. Lung cancer is more common in workers exposed to tar and soot, such as coke oven workers [3]. Organic dust exposure at work increases the risk of lung cancer, while silicosis is linked to increased lung cancer mortality [8, 9]. Exposure to asbestos and radon, as well as indoor air pollution resulting from the burning of biomass, are associated with elevated lung cancer risk [3, 10]. Among nonmodifiable risk factors, a family history of lung cancer was linked to a higher risk of developing lung cancer [11]. Linkage studies and GWAS have identified several candidate gene loci associated with the onset of lung cancer, namely 5p15, 6p21, 15q25, 3q28, etc. [12]. Previous respiratory diseases such as chronic bronchitis, pneumonia, asthma, and emphysema were also associated with an increased risk [4].

1.1.3 Screening and Diagnosis

In the 1970s, chest radiography and sputum cytology were the main screening strategies for diagnosing lung cancer [13, 14]. It has been reported that 80% of lung cancer patients who were diagnosed at late nonsurgical stages die soon after diagnosis [15]. Radiology and sputum cytology were used for early diagnosis of lung cancer, but there was no reduction in disease-specific mortality [16]. The low-dose helical computed tomography (LDCT) scan detects early-stage cancer far more successfully than traditional chest radiographs [16, 17]. However, this method suffers from a decreased sensitivity in detecting most squamous cell lung cancers and soft tissue abnormalities that are located in the central regions of the lung and middle of the thorax, respectively [18]. The risk of hemorrhage is 1% for transbronchial biopsy and 15% for pneumothorax [19]. FDG-PET screening is useful in avoiding biopsies for benign lesions [16].

Immunohistochemistry (IHC) is used for diagnosing and classifying lung cancer based on histology [20]. Thyroid transcription factor 1 (TTF-1) for adenocarcinoma and p40 for squamous cell carcinoma are the best markers for the classification of NSCLC [20]. The elevated levels of cytokeratin 19 fragment, carcinoembryonic antigen, and carbohydrate antigen 125 in the blood/serum are used as diagnostic markers for lung cancer [21]. Lung cancer enhances the stimulation of the complement system, resulting in increased C4d levels in body fluids [22]. Squamous cell lung cancer has been linked to increased expression of miR-93 and miR-221, while adenocarcinoma has been linked to high levels of miR-100 [20]. Recently, long noncoding RNAs such as *MALAT1*, *H19*, *HOTAIR*, *ANRIL*, and *UCA1* were reported to be overexpressed, while *MEG3*, *TUG1*, and *GAS5* showed down-regulation and correlated significantly with cancer stage, metastasis, and patient survival, indicating their clinical potential as markers of lung cancer prognosis and therapy [23].

1.2 Classification

Different types of classifications include anatomical, histological, and staging. Anatomical classification: based on the anatomic site, lung cancer is divided into two subtypes according to their location: (1) central lung cancer, mostly squamous cell carcinoma and small cell lung carcinoma, and (2) peripheral lung cancer, mostly adenocarcinoma.

1.2.1 Histological Classification

Based on histology, there are two subtypes: (1) small cell lung cancer (SCLC) and (2) non-small cell lung cancer (NSCLC) (Fig. 1.1). (1) SCLC is further classified into (a) pure SCLC (P-SCLC), accounting for 85% and (b) combined SCLC (C-SCLC), accounting for 15% of SCLCs (Fig. 1.1) [24]. (2) NSCLC includes (a) squamous cell carcinoma (SCC), accounting for 20%, (b) large cell carcinoma (LCC), accounting for 3%, and (c) adenocarcinoma, accounting for 40% of lung cancers (Fig. 1.1) [25–27].

1.2.2 Staging

TNM system: The TNM system denotes tumor size (T), involvement of adjacent lymph nodes (N), and metastasis (M) [28, 29]. Tx defines a primary tumor with malignant cells in sputum or bronchial washings [30]. T_0 indicates no evidence of a primary tumor, and Tis refers to carcinoma in situ [30]. T1 specifies tumors with a size <3 cm, surrounded by lung or visceral pleura [31]. T1 is further classified into T1a (minimal invasive adenocarcinoma with a tumor size of ≤1 cm), T1b (tumor with a size >1 cm but ≤2 cm), and T1c (tumor with a size >2 cm but ≤3 cm) [32].

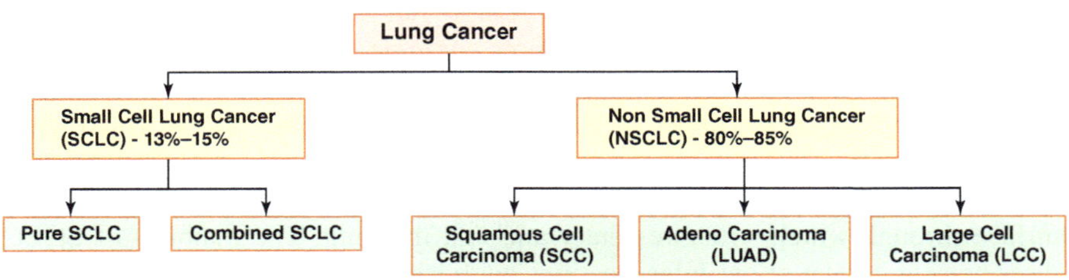

Fig. 1.1 Classification of lung cancers

T2 defines a tumor with a size of >3 cm but ≤5 cm along with the involvement of the main bronchus [31]. T2 is classified into T2a (tumor with a size >3 cm but ≤4 cm) and T2b (tumor with a size >4 cm but ≤5 cm) [30, 32]. T3 indicates a tumor with a size of >5 cm but ≤7 cm and may associate with separate tumor nodule(s) in the same lobe as the primary tumor or directly invades the chest wall [31]. T4 refers to the tumor with a size of >7 cm [30, 31]. Nx specifies that lymph nodes cannot be assessed, N_0 indicates no evidence of regional lymph node metastasis, N1 denotes metastasis in the ipsilateral peribronchial and/or ipsilateral hilar lymph nodes, N2 refers to metastasis in the mediastinal and/or subcarinal lymph nodes on the ipsilateral side, and N3 represents tumor metastasis in contralateral mediastinal and/or hilar, ipsilateral, or contralateral scalene or supraclavicular lymph nodes [33]. M_0 and M1 indicate the absence or presence of distant metastasis, respectively. M1 is further classified into M1a, which indicates a separate tumor module in a contralateral lobe, M1b indicates single extrathoracic metastasis, and M1c specifies multiple extrathoracic metastases [30]. Based on the TNM, stages IA1 till IIA represent N0M0 but vary in T: IA1 with T1a, IA2 with T1b, IA3 with T1c, IB with T2a, and IIA with T2b. Stages IIB to IIIC are M0 but with varying T and N: stage IIB has T1a–c/T2a/T2b with N1 or T3 with N0; stage IIIA has T1a–c/T2a–b with N2 or T3 with N1 or T4 with N0/N1; stage IIIB has T1a–c/T2a–b with N3 or T3/T4 with N2; stage IIIC has T3/T4 with N3. Stage IVA has any T and any N combined with either M1a or M1b, while stage IVB has any T and any N combined with M1c [30].

1.3 Pathophysiology

1.3.1 Anatomy and Histology

The lungs are a pair of spongy organs located on either side of the thorax. Inhaled air is conducted by the trachea or windpipe, which is a solid tube that passes anterior to the esophagus and is roughly 12 cm long and 2.5 cm wide, into the lungs by tubular branches called bronchi [34]. The inner lining of the tracheal and bronchial mucosa is made up of a pseudostratified ciliated columnar epithelium interspersed with goblet cells that lie on top of a basement membrane [35]. In an adult, the right lung weighs 155–720 g, and the left lung weighs 112–675 g [36]. The volume ratio of the right lung is slightly larger (53%) than that of the left lung (47%) [37]. Lung volume ranges from 3.5 to 8.5 L [38, 39]. The pleura is a two-layered membranous structure that forms the pleural sac [40]. Large cell lung carcinoma (LCLC) can develop in any part of the lung, but it is more common on the lung's periphery.

The right lung and the left lung are subdivided into three lobes (upper, middle, and lower) and two lobes (upper and lower lobe), respectively [37, 41]. The trachea divides at the sternal angle into the right and left major bronchi [34]. The primary bronchi enter the lungs at the hilum, which is the area on the lung's mediastinal surface through which structures enter and exit the lung. The majority of SCLC cases present in hilar or perihilar locations, with less than 5% occurring in the pleural area [42]. These primary bronchi branch into lobar bronchi, which supply air to each lobe [37]. Squamous cell carcinomas (SCC) typically develop in the lung's intermediate structures, such as the bronchi. Furthermore, secondary bronchi are divided into tertiary bronchi that supply air to bronchopulmonary segments, which are the lobe subdivisions. Each bronchiole is subdivided into terminal bronchioles [34]. In the terminal bronchiole, smooth muscle decreases and becomes scarce [37]. Terminal bronchioles lack mucous glands or goblet cells [34]. Each terminal bronchiole produces two or many smaller respiratory bronchioles with alveoli budding on their walls [34]. The scanty lining of smooth muscle is present on the walls of the respiratory bronchioles [34].

Ciliated cells, goblet cells, basal cells, and neuroendocrine cells are the major types of cells of the bronchial epithelium (Fig. 1.2) [36]. Ciliated epithelial cells make up 50–80% of the airway epithelium and function in propelling foreign particles [43, 44]. Goblet cells are present in both larger and smaller bronchi but not in the bronchioles (Fig. 1.2). In the proximal airways, goblet cells account for 5–15% of the epithelial cell lining [45]. The layer of protective mucus that coats the airway epithelium is produced by mucus-secreting goblet cells and ciliated cells [46]. Basal cells are found in 34% of the trachea, 27% of the big airways, and 10% of the small airways [47]. The basal cell, unlike the other bronchial epithelial cells, usually survives mucosal lesions to facilitate complete bronchial mucosa repair (Fig. 1.2) [36]. Acute lesions to the respiratory epithelium can result in the loss of ciliated cells and a reparative response in which the wounded area is covered by a thin, undifferentiated epithelial cell lining. When irritation becomes recurrent or persistent, the airway lining undergoes a change to differentiated metaplastic squamous epithelium. Squamous cell cancer of the lung is thus thought to emerge not from the initial respiratory epithelium but rather from areas of injury, repair, and squamous metaplasia and dysplasia that are produced in the bronchial epithelium.

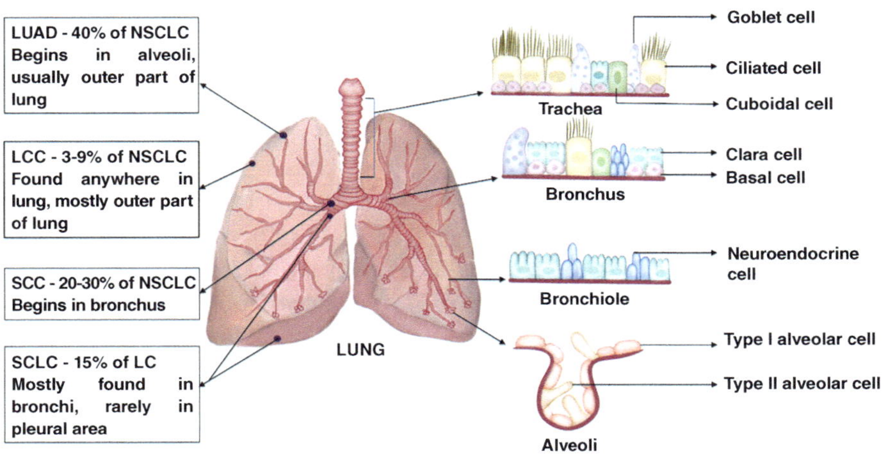

Fig. 1.2 Cell types and origins of lung cancer. *BCC* basal cell, *NE* neuroendocrine, *ATII* alveolar type II, *LC* lung cancer, *NSCLC* non-small cell lung cancer, *SCC* squamous cell carcinoma, *LUAD* adenocarcinoma, *LCC* large cell carcinoma

Each respiratory bronchiole is divided into 2–10 alveolar ducts, which are long, thin-walled airways with alveoli along their walls [34]. The ducts terminate in alveolar sacs, which are groups of alveoli arranged around a central region known as the atrium [34]. Nonciliated simple squamous epithelium covers the alveolar ducts [34]. An alveolus is a small pouch that constitutes squamous and round to cuboidal large (type II) alveolar cells (Fig. 1.2) [48]. Type I alveolar cells are thin, wide cells that cover roughly 95% of the alveolar surface area, whereas type II alveolar cells cover the remaining 5% [48]. Adenocarcinoma develops from cells that coat alveoli that are found throughout the lungs. Alveolar macrophages (dust cells) are the most abundant cells in the lung, wandering the lumens of the alveoli and connective tissue [34].

1.3.2 SCLC

SCLC accounts for roughly 15% of all lung cancers and is more aggressive than NSCLC [24, 49, 50]. Deletion of the retinoblastoma 1 gene (*RB1*) was found in 95% of tumors, while more than 65% of tumors contain mutations in the *TP53* gene [51–54]. This simultaneous inactivation of tumor suppressors differentiates SCLC from NSCLC, in which activating oncogenic mutations are the major drivers of tumorigenesis [55]. In addition, deletion of chromosome 3p has been identified in about 90% of SCLC cancers [56]. Inactivating tumor suppressor mutations were observed in *KMT2D* (13%), *PTEN* (7%), *NOTCH1* (6%), *CREBBP* (5%), *FAT1* (4%), *NF1* (4%), *APC* (4%), *NOTCH3* (2.9%), *ARID1A* (2.9%), *PTPRD* (2.7%), *ATRX* (2.4%), *TSC2* (2.3%), and *EP300* (2.1%) genes. In addition, increased expression of *PIK3CA* (7%), *EGFR* (4%), and *KRAS* (3%) were observed [55]. SCLC cells migrate and survive better when they have high levels of *CXCR4* [57–59]. Interestingly, $\alpha 3\beta 1$ promotes the development of axon-like growth on SCLC cells [60], which increases their ability to metastasize [61].

1.3.3 NSCLC

Lung adenocarcinoma progresses through four stages [62]. Atypical adenomatous hyperplasia (AAH) is the most frequent, followed by adenocarcinoma in situ (AIS), minimally invasive adenocarcinoma (MIA), and fully invasive adenocarcinoma [62]. While all subtypes of NSCLC carry *TP53* and *LRP1B* mutations, adenocarcinoma has a higher incidence of actionable somatic mutations in *KRAS*, *EGFR*, *KEAP1*, *STK11*, *MET*, and *BRAF* than SCC [62–66]. The RAS-RAF-MAPK and PIK3CA-AKT pathways are predominantly disrupted in adenocarcinoma, and the most prevalent chromosomal deletions are on 9p21.3 [64–66].

1.3.4 SCC

Recurring somatic mutations in SCCs were found in *TP53*, *LRP1B*, *CDKN2A*, *KEAP1*, *MLL2*, *HLA-A*, *NFE2L2*, *NOTCH1*, *RB1*, and *PDYN* genes [63]. Furthermore, SCC has a higher frequency of amplification events, particularly in the 3q26–3q29 area of chromosome 3 [63]. *SOX2*, *PIK3-CA*, *TP63*, *MAP3K13*, and *KLH6* are among the several genes in this region that encounter copy number gain or amplification [67, 68]. Furthermore, compared to lung adenocarcinoma (10%), SCC (40–45%) has a high frequency of loss of chromosome 9p21.3 [64, 69]. In SCC, somatic mutations in *KEAP1* and *NFE2L2* genes are linked to oxidative stress response, while copy number alterations in *SOX2* and *TP63* genes are associated with squamous differentiation [70]. Mutations in *PTEN*, *PIK3CA*, and copy number changes within the genes of the PI3K RTK-RAS signaling pathway might be present in up to 70% of SCC cases [63].

1.3.5 LCC

The third-most prevalent subtype of NSCLC is pulmonary LCC, which contributes to 3–9% of all NSCLCs [63]. *PLAUR*, *CTSL*, *VEGFC*, and *PPARG* genes that are involved in tissue remodeling and angiogenesis were overexpressed in large-cell lung carcinoma and metastatic adenocarcinoma [71]. Amplification of the *TP73L* gene was reported in 88% of SCCs, 42% of large cell carcinomas, and 11% of lung adenocarcinomas [72]. Additionally, microdeletion in the *MEN1A* gene and a Lys122Asn missense mutation in the *ACTN4* gene were found [73]. The *BCL2* promoter was aberrantly methylated in about a quarter of NSCLC but not in SCLC [71].

1.4 Treatment

Stage I–IIA SCLC patients typically have a surgical resection, but the prognosis remains poor [74]. Following surgical resection, adjuvant treatment with cisplatin/carboplatin and etoposide is suggested [74]. Chemotherapy is the primary therapeutic choice for SCLC, and irinotecan/cisplatin is effective for extensive disease SCLC [75–77]. Atezolizumab, along with chemotherapy, was reported to be effective in treating advanced-stage SCLC [78]. The overall response rate (ORR) for nivolumab was 11.9% and was approved for use in ES-SCLC patients who didn't respond to platinum-based chemotherapy [79]. The FDA approved Atezolizumab plus carboplatin and etoposide for the treatment of ES-SCLC [79]. Similarly, durvalumab plus etoposide and either carboplatin/cisplatin were approved for ES-SCLC treatment. Pembrolizumab was approved for ES-SCLC patients who had relapsed after platinum-based chemotherapy [79].

Early-stage NSCLC can be treated surgically [80]. Adjuvant platinum-based treatment reduces the risk of death by 5.4% in stages II–IIIA patients [80]. Most patients with stage III NSCLC do not require surgery; a combination of chemoradiotherapy followed by immunotherapy is prescribed [81]. Targeted therapies are recommended for patient-specific oncogenic drivers: EGFR (erlotinib, gefitinib, afatinib, and dacomitinib), ALK and ROS1 (crizotinib, ceritinib, and lorlatinib), ALK and RET (alectinib), ALK (brigatinib), BRAF-V600E (dabrafenib), MEK (trametinib), TRK (entrectinib and larotrectinib), MET (capmatinib and tepotinib), and RET (selpercatinib, pralsetinib, and cabozantinib) [82–94]. The phase 3 study, which compared alectinib to crizotinib, revealed a significant improvement in PFS of 24 months. Brigatinib, Crizotinib, and ceritinib are FDA-approved front-line treatments [81]. In 1–2% of NSCLC cases, *ROS1* rearrangement is an oncogenic driver. These *ROS1*-positive patients respond extremely well to treatment with ceritinib, crizotinib, and entrectinib [83, 93, 95]. Lorlatinib is an option in patients with progressed cancer [84]. Ipilimumab plus nivolumab, a recently approved combination, has a 2.2-month increase in OS [96]. Single-agent pembrolizumab, atezolizumab, or cemiplimab-rwlc are first-line therapy options for eligible patients with metastatic NSCLC regardless of histology, and absence of actionable driver mutations that have recommended first-line targeted therapies.

1.5 Conclusion

Based on histology, lung cancer is broadly divided into SCLC and NSCLC. NSCLC encompasses adenocarcinoma, SCC, and LCC. The invention of LDCT scan was a step forward in the development of lung cancer screening methods. Over the past decade, there have been substantial changes in the treatment of lung cancer. A deeper comprehension of the biology behind lung cancer has led to the development of effective targeted therapies, including immunotherapy. With a considerable improvement in OS, ICIs have replaced other treatments as the preferred option for NSCLC. ICI's therapeutic effect in SCLC is limited to first-line management of extensive-stage disease with small OS improvement. Novel therapeutic strategies, including the sequencing and combining of immune checkpoint inhibitors and other chemotherapeutics, are under clinical trials.

References

1. Sung H, Ferlay J, Siegel RL, Laversanne M, Soerjomataram I, Jemal A, Bray F. Global Cancer Statistics 2020: GLOBOCAN estimates of incidence and mortality worldwide for 36 cancers in 185 countries. CA Cancer Clin. 2021;71:209–49.
2. Minna JD, Roth JA, Gazdar AF. Focus on lung cancer. Cancer Cell. 2002;1:49–52.
3. Alberg AJ, Brock MV, Ford JG, Samet JM, Spivack SD. Epidemiology of lung cancer. Chest. 2013;143(5):e1S–29S.
4. Denholm R, Schüz J, Straif K, Stücker I, Jöckel KH, Brenner DR, De Matteis S, Boffetta P, Guida F, Brüske I, Wichmann HE. Is previous respiratory disease a risk factor for lung cancer? Am J Respir Crit Care Med. 2014;190(5):549–59.

5. Chao C, Li Q, Zhang F, White E. Alcohol consumption and risk of lung cancer in the VITamins and Lifestyle Study. Nutr Cancer. 2011;63(6):880–8.
6. Sun JY, Shi L, Gao XD, Xu SF. Physical activity and risk of lung cancer: a meta-analysis of prospective cohort studies. Asian Pac J Cancer Prev. 2012;13(7):3143–7.
7. Brenner DR, Yannitsos DH, Farris MS, Johansson M, Friedenreich CM. Leisure-time physical activity and lung cancer risk: a systematic review and meta-analysis. Lung Cancer. 2016;95:17–27.
8. Peters S, Kromhout H, Olsson AC, Wichmann HE, Brüske I, Consonni D, Landi MT, Caporaso N, Siemiatycki J, Richiardi L, Mirabelli D. Occupational exposure to organic dust increases lung cancer risk in the general population. Thorax. 2012;67(2):111–6.
9. Lacasse Y, Martin S, Simard S, Desmeules M. Meta-analysis of silicosis and lung cancer. Scand J Work Environ Health. 2005;31:450–8.
10. Szabo E. Lung cancer prevention. In: Fundamentals of cancer prevention. Springer; 2019. p. 511–42.
11. Lissowska J, Foretova L, Dąbek J, Zaridze D, Szeszenia-Dabrowska N, Rudnai P, Fabianova E, Cassidy A, Mates D, Bencko V, Janout V. Family history and lung cancer risk: international multicentre case–control study in eastern and Central Europe and meta-analyses. Cancer Causes Control. 2010;21:1091–104.
12. Musolf AM, Simpson CL, De Andrade M, Mandal D, Gaba C, Yang P, Li Y, You M, Kupert EY, Anderson MW, Schwartz AG. Parametric linkage analysis identifies five novel genome-wide significant loci for familial lung cancer. Hum Hered. 2017;82(1–2):64–74.
13. Vachani A, Sequist LV, Spira A. AJRCCM: 100-year anniversary. The shifting landscape for lung cancer: past, present, and future. Am J Respir Crit Care Med. 2017;195(9):1150–60.
14. Kadara H, Tran LM, Liu B, Vachani A, Li S, Sinjab A, Zhou XJ, Dubinett SM, Krysan K. Early diagnosis and screening for lung cancer. Cold Spring Harb Perspect Med. 2021;11(9):a037994.
15. Mulshine JL, Sullivan DC. Clinical practice. Lung cancer screening. N Engl J Med. 2005;352(26):2714–20.
16. Bastarrika G, García-Velloso MJ, Lozano MD, Montes U, Torre W, Spiteri N, Campo A, Seijo L, Alcaide AB, Pueyo J, Cano D. Early lung cancer detection using spiral computed tomography and positron emission tomography. Am J Respir Crit Care Med. 2005;171(12):1378–83.
17. Luís Duarte M, Dos Santos LR, Oliveira AS, Iared W, Peccin MS. Computed tomography with low-dose radiation versus standard-dose radiation for diagnosing fractures: systematic review and meta-analysis. Sao Paulo Med J. 2021;139:388–97.
18. Nanavaty P, Alvarez MS, Alberts WM. Lung cancer screening: advantages, controversies, and applications. Cancer Control. 2014;21(1):9–14.
19. Jemal A, Clegg LX, Ward E, Ries LA, Wu X, Jamison PM, Wingo PA, Howe HL, Anderson RN, Edwards BK. Annual report to the nation on the status of cancer, 1975–2001, with a special feature regarding survival. Cancer. 2004;101(1):3–27.
20. Šutić M, Vukić A, Baranašić J, Försti A, Džubur F, Samaržija M, Jakopović M, Brčić L, Knežević J. Diagnostic, predictive, and prognostic biomarkers in non-small cell lung cancer (NSCLC) management. J Pers Med. 2021;11:1102.
21. Chen F, Wang XY, Han XH, Wang H, Qi J. Diagnostic value of Cyfra21-1, SCC and CEA for differentiation of early-stage NSCLC from benign lung disease. Int J Clin Exp Med. 2015;8(7):11295.
22. Seijo LM, Peled N, Ajona D, Boeri M, Field JK, Sozzi G, Pio R, Zulueta JJ, Spira A, Massion PP, Mazzone PJ. Biomarkers in lung cancer screening: achievements, promises, and challenges. J Thorac Oncol. 2019;14(3):343–57.
23. Gao X, Wang Y, Zhao H, Wei F, Zhang X, Su Y, Wang C, Li H, Ren X. Plasma miR-324-3p and miR-1285 as diagnostic and prognostic biomarkers for early stage lung squamous cell carcinoma. Oncotarget. 2016;7(37):59664.
24. Guo Y, Yang L, Liu L, Wei J, Teng F, Zhang J, Zhu Y, Xing P, Li J. Comparative study of clinicopathological characteristics and prognosis between combined and pure small cell lung cancer (SCLC) after surgical resection. Thorac Cancer. 2020;11(10):2782–92.
25. Zheng M. Classification and pathology of lung cancer. Surg Oncol Clin. 2016;25(3):447–68.

26. Lewis DR, Check DP, Caporaso NE, Travis WD, Devesa SS. US lung cancer trends by histologic type. Cancer. 2014;120(18):2883–92.
27. Travis WD, Brambilla E, Noguchi M, Nicholson AG, Geisinger K, Yatabe Y, Ishikawa Y, Wistuba I, Flieder DB, Franklin W, Gazdar A. Diagnosis of lung adenocarcinoma in resected specimens: implications of the 2011 International Association for the Study of Lung Cancer/American Thoracic Society/European Respiratory Society classification. Arch Pathol Lab Med. 2013;137(5):685–705.
28. Rami-Porta R, Bolejack V, Crowley J, Ball D, Kim J, Lyons G, Rice T, Suzuki K, Thomas CF Jr, Travis WD, Wu YL. The IASLC lung cancer staging project: proposals for the revisions of the T descriptors in the forthcoming eighth edition of the TNM classification for lung cancer. J Thorac Oncol. 2015;10(7):990–1003.
29. Groome PA, Bolejack V, Crowley JJ, Kennedy C, Krasnik M, Sobin LH, Goldstraw P, IASLC International Staging Committee; Cancer Research and Biostatistics; Observers to the Committee; Participating Institutions. The IASLC Lung Cancer Staging Project: validation of the proposals for revision of the T, N, and M descriptors and consequent stage groupings in the forthcoming (seventh) edition of the TNM classification of malignant tumours. J Thorac Oncol. 2007;2(8):694–705.
30. Goldstraw P, Chansky K, Crowley J, Rami-Porta R, Asamura H, Eberhardt WE, Nicholson AG, Groome P, Mitchell A, Bolejack V, Rami-Porta R. The IASLC lung cancer staging project: proposals for revision of the TNM stage groupings in the forthcoming (eighth) edition of the TNM classification for lung cancer. J Thorac Oncol. 2016;11(1):39–51.
31. Rami-Porta R, Ball D, Crowley J, Giroux DJ, Jett J, Travis WD, Tsuboi M, Vallieres E, Goldstraw P, IASLC International Staging Committee; Cancer Research and Biostatistics; Observers to the Committee; Participating Institutions. The IASLC lung cancer staging project: proposals for the revision of the T descriptors in the forthcoming (seventh) edition of the TNM classification for lung cancer. J Thorac Oncol. 2007;2(7):593–602.
32. Goldstraw P. The 7th edition of TNM in lung cancer: what now? J Thorac Oncol. 2009;4(6):671–3.
33. Rusch VW, Asamura H, Watanabe H, Giroux DJ, Rami-Porta R, Goldstraw P. The IASLC lung cancer staging project: a proposal for a new international lymph node map in the forthcoming seventh edition of the TNM classification for lung cancer. J Thorac Oncol. 2009;4(5):568–77.
34. Saladin KS, McFarland R, Gan CA, Cushman HN. Essentials of anatomy and physiology. McGraw-Hill Education; 2014.
35. Prange T. Chapter 48: Trachea. In: Equine surgery. 5th ed. Missouri: Elsevier; 2019. p. 797–804.
36. Tomashefski JF Jr, Farver CF. Anatomy and histology of the lung. In: Dail DH, Hammar SP, editors. Dail and Hammar's pulmonary pathology: volume I: nonneoplastic lung disease. New York: Springer; 2008. p. 20–48.
37. Molina DK, DiMaio VJ. Normal organ weights in men: part II—the brain, lungs, liver, spleen, and kidneys. Am J Forensic Med Pathol. 2012;33(4):368–72.
38. Sobonya RE. Normal anatomy and development of the lung. In: Baum GL, Wolinsky E, editors. Textbook of pulmonary diseases. 4th ed. Boston: Little, Brown; 1989. p. 3–20.
39. Thurlbeck WM. Post-mortem lung volumes. Thorax. 1979;34(6):735–9.
40. Mahabadi N, Goizueta AA, Bordoni B. Anatomy, thorax, lung pleura and mediastinum. In: StatPearls [Internet]. Treasure Island (FL): StatPearls Publishing; 2018.
41. Felson B. Chest roentgenology. Philadelphia: WB Saunders; 1973.
42. Touman AA, Vitsas VV, Koulouris NG, Stratakos GK. Gaining access to the periphery of the lung: bronchoscopic and transthoracic approaches. Ann Thorac Med. 2017;12(3):162.
43. Yaghi A, Dolovich MB. Airway epithelial cell cilia and obstructive lung disease. Cells. 2016;5(4):40.
44. Park KS, Wells JM, Zorn AM, Wert SE, Laubach VE, Fernandez LG, Whitsett JA. Transdifferentiation of ciliated cells during repair of the respiratory epithelium. Am J Respir Cell Mol Biol. 2006;34(2):151–7.

45. Gohy S, Carlier FM, Fregimilicka C, Detry B, Lecocq M, Ladjemi MZ, Verleden S, Hoton D, Weynand B, Bouzin C, Pilette C. Altered generation of ciliated cells in chronic obstructive pulmonary disease. Sci Rep. 2019;9(1):1–2.
46. Boucherat O, Boczkowski J, Jeannotte L, Delacourt C. Cellular and molecular mechanisms of goblet cell metaplasia in the respiratory airways. Exp Lung Res. 2013;39(4–5):207–16.
47. Crystal RG. Airway basal cells. The "smoking gun" of chronic obstructive pulmonary disease. Am J Respir Crit Care Med. 2014;190(12):1355–62.
48. Knudsen L, Ochs M. The micromechanics of lung alveoli: structure and function of surfactant and tissue components. Histochem Cell Biol. 2018;150:661–76.
49. Varricchio CG, editor. A cancer source book for nurses. Jones & Bartlett Learning; 2004.
50. Yoder LH. An overview of lung cancer symptoms, pathophysiology, and treatment. Medsurg Nurs. 2006;15(4):231.
51. D'amico D, Carbone D, Mitsudomi T, Nau M, Fedorko J, Russell E, Johnson B, Buchhagen D, Bodner S, Phelps R. High frequency of somatically acquired p53 mutations in small-cell lung cancer cell lines and tumors. Oncogene. 1992;7(2):339–46.
52. Helin K, Holm K, Niebuhr A, Eiberg H, Tommerup N, Hougaard S, Poulsen HS, Spang-Thomsen M, Nørgaard P. Loss of the retinoblastoma protein-related p130 protein in small cell lung carcinoma. Proc Natl Acad Sci. 1997;94(13):6933–8.
53. George J, Lim JS, Jang SJ, Cun Y, Ozretić L, Kong G, Leenders F, Lu X, Fernández-Cuesta L, Bosco G, Müller C. Comprehensive genomic profiles of small cell lung cancer. Nature. 2015;524(7563):47–53.
54. Meder L, König K, Ozretić L, Schultheis AM, Ueckeroth F, Ade CP, Albus K, Boehm D, Rommerscheidt-Fuss U, Florin A, Buhl T. NOTCH, ASCL1, p53 and RB alterations define an alternative pathway driving neuroendocrine and small cell lung carcinomas. Int J Cancer. 2016;138(4):927–38.
55. Rudin CM, Brambilla E, Faivre-Finn C, Sage J. Small-cell lung cancer. Nat Rev Dis Primers. 2021;7(1):3.
56. Wistuba II, Gazdar AF, Minna JD. Molecular genetics of small cell lung carcinoma. In: Seminars in oncology, vol. 28. WB Saunders; 2001. p. 3–13.
57. Burger H, Den Bakker MA, Stoter G, Verweij J, Nooter K. Lack of c-KIT exon 11 activating mutations in c-KIT/CD117-positive SCLC tumour specimens. Eur J Cancer. 2003;39(6):793–9.
58. Hartmann TN, Burger JA, Glodek A, Fujii N, Burger M. CXCR4 chemokine receptor and integrin signaling co-operate in mediating adhesion and chemoresistance in small cell lung cancer (SCLC) cells. Oncogene. 2005;24(27):4462–71.
59. Burger JA, Stewart DJ, Wald O, Peled A. Potential of CXCR4 antagonists for the treatment of metastatic lung cancer. Expert Rev Anticancer Ther. 2011;11(4):621–30.
60. Guo NH, Templeton NS, Al-Barazi H, Cashel J, Sipes JM, Krutzsch HC, Roberts DD. Thrombospondin-1 promotes α3β1 integrin-mediated adhesion and neurite-like outgrowth and inhibits proliferation of small cell lung carcinoma cells. Cancer Res. 2000;60(2):457–66.
61. Yang S, Zhang Z, Wang Q. Emerging therapies for small cell lung cancer. J Hematol Oncol. 2019;12:1–1.
62. Succony L, Rassl DM, Barker AP, McCaughan FM, Rintoul RC. Adenocarcinoma spectrum lesions of the lung: detection, pathology and treatment strategies. Cancer Treat Rev. 2021;99:102237.
63. Suster DI, Mino-Kenudson M. Molecular pathology of primary non-small cell lung cancer. Arch Med Res. 2020;51(8):784–98.
64. Jordan EJ, Kim HR, Arcila ME, Barron D, Chakravarty D, Gao J, Chang MT, Ni A, Kundra R, Jonsson P, Jayakumaran G. Prospective comprehensive molecular characterization of lung adenocarcinomas for efficient patient matching to approved and emerging therapies. Cancer Discov. 2017;7(6):596–609.
65. Ding L, Getz G, Wheeler DA, Mardis ER, McLellan MD, Cibulskis K, Sougnez C, Greulich H, Muzny DM, Morgan MB, Fulton L. Somatic mutations affect key pathways in lung adenocarcinoma. Nature. 2008;455(7216):1069–75.

66. Seo JS, Ju YS, Lee WC, Shin JY, Lee JK, Bleazard T, Lee J, Jung YJ, Kim JO, Shin JY, Yu SB. The transcriptional landscape and mutational profile of lung adenocarcinoma. Genome Res. 2012;22(11):2109–19.
67. Tonon G, Wong KK, Maulik G, Brennan C, Feng B, Zhang Y, Khatry DB, Protopopov A, You MJ, Aguirre AJ, Martin ES. High-resolution genomic profiles of human lung cancer. Proc Natl Acad Sci. 2005;102(27):9625–30.
68. Hussenet T, Dali S, Exinger J, Monga B, Jost B, Dembelé D, Martinet N, Thibault C, Huelsken J, Brambilla E, du Manoir S. SOX2 is an oncogene activated by recurrent 3q26.3 amplifications in human lung squamous cell carcinomas. PLoS One. 2010;5(1):e8960.
69. Kashima J, Kitadai R, Okuma Y. Molecular and morphological profiling of lung cancer: a foundation for "next-generation" pathologists and oncologists. Cancers. 2019;11(5):599.
70. Sato T, Yoo S, Kong R, Sinha A, Chandramani-Shivalingappa P, Patel A, Fridrikh M, Nagano O, Masuko T, Beasley MB, Powell CA. Epigenomic profiling discovers trans-lineage SOX2 partnerships driving tumor heterogeneity in lung squamous cell carcinoma. Cancer Res. 2019;79(24):6084–100.
71. Cooper DN. The molecular genetics of lung cancer. Heidelberg: Springer; 2005. p. 410.
72. Massion PP, Taflan PM, Jamshedur Rahman SM, Yildiz P, Shyr Y, Edgerton ME, Westfall MD, Roberts JR, Pietenpol JA, Carbone DP, Gonzalez AL. Significance of p63 amplification and overexpression in lung cancer development and prognosis. Cancer Res. 2003;63(21):7113–21.
73. Echchakir H, Mami-Chouaib F, Vergnon I, Baurain JF, Karanikas V, Chouaib S, Coulie PG. A point mutation in the α-actinin-4 gene generates an antigenic peptide recognized by autologous cytolytic T lymphocytes on a human lung carcinoma. Cancer Res. 2001;61(10):4078–83.
74. Iyoda A, Azuma Y, Sano A. Neuroendocrine tumors of the lung: clinicopathological and molecular features. Surg Today. 2020;50:1578–84.
75. Noda K, Nishiwaki Y, Kawahara M, Negoro S, Sugiura T, Yokoyama A, Fukuoka M, Mori K, Watanabe K, Tamura T, Yamamoto S. Irinotecan plus cisplatin compared with etoposide plus cisplatin for extensive small-cell lung cancer. N Engl J Med. 2002;346(2):85–91.
76. Jiang J, Liang X, Zhou X, Huang L, Huang R, Chu Z, Zhan Q. A meta-analysis of randomized controlled trials comparing irinotecan/platinum with etoposide/platinum in patients with previously untreated extensive-stage small cell lung cancer. J Thorac Oncol. 2010;5(6):867–73.
77. Lima JP, dos Santos LV, Sasse EC, Lima CS, Sasse AD. Camptothecins compared with etoposide in combination with platinum analog in extensive stage small cell lung cancer: systematic review with meta-analysis. J Thorac Oncol. 2010;5(12):1986–93.
78. Horn L, Mansfield AS, Szczęsna A, Havel L, Krzakowski M, Hochmair MJ, Huemer F, Losonczy G, Johnson ML, Nishio M, Reck M. First-line atezolizumab plus chemotherapy in extensive-stage small-cell lung cancer. N Engl J Med. 2018;379(23):2220–9.
79. Saltos A, Shafique M, Chiappori A. Update on the biology, management, and treatment of small cell lung cancer (SCLC). Front Oncol. 2020;10:1074.
80. Alexander M, Kim SY, Cheng H. Update 2020: management of non-small cell lung cancer. Lung. 2020;198:897–907.
81. Brierley JGM, Wittekind C. TNM classification of malignant tumours. 8th ed. Hoboken: Wiley; 2017.
82. Rosell R, Carcereny E, Gervais R, Vergnenegre A, Massuti B, Felip E, Palmero R, Garcia-Gomez R, Pallares C, Sanchez JM, Porta R. Erlotinib versus standard chemotherapy as first-line treatment for European patients with advanced EGFR mutation-positive non-small-cell lung cancer (EURTAC): a multicentre, open-label, randomised phase 3 trial. Lancet Oncol. 2012;13(3):239–46.
83. Shaw AT, Solomon BJ, Chiari R, Riely GJ, Besse B, Soo RA, Kao S, Lin CC, Bauer TM, Clancy JS, Thurm H. Lorlatinib in advanced ROS1-positive non-small-cell lung cancer: a multicentre, open-label, single-arm, phase 1–2 trial. Lancet Oncol. 2019;20(12):1691–701.
84. Shaw AT, Solomon BJ, Besse B, Bauer TM, Lin CC, Soo RA, Riely GJ, Ou SH, Clancy JS, Li S, Abbattista A. ALK resistance mutations and efficacy of lorlatinib in advanced anaplastic lymphoma kinase-positive non-small-cell lung cancer. J Clin Oncol. 2019;37(16):1370.

85. Lin JJ, Kennedy E, Sequist LV, Brastianos PK, Goodwin KE, Stevens S, Wanat AC, Stober LL, Digumarthy SR, Engelman JA, Shaw AT. Clinical activity of alectinib in advanced RET-rearranged non-small cell lung cancer. J Thorac Oncol. 2016;11(11):2027–32.
86. Sabari JK, Santini FC, Schram AM, Bergagnini I, Chen R, Mrad C, Lai WV, Arbour KC, Drilon A. The activity, safety, and evolving role of brigatinib in patients with ALK-rearranged non-small cell lung cancers. Onco Targets Ther. 2017;10:1983.
87. Planchard D, Besse B, Groen HJ, Souquet PJ, Quoix E, Baik CS, Barlesi F, Kim TM, Mazieres J, Novello S, Rigas JR. Dabrafenib plus trametinib in patients with previously treated BRAFV600E-mutant metastatic non-small cell lung cancer: an open-label, multicentre phase 2 trial. Lancet Oncol. 2016;17(7):984–93.
88. Drilon A, Laetsch TW, Kummar S, DuBois SG, Lassen UN, Demetri GD, Nathenson M, Doebele RC, Farago AF, Pappo AS, Turpin B. Efficacy of larotrectinib in TRK fusion-positive cancers in adults and children. N Engl J Med. 2018;378(8):731–9.
89. Doebele RC, Drilon A, Paz-Ares L, Siena S, Shaw AT, Farago AF, Blakely CM, Seto T, Cho BC, Tosi D, Besse B. Entrectinib in patients with advanced or metastatic NTRK fusion-positive solid tumours: integrated analysis of three phase 1–2 trials. Lancet Oncol. 2020;21(2):271–82.
90. Le X, Paz-Ares LG, Van Meerbeeck J, Viteri S, Cabrera Galvez C, Vicente Baz D, Kim YC, Kang JH, Schumacher KM, Karachaliou N, Adrian S. Tepotinib in patients (pts) with advanced non-small cell lung cancer (NSCLC) with MET amplification (MET amp).
91. Wolf J, Seto T, Han JY, Reguart N, Garon EB, Groen HJ, Tan DS, Hida T, de Jonge M, Orlov SV, Smit EF. Capmatinib in MET exon 14-mutated or MET-amplified non-small-cell lung cancer. N Engl J Med. 2020;383(10):944–57.
92. Gainor JF, Curigliano G, Kim DW, Lee DH, Besse B, Baik CS, Doebele RC, Cassier PA, Lopes G, Tan DS, Garralda E. Pralsetinib for RET fusion-positive non-small-cell lung cancer (ARROW): a multi-cohort, open-label, phase 1/2 study. Lancet Oncol. 2021;22(7):959–69.
93. Drilon A, Oxnard GR, Tan DS, Loong HH, Johnson M, Gainor J, McCoach CE, Gautschi O, Besse B, Cho BC, Peled N. Efficacy of selpercatinib in RET fusion-positive non-small-cell lung cancer. N Engl J Med. 2020;383(9):813–24.
94. Drilon A, Rekhtman N, Arcila M, Wang L, Ni A, Albano M, Van Voorthuysen M, Somwar R, Smith RS, Montecalvo J, Plodkowski A. Cabozantinib in patients with advanced RET-rearranged non-small-cell lung cancer: an open-label, single-centre, phase 2, single-arm trial. Lancet Oncol. 2016;17(12):1653–60.
95. Lim SM, Kim HR, Lee JS, Lee KH, Lee YG, Min YJ, Cho EK, Lee SS, Kim BS, Choi MY, Shim HS. Open-label, multicenter, phase II study of ceritinib in patients with non-small-cell lung cancer harboring ROS1 rearrangement. J Clin Oncol. 2017;35(23):2613–8.
96. Dafni U, Tsourti Z, Vervita K, Peters S. Immune checkpoint inhibitors, alone or in combination with chemotherapy, as first-line treatment for advanced non-small cell lung cancer. A systematic review and network meta-analysis. Lung Cancer. 2019;134:127–40.

Breast Cancer

2

Sai Charitha Mullaguri, Sathish Kumar Mungamuri, Krishna Chaitanya Puligundla, Sandhya Annamaneni, and Rama Krishna Kancha

2.1 Introduction

2.1.1 Epidemiology

Globally, breast cancer ranked first in incidence in the year 2020 with 22,61,419 new cases contributing to 11.7% of all cancers diagnosed and fifth in mortality with 6,84,996 deaths accounting for 6.9% of all cancer-related deaths [1]. According to GLOBOCAN, the incidence and mortality rates were high in Asia (10,26,171 new cases and 3,46,009 deaths), contributing to 45.4% and 50.5% of breast cancer incidence and mortality, respectively [2]. In Europe, breast cancer accounted for 23.5% (5,31,086 new cases) and 20.7% (1,41,765 deaths) of all global breast cancer incidence and deaths, respectively. According to the SEER database for the year 2022, the estimated new breast cancer cases and deaths were 2,90,560 and 43,780, respectively [3]. Based on combined data from the SEER database and the National Program of Cancer Registries of the United States for the year 2022, the number of new cases of invasive breast cancer and ductal carcinoma in situ were 2,87,850 and 51,400, respectively [4]. The 5-year survival rate varied according to clinical

S. C. Mullaguri · R. K. Kancha (✉)
Molecular Medicine and Therapeutics Laboratory, CPMB, Osmania University, Hyderabad, India
e-mail: ramakancha@osmania.ac.in

S. K. Mungamuri
ICMR-National Institute of Nutrition, Hyderabad, India

K. C. Puligundla
Department of Medical Oncology, MNJ Institute of Oncology and Regional Cancer Centre, Hyderabad, India

S. Annamaneni (✉)
Department of Genetics, Osmania University, Hyderabad, India

R. K. Kancha (ed.), *Biomedical Aspects of Solid Cancers*,
https://doi.org/10.1007/978-981-97-1802-3_2

subtype and size of the tumor but mainly varied based on the cancer stage at which the patient is diagnosed; the highest 5-year survival rate (99%) was in patients with localized cancer, and the lowest (29%) was observed in patients with metastatic cancer [3]. The 5-year survival rates for localized, regional metastatic, and distant metastatic stages were 96%, 78%, and 20%, respectively, for women belonging to black race and Hispanic ethnicity, and were >99%, 87%, and 30% for the women belonging to white race [3]. In Europe, the incidence rates were 34.8%, 34.3%, and 22.5%, and mortality rates were 25.1%, 19.3%, and 15.1% for the age groups 0–44 years, 45–64 years, and 65 years or above, respectively [5]. Among women across 185 countries in the age group of 0–39 years, the mortality rates varied to a greater extent than incidence across countries [6]. Based on the cancer data in 2020, the incidence rates were 0.1%, 5.7%, and 46.6%, and mortality rates were 0%, 0.4%, and 4.8% for the age groups 15–19, 20–29, and 30–39, respectively [7].

2.1.2 Risk Factors

Main risk factors are family history of any breast malignancy, sporadic alterations in genes, high levels of estrogen, poor diet and nutrition, excessive alcohol and dietary fat intake, reproductive aspects such as early menarche, late menopause, as well as the use of oral contraceptives [8]. A cohort study of 1,13,000 women from the general UK population concluded that first-degree female relatives of breast cancer patients have a 2.5-fold risk of developing breast cancer [9]. Additionally, a meta-analysis of epidemiological data from 117 case-control studies and cohort studies, including 1,18,964 women, revealed that the menarcheal age is inversely proportional to the risk of developing breast cancer [10]. Another cohort study that included women in the age group 15–49 years in Denmark revealed that women on hormonal contraceptives have a relative breast cancer risk of 1.20 more than women who never used hormonal contraceptives [11].

2.1.3 Diagnosis

The usual methods for detecting breast cancer are screening (mammography and ultrasonography) or the presence of symptoms that include pain or a palpable tumor, which require further diagnostic evaluation [12]. When healthy women are screened, smaller tumors are more likely to be found, which makes them more responsive to lumpectomy and limited axillary surgery, and the patients are less likely to require chemotherapy [13]. Mammography is the only screening method that has been shown to lower deaths due to breast cancer [14, 15]. Breast cancer mortality rate has been reduced by 19% as a result of screening through mammography, with women in their 40s and 60s benefiting less (15%) and more (32%), respectively [16]. A study of 4384 breast cancer patients revealed that ultrasonography has a sensitivity of 100% and specificity of 89.1% [17]. In a meta-analysis of 12 population studies comprising 32,247 patients, the annual mammography in women aged 40–74 years reduced deaths by 36–39%, while additional annual MRI starting at ages 30–35 years reduced mortality due to breast cancer by 54–60% [18].

2.2 Classification

Different classifications have been made based on (1) the site of the tumor, (2) histology, (3) molecular markers, and (4) staging. (1) Based on the site of the tumor, breast cancer is divided into three types: (a) noninvasive: the tumor is present within the lobules and ducts [19], (b) invasive: the tumor has spread to the surrounding regions of the breast tissue [20], and (c) metastatic: the tumor spreads to distant parts (Fig. 2.1) [21].

(2) Based on histology, breast cancer is classified into ductal, lobular, medullary, mucinous, and tubular carcinoma (Fig. 2.1) [22]. (a) Ductal carcinoma (80%) arises in the milk ducts and includes ductal carcinoma in situ (DCIS), which is limited to the mammary ducts [23, 24], and infiltrating ductal carcinoma (IDC), which has spread to the duct walls, breast fatty tissues, and then to the surrounding regions of the breast [25]. (b) Lobular carcinoma (10%) arises in the lobules of the breast and is further divided into two types: lobular carcinoma in situ (LCIS), which is limited to mammary lobules [26], and infiltrating lobular carcinoma (ILC), which has spread to the surrounding regions of the breast [27]. (c) Medullary carcinoma (3–5%) has prominent syncytial growth (a single cell with several nuclei), clearly distinguished margins, and infiltrates into surrounding lymph nodes [28]. (d) Mucinous carcinoma (1–7%), also called colloid carcinoma, is categorized into two types, namely mixed and pure mucinous carcinomas, based on the mucinous

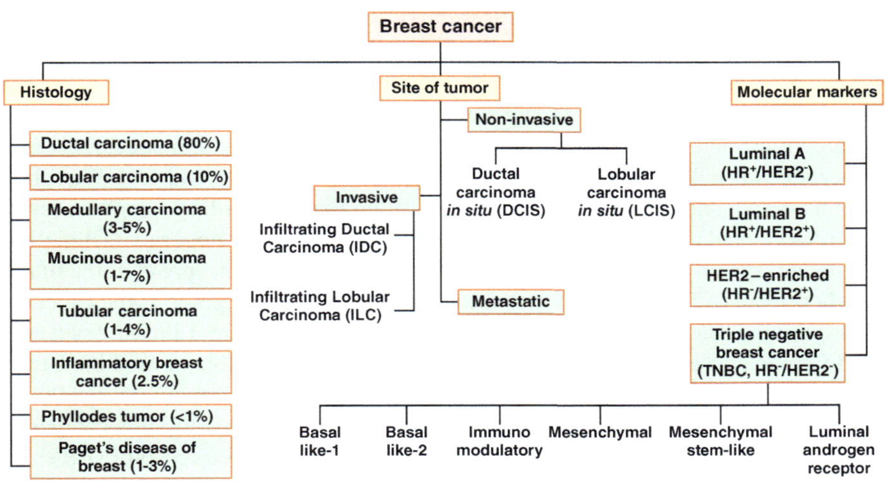

Fig. 2.1 Classification of breast cancer based on histology, site of tumor, and molecular markers

content [29]. Pure mucinous carcinomas have a better prognosis and lesser metastasis to axillary lymph nodes when compared to mixed mucinous carcinomas [30, 31]. (e) Tubular carcinoma (1–4%) consists of cells that are small, have less nodal involvement, and have a better prognosis [32, 33]. DCIS and LCIS are categorized as noninvasive carcinomas, whereas IDC, ILC, medullary, mucinous, and tubular are categorized as invasive carcinomas (Fig. 2.1) [22]. Loss of E-cadherin, a cell-adhesion molecule, is usually observed in ILC, whereas it is expressed in IDC [34]. Other rare subtypes are inflammatory breast cancer (IBC), phyllodes tumor, and Paget's disease of the breast (Fig. 2.1) [22]. IBC is highly aggressive and occurs in about 2.5% of breast cancer patients [35]. Phyllode tumors occur in less than 1% of patients with breast cancer and develop in the connective tissues (stroma) of the breast [36, 37]. Paget's disease of the breast occurs in 1–3% of breast cancer patients and is characterized by visual changes such as red, itchy rashes on the nipple of the breast [38, 39].

(3) Molecular subtypes include (1) HR (hormone receptor) positive (70%) tumors expressing either estrogen receptor (ER) or progesterone receptor (PR) in at least 1% of the tumor cells and (2) *HER2* positive (20%), also called as *ERBB2* positive, which include tumors with overexpression or amplification of the *ERBB2* gene (Fig. 2.1) [15, 40]. Breast cancer can be classified into four subtypes based on the presence or absence of these molecular markers. (a) luminal A, which are HR^+/$HER2^-$, (b) luminal B, which are HR^+/$HER2^+$, (c) HER2-enriched, which are HR^-/$HER2^+$, and (d) triple-negative, which are HR^-/$HER2^-$ (Fig. 2.1) [40, 41]. Based on gene expression analysis of samples present in 21 breast cancer datasets, triple-negative breast cancer (TNBC) was further classified into subtypes that include basal-like 1 (BL-1), basal-like 2 (BL-2), mesenchymal, immunomodulatory (IM), mesenchymal stem-like (MSL), and luminal androgen receptor (LAR) (Fig. 2.1) [42].

(4) According to the eighth edition of the AJCC TNM staging system, breast cancer is classified into different stages [43, 44]. The T categories include T0 (absence of a primary tumor), Tis (the tumor is restricted to the breast tissue and the size is less than 2 cm), T1 (the size of the tumor is less than or equal to 2 cm), T2 (the size of the tumor is between 2 and 5 cm), T3 (the size of the tumor is greater than 5 cm), and T4 (a tumor of any size that grows into the wall of the chest). The N categories include N0 (no spread of the tumor to regional lymph nodes), N1 (the tumor spread to 1–3 axillary lymph nodes), N2 (the tumor spread to 4–9 axillary lymph nodes), and N3 (the tumor spread to more than 10 axillary lymph nodes or the infraclavicular nodes or supraclavicular nodes). The M categories include M0 (no distant spread of the tumor to other organs) and M1 (distant spread of the tumor to other organs). The grades of breast cancer cells include (1) grade 1: the cancer is slow-growing, and the tumor cells resemble the cells of normal breast tissue, (2) grade 2: the cancer is fast-growing, but the tumor cells resemble normal breast tissue cells, and (3) grade 3: faster-growing cancer, and the abnormal tumor cells are more likely to spread to different organs of the body. Combining different categories of TNM, as well as the grades and the status of *HER2*, estrogen receptor (ER), and progesterone receptor (PR), AJCC classifies breast cancer into 0, IA, IB, IIA, IIB, IIIA, IIIB, IIIC, and IV stages.

2.3 Pathophysiology

2.3.1 Anatomy

The female mammary gland consists of two regions, namely stroma and parenchyma. The stroma is further divided into four subregions as follows: (a) adipose tissue, (b) dense interlobular fibrous stroma, (c) periductal stroma, and (d) intralobular mantle stroma. Collagenous connective tissue, circular and longitudinal smooth muscle bundles, and sporadic elastic fibers make up the mammary stroma. The collagenous connective tissue is histologically poor in cells, fibrocytes and (myo)fibroblasts. In the surface stroma of the mammary glands, sebaceous and apocrine glands are present. The parenchyma, which is also known as segments, is made up of 15–25 distinct glands (Fig. 2.2). The milk duct system (ducts) and terminal duct segments with lobules make up each gland, called as a terminal ductulo-lobular unit (TDLU) (Fig. 2.2). The lobules are secretory units with an average diameter of 0.5 mm, and on average, each lobule comprises 40–80 ductules or acini. The entire parenchyma is made up of luminal tissue bordered by a glandular epithelium, which is composed of single-row cubic cells with monomorphic morphology in the interlobular ducts and lobules, and two or more rows of cubic cells in the bigger milk ducts. The entire glandular parenchyma is covered by a basal myoepithelial cell layer, which is encircled by a basement membrane (Fig. 2.2). A distinct, loose mantle tissue covers the parenchyma. The mantle tissue has type III collagen (reticulin fibers) and a dense capillary network. Mast cells, plasma cells, and lymphocytes are the most prevalent cell types in the lobular mantle tissue. The Cooper

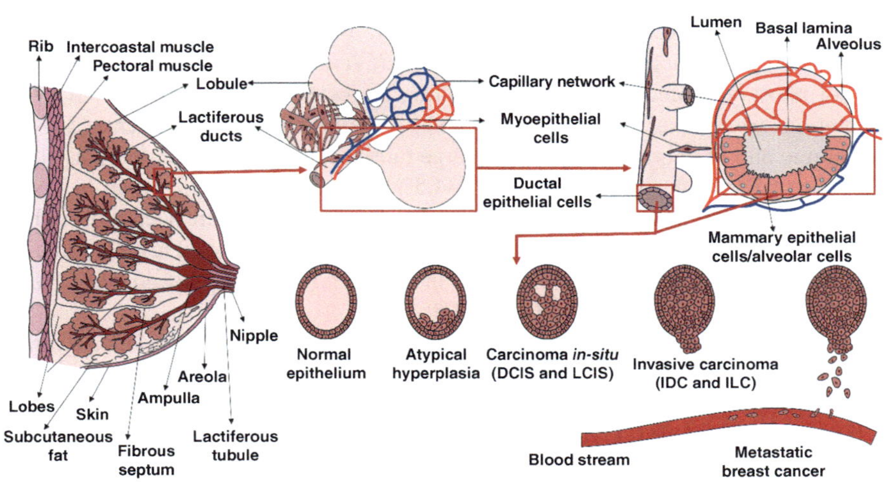

Fig. 2.2 Pathophysiology of breast cancer. The basic anatomy of the breast is depicted along with the progression of breast cancer. *DCIS* ductal carcinoma in situ, *LCIS* lobular carcinoma in situ, *IDC* infiltrating ductal carcinoma, *ILC* infiltrating lobular carcinoma

ligaments, also known as suspensory ligaments, and the connective tissue skeleton of the mammary gland gives consistency in the glandular body (Fig. 2.2).

2.3.2 Cell of Origin

Carcinoma usually arises from the epithelial cells lining the glandular breast tissue (Fig. 2.2). When tumor cells are confined to the epithelial compartment, they increase in number (hyperplasia), leading to either benign breast lesions or carcinoma in situ. Atypical hyperplasia (proliferation of abnormal cells) occurs in ducts and lobules, known as atypical ductal hyperplasia (ADH) as well as atypical lobular hyperplasia (ALH) (Fig. 2.2). The ADH and ALH further lead to the DCIS and LCIS, respectively (Fig. 2.2). The DCIS and LCIS eventually progress into invasive breast carcinoma, i.e., IDC and ILC, respectively (Fig. 2.2). The invasive breast carcinoma is devoid of myoepithelial cells, whereas carcinoma in situ always has a layer of myoepithelial cells attached to the tumor cells.

2.3.3 Genetics

Mutations in *PIK3CA* were commonly observed in metastatic breast cancer (MBC), accounting for 20–35% of breast cancer patients [45–47]. Among TNBC subtypes, mutations in *PIK3CA* were frequently observed in LAR (33.3%) and unclassified (31.5%), followed by mesenchymal (10.5%) and BL-1 (5%) [48]. In a cohort study, patients with *HER2*-enriched, *PIK3CA* mutated tumors had a higher number of tumor-infiltrating lymphocytes (TILs) and upregulated immune genes when compared to patients with wildtype *PIK3CA* [49]. In addition, *ERBB2* was mutated in 2–3% of breast cancers, predominantly in *HER2*$^+$ breast cancers [50]. Tumors of the LAR subtype had activating mutations in *PIK3CA* and *ERBB2*, leading to high levels of phosphorylated downstream signaling molecules [51]. *MAP3K1* and *PTEN* mutations were observed in about 6% and 2.2% of breast cancer patients [52, 53]. Genomic and proteomic analysis of a large number of samples reported a high frequency of *PIK3CA* mutations in *HR*$^+$ (34.5%) and *HER2*$^+$ (22.7%) than in TNBC (8.3%), while mutations in *AKT1* (1.4%) and *PTEN* (2.3%) were seen only in HR$^+$ cancers [54]. Analysis of germline DNA from 2595 MBC patients revealed that the frequencies of mutations were higher in *BRCA2* (2.9%), followed by *CHEK2* (2.2%), *BRCA1* (2.0%), and *PALB2* (1.1%) [55].

Sequencing analysis of samples from 1,13,927 women (60,466 breast cancer patients and 53,461 healthy women) revealed the association of BC risk with protein-truncating variants in *ATM*, *CHEK2*, *PALB2*, *BRCA1*, and *BRCA2* (*P* value <0.0001), *BARD1*, *RAD51C*, *RAD51D*, and *TP53* (*P* value <0.05), and rare missense variants in *ATM*, *TP53*, and *CHEK2* (*P* value <0.001) [56]. Another study revealed the association between germline genetic variants and breast cancer subtypes: (1) *RAD51C*, *RAD51D*, *BARD1*, *BRCA2*, and *PALB2* with TNBC, (2) *ATM* with HR$^+$/ERBB2$^-$ high-grade as well as low-grade tumors, (3) *CHEK2* with HR$^+$,

$HR^-/ERBB2^+$ but not TNBC, (4) *BRCA1* with all molecular subtypes, and (5) *TP53* with $HR^+/ERBB2^+$ and $HR^-/ERBB2^+$ subtypes [57]. In IBC patients, activated *PDGFRA* was frequently observed when compared to non-IBC patients [58]. Cytogenetic abnormalities, namely 1q gain and 16q loss, were found to be recurrent in breast cancer malignancies. 16q loss was observed in 77% of lobular carcinomas [59], while in tubular breast cancers, a higher frequency of loss of 16q was observed [60].

The Oncotype DX assay, which involves a panel of 21 genes (16 were cancer-related and 5 were reference genes), has been used in various studies to categorize patients into three risk categories, namely low, intermediate, and high [61]. Additionally, based on ChIP-seq and GWAS, 22 breast cancer risk-associated transcription factors were identified, of which the interaction of FOXA1 with ESR1 and E2F1 plays a major role in breast cancer susceptibility [62]. In a trial testing the relation of germline variant status of *BRCA1/2* with treatment response in high-risk early breast cancer (EBC) patients, the pathologic complete response (pCR) was higher (60.4%) in patients with *gBRCA1/2* variants than in patients without *gBRCA1/2* variants (46.7%) [63].

2.4 Treatment

The first-line treatment for patients with tumors confined to the breast tissues includes surgeries such as (1) lumpectomy, also called breast-conserving surgery, where the tumor-containing part of the breast along with surrounding lymph nodes is removed [64], and (2) bilateral prophylactic mastectomy is the total removal of breast tissue to decrease the recurrence of breast cancer [65]. In a multicentered study carried out among 3536 women with stage I/II breast cancer who had undergone either lumpectomy or mastectomy, the 5-year survival rates were 94.9% and 92.9% among patients who had undergone lumpectomy and mastectomy, respectively [66]. Additional therapies include radiotherapy to the regions including both the site of the tumor and regional lymph nodes, neoadjuvant systemic therapies, and postoperative systemic adjuvant therapies [67, 68]. In TNBC and *$HER2^+$* breast cancer, tumor-infiltrating lymphocytes in the tumor and stroma have been detected and predict the response to chemotherapies such as anthracycline-based chemotherapy with or without the combination of taxanes [69] and neoadjuvant combination chemotherapy [70]. In premenopausal women with a recurrence score of $\leq$25 based on a 21-gene breast cancer assay, the 5-year invasive disease-free survival (DFS) was higher in the chemo-endocrine group (93.9%) than in the endocrine group (89.0%) [71].

In $HR^+/HER2^-$ advanced stage patients, treatment with ribociclib and letrozole resulted in higher overall survival (OS) of 63.9 months compared to the placebo and letrozole group (51.4 months) [72]. In a randomized trial of $HR^+/HER2^-$ advanced breast cancer patients with *PIK3CA* gene mutations, the progression-free survival (PFS) and overall response rate (ORR) were high (PFS: 11.0 months; ORR: 26.6%) in patients treated with alpelisib plus fulvestrant than the placebo-fulvestrant group

(PFS: 5.7 months; ORR: 12.8%) [73]. In ER^+/$HER2^-$ patients, treatment with elacestrant, a novel oral selective ER degrader, resulted in better PFS (6 months PFS: 34.3%, 12 months PFS: 22.3%) than in patients treated with standard endocrine therapy (6 months PFS: 20.4%, 12 months PFS: 9.4%) [74]. In a phase-II trial of ER^+/HER2-mutated or HER2 nonamplified MBC patients, the clinical benefit rate (CBR) was 38% in fulvestrant-treated, 30% in fulvestrant-naïve, and 25% in ER^- MBC patients [75]. In *HER2*$^+$ EBC, pertuzumab when combined with standard adjuvant chemotherapy resulted in a higher 3-year rate of invasive DFS (94.1%) than in patients in the placebo group (93.2%) [76]. In a phase III trial of patients with residual invasive *HER2*$^+$ breast cancer, the 3-year invasive DFS was higher in the trastuzumab emtansine group (88.3%) than in the trastuzumab alone group (77.0%) [77]. In *HER2*$^+$ BC, resistance to targeted therapies is frequently observed due to the presence of pre-drug-tolerant persisters (pre-DTPs) that give rise to drug-tolerant persisters (DTPs) upon exposure to HER2 tyrosine kinase inhibitors (TKIs) [78].

In a phase 3 trial of 1836 patients with *HER2*$^-$ EBC and germline *BRCA1/2* mutations, the 3-year invasive DFS was higher in the olaparib-treated group (85.9%) than in the placebo group (77.1%) [79]. In a clinical trial among patients with *HER2*$^-$ invasive breast cancer, the DFS and ORR were higher in patients who received capecitabine after neoadjuvant chemotherapy (DFS: 74.1%; ORR: 89.2%) than in the control group (DFS: 67.6%; ORR: 83.6%) [80]. In a phase III trial of 1174 patients with early TNBC, complete response was seen in 64.8% of TNBC patients receiving pembrolizumab and neoadjuvant chemotherapy, and 51.2% of patients under the placebo and neoadjuvant chemotherapy group [81]. A meta-analysis including a total of six clinical trials concluded that the ORR is higher in atezolizumab/pembrolizumab plus chemotherapy-treated patients than in the placebo group [82]. In an intention-to-treat study, 112 patients (60.9%) out of 184 patients showed a response to trastuzumab deruxtecan treatment [83]. In a clinical trial of MBC patients with *gBRCA* mutations, the PFS and ORR were higher in patients treated with olaparib (PFS: 7.0 months; ORR: 59.9%) than in patients who had undergone standard therapy (PFS: 4.2 months; ORR: 28.8%) [84]. The fatty acid synthesis was higher in tumors of MBC that were metastasized to the brain, suggesting that fatty acid synthase inhibition could be a potential strategy to reduce the metastasis of breast tumors to the brain [85]. In preclinical *HER2*-low models of breast cancer with a loss of 17p, α-amanitin-conjugated trastuzumab treatment has greater efficacy in combination therapy, resulting in immune checkpoint blockade [86]. In IBC cells expressing active *PDGFRA*, crenolanib showed an inhibitory effect in vitro [58].

2.5 Conclusion

The incidence of breast cancer varies across countries and can likely be attributed to differences in prevalence, screening programs, early detection, and prevailing major risk factors such as obesity, reproductive factors, etc. Breast cancer exhibits remarkable genetic heterogeneity and variability concerning clinical subtype, tumor stage, age, race, and population. Clinically, subtypes such as TNBC and aggressive phenotypes exhibit a greater risk for metastasis, which is a major clinical challenge owing to treatment failure or death. Most cases are sporadic, while only 10–30% are hereditary, involving genetic mutations in *BRCA1/2*, *PIK3CA*, and *PTEN*, etc. Apart from conventional treatment options, existing molecular therapies have contributed to better survival and prognosis. However, drug resistance and relapse are the major concerns, posing the need for the identification of specific molecular signatures as well as early diagnostic/prognostic indicators so that novel therapeutic approaches or combinational therapies can be designed.

References

1. Sung H, Ferlay J, Siegel RL, Laversanne M, Soerjomataram I, Jemal A, Bray F. Global cancer statistics 2020: GLOBOCAN estimates of incidence and mortality worldwide for 36 cancers in 185 countries. CA Cancer J Clin. 2021;71(3):209–49.
2. Lei S, Zheng R, Zhang S, Wang S, Chen R, Sun K, Zeng H, Zhou J, Wei W. Global patterns of breast cancer incidence and mortality: a population-based cancer registry data analysis from 2000 to 2020. Cancer Commun. 2021;41(11):1183–94.
3. Siegel RL, Miller KD, Fuchs HE, Jemal A. Cancer statistics, 2022. CA Cancer J Clin. 2022;72(1):7–33.
4. Giaquinto AN, Sung H, Miller KD, Kramer JL, Newman LA, Minihan A, Jemal A, Siegel RL. Breast cancer statistics, 2022. CA Cancer J Clin. 2022;72(6):524–41.
5. Dyba T, Randi G, Bray F, Martos C, Giusti F, Nicholson N, Gavin A, Flego M, Neamtiu L, Dimitrova N, Carvalho RN. The European cancer burden in 2020: incidence and mortality estimates for 40 countries and 25 major cancers. Eur J Cancer. 2021;157:308–47.
6. Sopik V. International variation in breast cancer incidence and mortality in young women. Breast Cancer Res Treat. 2021;186:497–507.
7. Miller KD, Fidler-Benaoudia M, Keegan TH, Hipp HS, Jemal A, Siegel RL. Cancer statistics for adolescents and young adults, 2020. CA Cancer J Clin. 2020;70(6):443–59.
8. Sun YS, Zhao Z, Yang ZN, Xu F, Lu HJ, Zhu ZY, Shi W, Jiang J, Yao PP, Zhu HP. Risk factors and preventions of breast cancer. Int J Biol Sci. 2017;13(11):1387.
9. Brewer HR, Jones ME, Schoemaker MJ, Ashworth A, Swerdlow AJ. Family history and risk of breast cancer: an analysis accounting for family structure. Breast Cancer Res Treat. 2017;165:193–200.
10. Collaborative Group on Hormonal Factors in Breast Cancer. Menarche, menopause, and breast cancer risk: individual participant meta-analysis, including 118,964 women with breast cancer from 117 epidemiological studies. Lancet Oncol. 2012;13(11):1141–51.
11. Mørch LS, Skovlund CW, Hannaford PC, Iversen L, Fielding S, Lidegaard Ø. Contemporary hormonal contraception and the risk of breast cancer. N Engl J Med. 2017;377(23):2228–39.
12. McDonald ES, Clark AS, Tchou J, Zhang P, Freedman GM. Clinical diagnosis and management of breast cancer. J Nucl Med. 2016;57(Supplement 1):9S–16S.
13. Fuller MS, Lee CI, Elmore JG. Breast cancer screening: an evidence-based update. Med Clin. 2015;99(3):451–68.
14. Berry DA, Cronin KA, Plevritis SK, Fryback DG, Clarke L, Zelen M, Mandelblatt JS, Yakovlev AY, Habbema JD, Feuer EJ. Effect of screening and adjuvant therapy on mortality from breast cancer. N Engl J Med. 2005;353(17):1784–92.
15. Waks AG, Winer EP. Breast cancer treatment: a review. JAMA. 2019;321(3):288–300.
16. Pace LE, Keating NL. A systematic assessment of benefits and risks to guide breast cancer screening decisions. JAMA. 2014;311(13):1327–35.

17. Zanello PA, Robim AF, Oliveira TM, Elias Junior J, Andrade JM, Monteiro CR, Sarmento Filho JM, Carrara HH, Muglia VF. Breast ultrasound diagnostic performance and outcomes for mass lesions using breast imaging reporting and data system category 0 mammogram. Clinics. 2011;66:443–8.
18. Lowry KP, Geuzinge HA, Stout NK, Alagoz O, Hampton J, Kerlikowske K, De Koning HJ, Miglioretti DL, Van Ravesteyn NT, Schechter C, Sprague BL. Breast cancer screening strategies for women with ATM, CHEK2, and PALB2 pathogenic variants: a comparative modeling analysis. JAMA Oncol. 2022;8(4):587–96.
19. West AK, Wullkopf L, Christensen A, Leijnse N, Tarp JM, Mathiesen J, Erler JT, Oddershede LB. Division induced dynamics in non-invasive and invasive breast cancer. Biophys J. 2017;112(3):123a.
20. Harris LN, Ismaila N, McShane LM, Andre F, Collyar DE, Gonzalez-Angulo AM, Hammond EH, Kuderer NM, Liu MC, Mennel RG, Van Poznak C. Use of biomarkers to guide decisions on adjuvant systemic therapy for women with early-stage invasive breast cancer: American Society of Clinical Oncology clinical practice guideline. J Clin Oncol. 2016;34(10):1134.
21. Jones SE. Metastatic breast cancer: the treatment challenge. Clin Breast Cancer. 2008;8(3):224–33.
22. Akram M, Iqbal M, Daniyal M, Khan AU. Awareness and current knowledge of breast cancer. Biol Res. 2017;50:1–23.
23. Burstein HJ, Polyak K, Wong JS, Lester SC, Kaelin CM. Ductal carcinoma in situ of the breast. N Engl J Med. 2004;350(14):1430–41.
24. van Seijen M, Lips EH, Thompson AM, Nik-Zainal S, Futreal A, Hwang ES, Verschuur E, Lane J, Jonkers J, Rea DW, Wesseling J. Ductal carcinoma in situ: to treat or not to treat, that is the question. Br J Cancer. 2019;121(4):285–92.
25. Somiari RI, Sullivan A, Russell S, Somiari S, Hu H, Jordan R, George A, Katenhusen R, Buchowiecka A, Arciero C, Brzeski H. High-throughput proteomic analysis of human infiltrating ductal carcinoma of the breast. Proteomics. 2003;3(10):1863–73.
26. Chuba PJ, Hamre MR, Yap J, Severson RK, Lucas D, Shamsa F, Aref A. Bilateral risk for subsequent breast cancer after lobular carcinoma-in-situ: analysis of surveillance, epidemiology, and end results data. J Clin Oncol. 2005;23(24):5534–41.
27. Arpino G, Bardou VJ, Clark GM, Elledge RM. Infiltrating lobular carcinoma of the breast: tumor characteristics and clinical outcome. Breast Cancer Res. 2004;6(3):1–8.
28. Ridolfi RL, Rosen PP, Port A, Kinne D, Miké V. Medullary carcinoma of the breast. A clinicopathologic study with 10 year follow-up. Cancer. 1977;40(4):1365–85.
29. Matsuda M, Yoshimoto M, Iwase T, Takahashi K, Kasumi F, Akiyama F, Sakamoto G. Mammographic and clinicopathological features of mucinous carcinoma of the breast. Breast Cancer. 2000;7:65–70.
30. Ishikawa T, Hamaguchi Y, Ichikawa Y, Shimura M, Kawano N, Nakatani Y, Ohnishi H, Maegawa J, Ogino I, Shimada H. Locally advanced mucinous carcinoma of the breast with sudden growth acceleration: a case report. Jpn J Clin Oncol. 2002;32(2):64–7.
31. Wilson TE, Helvie MA, Oberman HA, Joynt LK. Pure and mixed mucinous carcinoma of the breast: pathologic basis for differences in mammographic appearance. AJR Am J Roentgenol. 1995;165(2):285–9.
32. Diab SG, Clark GM, Osborne CK, Libby A, Allred DC, Elledge RM. Tumor characteristics and clinical outcome of tubular and mucinous breast carcinomas. J Clin Oncol. 1999;17(5):1442.
33. Rakha EA, Lee AH, Evans AJ, Menon S, Assad NY, Hodi Z, Macmillan D, Blamey RW, Ellis IO. Tubular carcinoma of the breast: further evidence to support its excellent prognosis. J Clin Oncol. 2010;28(1):99–104.
34. Fentiman IS, D'Arrigo C. Pathogenesis of breast carcinoma. Int J Clin Pract. 2004;58(1):35–40.
35. Robertson FM, Bondy M, Yang W, Yamauchi H, Wiggins S, Kamrudin S, Krishnamurthy S, Le-Petross H, Bidaut L, Player AN, Barsky SH. Inflammatory breast cancer: the disease, the biology, the treatment. CA Cancer J Clin. 2010;60(6):351–75.
36. Tse GM, Niu Y, Shi HJ. Phyllodes tumor of the breast: an update. Breast Cancer. 2010;17:29–34.

37. Sera T, Kashiwagi S, Takashima T, Asano Y, Goto W, Iimori N, Noda S, Onoda N, Ohsawa M, Hirakawa K, Ohira M. Multiple metastatic malignant phyllodes tumor of the breast with tonsillar metastasis: a case report. BMC Res Notes. 2017;10(1):1–4.
38. Ashikari R, Park K, Huvos AG, Urban JA. Paget's disease of the breast. Cancer. 1970;26(3):680–5.
39. Sandoval-Leon AC, Drews-Elger K, Gomez-Fernandez CR, Yepes MM, Lippman ME. Paget's disease of the nipple. Breast Cancer Res Treat. 2013;141:1–12.
40. Tsang J, Tse GM. Molecular classification of breast cancer. Adv Anat Pathol. 2020;27(1):27–35.
41. Andre F, Pusztai L. Molecular classification of breast cancer: implications for selection of adjuvant chemotherapy. Nat Clin Pract Oncol. 2006;3(11):621–32.
42. Lehmann BD, Bauer JA, Chen X, Sanders ME, Chakravarthy AB, Shyr Y, Pietenpol JA. Identification of human triple-negative breast cancer subtypes and preclinical models for selection of targeted therapies. J Clin Invest. 2011;121(7):2750–67.
43. Hortobagyi GN, Edge SB, Giuliano A. New and important changes in the TNM staging system for breast cancer. Am Soc Clin Oncol Educ Book. 2018;38:457–67.
44. Giuliano AE, Edge SB, Hortobagyi GN. Of the AJCC cancer staging manual: breast cancer. Ann Surg Oncol. 2018;25:1783–5.
45. Dieci MV, Prat A, Tagliafico E, Paré L, Ficarra G, Bisagni G, Piacentini F, Generali DG, Conte P, Guarneri V. Integrated evaluation of PAM50 subtypes and immune modulation of pCR in HER2-positive breast cancer patients treated with chemotherapy and HER2-targeted agents in the CherLOB trial. Ann Oncol. 2016;27(10):1867–73.
46. Guarneri V, Dieci MV, Bisagni G, Frassoldati A, Bianchi GV, De Salvo GL, Orvieto E, Urso L, Pascual T, Paré L, Galván P. De-escalated therapy for HR+/HER2+ breast cancer patients with Ki67 response after 2-week letrozole: results of the PerELISA neoadjuvant study. Ann Oncol. 2019;30(6):921–6.
47. Martínez-Sáez O, Chic N, Pascual T, Adamo B, Vidal M, González-Farré B, Sanfeliu E, Schettini F, Conte B, Brasó-Maristany F, Rodríguez A. Frequency and spectrum of PIK3CA somatic mutations in breast cancer. Breast Cancer Res. 2020;22(1):1–9.
48. Kumar S, Bal A, Das A, Loriya I, Khare S, Bhattacharya S, Singh G. Spectrum of PIK3CA/AKT mutations across molecular subtypes of triple-negative breast cancer. Breast Cancer Res Treat. 2021;187(3):625–33.
49. Guarneri V, Dieci MV, Bisagni G, Brandes AA, Frassoldati A, Cavanna L, Musolino A, Giotta F, Rimanti A, Garrone O, Bertone E. PIK3CA mutation in the ShortHER randomized adjuvant trial for patients with early HER2+ breast cancer: association with prognosis and integration with PAM50 SubtypePIK3CA in the ShortHER trial. Clin Cancer Res. 2020;26(22):5843–51.
50. Bose R, Kavuri SM, Searleman AC, Shen W, Shen D, Koboldt DC, Monsey J, Goel N, Aronson AB, Li S, Ma CX. Activating HER2 mutations in HER2 gene amplification negative breast cancer. Cancer Discov. 2013;3(2):224–37.
51. Lehmann BD, Colaprico A, Silva TC, Chen J, An H, Ban Y, Huang H, Wang L, James JL, Balko JM, Gonzalez-Ericsson PI. Multi-omics analysis identifies therapeutic vulnerabilities in triple-negative breast cancer subtypes. Nat Commun. 2021;12(1):6276.
52. Stephens PJ, Tarpey PS, Davies H, Van Loo P, Greenman C, Wedge DC, Nik-Zainal S, Martin S, Varela I, Bignell GR, Yates LR. The landscape of cancer genes and mutational processes in breast cancer. Nature. 2012;486(7403):400–4.
53. Zhang HY, Liang F, Jia ZL, Song ST, Jiang ZF. PTEN mutation, methylation and expression in breast cancer patients. Oncol Lett. 2013;6(1):161–8.
54. Stemke-Hale K, Gonzalez-Angulo AM, Lluch A, Neve RM, Kuo WL, Davies M, Carey M, Hu Z, Guan Y, Sahin A, Symmans WF. An integrative genomic and proteomic analysis of PIK3CA, PTEN, and AKT mutations in breast cancer. Cancer Res. 2008;68(15):6084–91.
55. Fasching PA, Yadav S, Hu C, Wunderle M, Häberle L, Hart SN, Rübner M, Polley EC, Lee KY, Gnanaolivu RD, Hadji P. Mutations in BRCA1/2 and other panel genes in patients with metastatic breast cancer—association with patient and disease characteristics and effect on prognosis. J Clin Oncol. 2021;39(15):1619.

56. Breast Cancer Association Consortium. Breast cancer risk genes—association analysis in more than 113,000 women. N Engl J Med. 2021;384(5):428–39.
57. Mavaddat N, Dorling L, Carvalho S, Allen J, González-Neira A, Keeman R, Bolla MK, Dennis J, Wang Q, Ahearn TU, Andrulis IL. Pathology of tumors associated with pathogenic germline variants in 9 breast cancer susceptibility genes. JAMA Oncol. 2022;8(3):e216744.
58. Joglekar-Javadekar M, Van Laere S, Bourne M, Moalwi M, Finetti P, Vermeulen PB, Birnbaum D, Dirix LY, Ueno N, Carter M, Rains J. Characterization and targeting of platelet-derived growth factor receptor alpha (PDGFRA) in inflammatory breast cancer (IBC). Neoplasia. 2017;19(7):564–73.
59. Ciriello G, Gatza ML, Beck AH, Wilkerson MD, Rhie SK, Pastore A, Zhang H, McLellan M, Yau C, Kandoth C, Bowlby R. Comprehensive molecular portraits of invasive lobular breast cancer. Cell. 2015;163(2):506–19.
60. Waldman FM, Hwang ES, Etzell J, Eng C, DeVries S, Bennington J, Thor A. Genomic alterations in tubular breast carcinomas. Hum Pathol. 2001;32(2):222–6.
61. Paik S, Shak S, Tang G, Kim C, Baker J, Cronin M, Baehner FL, Walker MG, Watson D, Park T, Hiller W. A multigene assay to predict recurrence of tamoxifen-treated, node-negative breast cancer. N Engl J Med. 2004;351(27):2817–26.
62. Wen W, Chen Z, Bao J, Long Q, Shu XO, Zheng W, Guo X. Genetic variations of DNA bindings of FOXA1 and co-factors in breast cancer susceptibility. Nat Commun. 2021;12(1):5318.
63. Pohl-Rescigno E, Hauke J, Loibl S, Moebus V, Denkert C, Fasching PA, Kayali M, Ernst C, Weber-Lassalle N, Hanusch C, Tesch H. Association of germline variant status with therapy response in high-risk early-stage breast cancer: a secondary analysis of the GeparOcto randomized clinical trial. JAMA Oncol. 2020;6(5):744–8.
64. Schnitt SJ, Moran MS, Giuliano AE. Lumpectomy margins for invasive breast cancer and ductal carcinoma in situ: current guideline recommendations, their implications, and impact. J Clin Oncol. 2020;38(20):2240–5.
65. Osborne MP, Borgen PI. Role of mastectomy in breast cancer. Surg Clin N Am. 1990;70(5):1023–46.
66. Sinnadurai S, Kwong A, Hartman M, Tan EY, Bhoo-Pathy NT, Dahlui M, See MH, Yip CH, Taib NA, Bhoo-Pathy N. Breast-conserving surgery versus mastectomy in young women with breast cancer in Asian settings. BJS Open. 2019;3(1):48–55.
67. Coates AS, Winer EP, Goldhirsch A, Gelber RD, Gnant M, Piccart-Gebhart M, Thürlimann B, Senn HJ, Members P, André F, Baselga J. Tailoring therapies—improving the management of early breast cancer: St Gallen international expert consensus on the primary therapy of early breast cancer 2015. Ann Oncol. 2015;26(8):1533–46.
68. Harbeck N, Gnant M. Interpretation of the evidence for the efficacy and safety of statin therapy. Lancet. 2017;389(10074):1134–50.
69. Loi S, Drubay D, Adams S, Pruneri G, Francis PA, Lacroix-Triki M, Joensuu H, Dieci MV, Badve S, Demaria S, Gray R. Tumor-infiltrating lymphocytes and prognosis: a pooled individual patient analysis of early-stage triple-negative breast cancers. J Clin Oncol. 2019;37(7):559.
70. Denkert C, von Minckwitz G, Darb-Esfahani S, Lederer B, Heppner BI, Weber KE, Budczies J, Huober J, Klauschen F, Furlanetto J, Schmitt WD. Tumour-infiltrating lymphocytes and prognosis in different subtypes of breast cancer: a pooled analysis of 3771 patients treated with neoadjuvant therapy. Lancet Oncol. 2018;19(1):40–50.
71. Kalinsky K, Barlow WE, Gralow JR, Meric-Bernstam F, Albain KS, Hayes DF, Lin NU, Perez EA, Goldstein LJ, Chia SK, Dhesy-Thind S. 21-Gene assay to inform chemotherapy benefit in node-positive breast cancer. N Engl J Med. 2021;385(25):2336–47.
72. Hortobagyi GN, Stemmer SM, Burris HA, Yap YS, Sonke GS, Hart L, Campone M, Petrakova K, Winer EP, Janni W, Conte P. Overall survival with ribociclib plus letrozole in advanced breast cancer. N Engl J Med. 2022;386(10):942–50.
73. André F, Ciruelos E, Rubovszky G, Campone M, Loibl S, Rugo HS, Iwata H, Conte P, Mayer IA, Kaufman B, Yamashita T. Alpelisib for PIK3CA-mutated, hormone receptor–positive advanced breast cancer. N Engl J Med. 2019;380(20):1929–40.

74. Bidard FC, Kaklamani VG, Neven P, Streich G, Montero AJ, Forget F, Mouret-Reynier MA, Sohn JH, Taylor D, Harnden KK, Khong H. Elacestrant (oral selective estrogen receptor degrader) versus standard endocrine therapy for estrogen receptor-positive, human epidermal growth factor receptor 2-negative advanced breast cancer: results from the randomized phase III EMERALD trial. J Clin Oncol. 2022;40(28):3246–56.
75. Ma CX, Luo J, Freedman RA, Pluard TJ, Nangia JR, Lu J, Valdez-Albini F, Cobleigh M, Jones JM, Lin NU, Winer EP. The phase II MutHER study of neratinib alone and in combination with fulvestrant in HER2-mutated, non-amplified metastatic breast cancer. Clin Cancer Res. 2022;28(7):1258–67.
76. Von Minckwitz G, Procter M, de Azambuja E, Zardavas D, Benyunes M, Viale G, Suter T, Arahmani A, Rouchet N, Clark E, Knott A. Adjuvant pertuzumab and trastuzumab in early HER2-positive breast cancer. N Engl J Med. 2017;377(2):122–31.
77. Von Minckwitz G, Huang CS, Mano MS, Loibl S, Mamounas EP, Untch M, Wolmark N, Rastogi P, Schneeweiss A, Redondo A, Fischer HH. Trastuzumab emtansine for residual invasive HER2-positive breast cancer. N Engl J Med. 2019;380(7):617–28.
78. Chang CA, Jen J, Jiang S, Sayad A, Mer AS, Brown KR, Nixon AM, Dhabaria A, Tang KH, Venet D, Sotiriou C. Ontogeny and vulnerabilities of drug-tolerant persisters in HER2+ breast cancer. Cancer Discov. 2022;12(4):1022–45.
79. Tutt AN, Garber JE, Kaufman B, Viale G, Fumagalli D, Rastogi P, Gelber RD, de Azambuja E, Fielding A, Balmaña J, Domchek SM. Adjuvant olaparib for patients with BRCA1-or BRCA2-mutated breast cancer. N Engl J Med. 2021;384(25):2394–405.
80. Masuda N, Lee SJ, Ohtani S, Im YH, Lee ES, Yokota I, Kuroi K, Im SA, Park BW, Kim SB, Yanagita Y. Adjuvant capecitabine for breast cancer after preoperative chemotherapy. N Engl J Med. 2017;376(22):2147–59.
81. Schmid P, Cortes J, Pusztai L, McArthur H, Kümmel S, Bergh J, Denkert C, Park YH, Hui R, Harbeck N, Takahashi M. Pembrolizumab for early triple-negative breast cancer. N Engl J Med. 2020;382(9):810–21.
82. Latif F, Bint Abdul Jabbar H, Malik H, Sadaf H, Sarfraz A, Sarfraz Z, Cherrez-Ojeda I. Atezolizumab and pembrolizumab in triple-negative breast cancer: a meta-analysis. Expert Rev Anticancer Ther. 2022;22(2):229–35.
83. Modi S, Saura C, Yamashita T, Park YH, Kim SB, Tamura K, Andre F, Iwata H, Ito Y, Tsurutani J, Sohn J. Trastuzumab deruxtecan in previously treated HER2-positive breast cancer. N Engl J Med. 2020;382(7):610–21.
84. Robson M, Im SA, Senkus E, Xu B, Domchek SM, Masuda N, Delaloge S, Li W, Tung N, Armstrong A, Wu W. Olaparib for metastatic breast cancer in patients with a germline BRCA mutation. N Engl J Med. 2017;377(6):523–33.
85. Ferraro GB, Ali A, Luengo A, Kodack DP, Deik A, Abbott KL, Bezwada D, Blanc L, Prideaux B, Jin X, Posada JM. Fatty acid synthesis is required for breast cancer brain metastasis. Nat Cancer. 2021;2(4):414–28.
86. Li Y, Sun Y, Kulke M, Hechler T, Van der Jeught K, Dong T, He B, Miller KD, Radovich M, Schneider BP, Pahl A. Targeted immunotherapy for HER2-low breast cancer with 17p loss. Sci Transl Med. 2021;13(580):eabc6894.

Esophageal Cancer

3

Meghana Korikani, Veena Akula, Ravikanth Vishnubhotla, and Rama Krishna Kancha

3.1 Introduction

3.1.1 Epidemiology

In 2020, Esophageal Cancer (EC) ranked seventh in incidence and sixth in overall mortality globally [1]. In the United States, the incidence (5.6/100,000) is lower than the global average (9.3/100,000) [2]. Among the two histological subtypes, esophageal squamous cell carcinoma (ESCC), which occurs most frequently in the proximal two-thirds region of the esophagus, constitutes 87%, while esophageal adenocarcinoma (EAC), mostly observed in the distal one-third of the esophagus, accounts for 11% of all cases [1, 2]. While ESCC was more prevalent in the past, the increased incidence of EAC in recent years has been reported as a result of increased occurrence of EAC-associated risk factors that include obesity and GERD combined with reduced ESCC risk factors such as lowered use of alcohol and tobacco [3]. The incidence of EC increases with aging: in the United States, the average age of diagnosis is 68 years, and 88% of all cases occur after the age of 55 years [2]. According to the SEER database for the year 2016, the age-adjusted incidence rates were 0.3, 8.0, 20.3, and 24.9 per 100,000, and mortality rates were 0.3, 6.9, 17.5, and 25 per 100,000 for the age groups 20–49, 50–64, 65–74, and 75 or above, respectively [2]. The highest risk of incidence is reported in the area between central Asia and North-Central China, which is considered the EC belt; approximately half of the deaths

M. Korikani · V. Akula · R. K. Kancha (✉)
Molecular Medicine and Therapeutics Laboratory, Centre for Plant Molecular Biology, Osmania University, Hyderabad, Telangana, India
e-mail: ramakancha@osmania.ac.in

R. Vishnubhotla
Department of Genomics and Molecular Biology, Institute of Translational Research, Asian Institute of Gastroenterology, Hyderabad, Telangana, India

R. K. Kancha (ed.), *Biomedical Aspects of Solid Cancers*,
https://doi.org/10.1007/978-981-97-1802-3_3

occur in China [4]. Least incidence rate of 0.98/100 was reported in Central America [2, 5]. Males make up to 70% of all cases, with a two- to threefold increased incidence and mortality rates compared to females [1, 5]. For men, incidence and mortality rates are higher in developed countries than in developing countries; however, for women, rates are comparable [1]. Moreover, white men have a high prevalence of EAC, which has increased by threefold between the years 1976 and 1990 [6].

3.1.2 Risk Factors

The major risk factors for EC include age, sex, genetics, family history, obesity, gastroesophageal reflux, tobacco, alcohol, diet, previous cholecystectomy, and *Helicobacter pylori*. In the United States, a history of smoking, gastroesophageal reflux, high BMI, and low intake of vegetables and fruits are associated with ESCC (90%) and EAC (80%) [7]. The rates of EC increase with age, attributed to the fact that this cancer takes several years to develop [2]. Males are more likely to develop EC than females [5]. EC, especially the EAC subtype, is associated with a family history of hiatal hernia [8]. Fanconi anemia is also associated with about a 1000-fold increased risk of developing EC [9]. Tylosis, an autosomal dominant disorder, is associated with a 90% cumulative risk of developing ESCC by the age of 70 years [10]. Obesity increases the risk of EAC [11], by a factor of 16 times in individuals with a BMI of $\geq$30 kg/m^2 when compared to individuals with a BMI of $\leq$22 [12]. Interestingly, independent of BMI, the risk for EAC increases with increasing waist circumference, thus explaining the possible high incidence of this cancer in males, as abdominal obesity is more prevalent in males [13]. A variety of benign and malignant gastrointestinal tract diseases are caused due to *Helicobacter pylori* infection (primary causative agent) [2]. Interestingly, *H. pylori* infection is inversely linked with EAC development [14]. Therefore, the increased incidence of EAC might be due to decreasing *H. pylori* seropositivity arising from improving socioeconomic conditions [15].

Preexisting esophageal diseases resulting in chronic injury of the mucosa are associated with an increased risk of EC. A condition where stomach acid flows back into the esophagus on a regular basis is called gastroesophageal reflux disease (GERD) and is associated with the EAC subtype only [16]. Weekly symptoms and daily symptoms of GERD were shown to increase the odds of developing EAC by fivefold and sevenfold, respectively [17]. According to population studies, Barrett's esophagus is a precursor to EAC in individuals who consume a diet that contains more meat [18]. The annual risk of developing EC is increased by 30% in individuals with Barrett esophagus [19]. A greater than tenfold and 1000-fold increase in EC were reported in patients suffering from achalasia [20] and caustic injury [21], respectively. Betel quid chewing, which is most common in India and Southeast Asia, is another risk factor for ESCC; the risk of developing ESCC is very high (41-fold) when betel quid chewing is combined with alcohol and tobacco [22]. According to observational studies, using aspirin or other nonsteroidal anti-inflammatory drugs (NSAID) decreases the risk of developing EC by 40–50% [23].

3.1.3 Diagnosis

EC can be diagnosed by certain tests such as (a) barium esophagram, (b) endoscopy, (c) biopsy, and (d) biomarkers. (a) Barium esophagram is a technique in which the patient swallows liquid barium, which sticks to the walls of the esophagus and reveals narrowing of the lumen and dilation proximal to the level of the tumor through an X-ray [24]. (b) Endoscopy is an invasive procedure in which an endoscope is inserted down the throat, passing through the esophagus and stomach, where the image is displayed on a monitor screen to determine if any malignancies exist [25]. There are different types of endoscopy such as (1) chromoendoscopy: detection of changes on the surface of the epithelium by staining the esophagus with Lugol dye or methylene blue, (2) narrow-band imaging is a technique that detects the mucosal surface in detail by using light of blue and green wavelengths, and (3) autofluorescence imaging: used to detect lesions in the pharynx and esophagus; the neoplastic area of the mucosal epithelium of the esophagus emits weaker autofluorescence (purple-colored) and nonneoplastic areas emit stronger autofluorescence (green-colored) [26]. (c) During the process of upper endoscopy, if any tumor is found, it is removed, which is called biopsy and sent for further examination [24]. (d) Biomarkers: high levels of H2RLN indicate distant metastasis of EC [27]. The *TP53* gene is a marker for ESCC, and higher concentrations of WDR66 in tumor specimens indicate the presence of ESCC [27]. Lower expression of PLA2G2A correlates to high-grade tumors and metastasis [27]. In EC tissues, modern proteomic approaches have proposed a variety of potential biomarkers, including HMGB3, LSD1, ANGPTL2, and EI24, among others [28].

3.2 Classification

EC is classified based on (A) histology and (B) staging. (A) According to WHO, ECs are classified into six types based on histology which include (1) EAC, (2) adenoid cystic carcinoma, (3) mucoepidemoid carcinoma and adenosquamous carcinoma, (4) ESCC, (5) undifferentiated carcinoma, and (6) neuroendocrine neoplasm (Fig. 3.1) [29]. ESCC and EAC are the two major histological subtypes of EC [15]. Additional subtypes include basal, transitional, and unspecified carcinomas, which account for 5% of all ECs [2]. In the United States, around 64% of EAC and 31% of ESCC of all EC cases were reported [2]. ESCC develops from epithelial cells of the upper 2/third of the esophagus, and EAC develops from the Barrett esophagus (where the squamous epithelium is replaced by the columnar epithelium intestinal mucosa) in the lower 1/third of the esophagus [15].

(1) *EAC* is the prevailing type of EC seen in Western populations. Barrett's esophagus, which causes EAC and typically develops in the lower esophagus or at the gastroesophageal junction, is the primary cause of gastroesophageal diseases with precursor lesions. (2) *Adenoid cystic carcinoma (ACC)* is made up of epithelial and myoepithelial tumor cells that are arranged in a cribriform, tubular, and solid architecture to form true glands and pseudo glands. ACC is a very rare subtype of

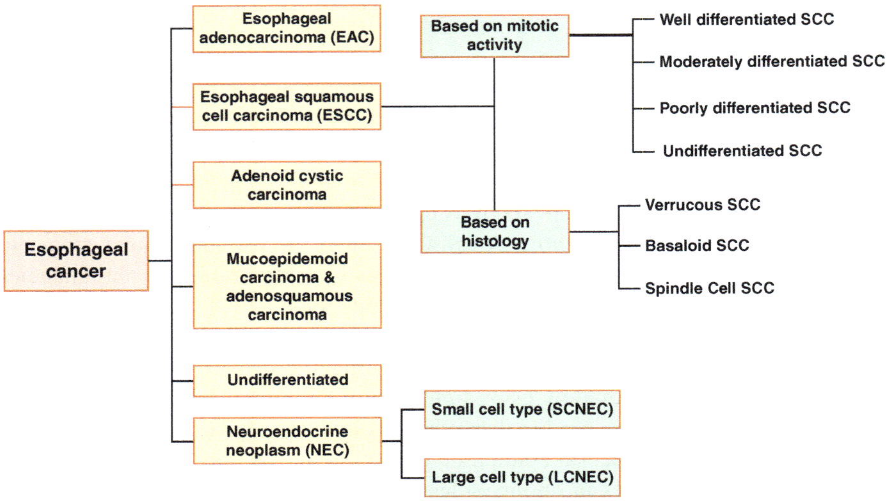

Fig. 3.1 WHO classification of esophageal cancer

EC which has been reported in less than a 100 cases in the literature. Generally, ACC is observed in the middle part of the esophagus. It is more common in men than in women and typically manifests at the age of 70 [29]. (3) *Mucoepidemoid and adenosquamous carcinomas* are made up of components such as mucinous (glandular) and squamous. Adenosquamous cancer has separate squamous and mucinous-containing components. However, mucoepidermoid cancer is made up of squamous, mucinous-containing, along with intermediate components. About 2% of esophageal carcinomas are of this type. These carcinomas are frequently found in the midsection of the esophagus, similar to squamous cell carcinoma [29]. (4) ESCC is the most common subtype of EC and is typically found in Asian populations. ESCC is classified into well- (grade 1), moderately- (grade 2), and poorly-differentiated SCC (grade 3), and undifferentiated SCC (grade 4) (Fig. 3.1) [30]. (5) Esophageal tumors that lack squamous, glandular, or neuroendocrine characteristics are referred to as *undifferentiated carcinoma*. A thorough histological investigation by using techniques such as histochemical stains (mucins) and immunohistochemical markers is conducted on samples to rule out the existence of squamous, glandular, or neuroendocrine differentiation. They can sometimes have the rhabdoid appearance of dispersed large atypical cells with the loss of *SMRCA2/SMARCA4* gene expression. (6) *Neuroendocrine neoplasms (NEC)* are of two types: (a) small cell type (SCNEC) and (b) large cell type (LCNEC) (Fig. 3.1). (a) SCNEC is a very uncommon and aggressive cancer, with a prevalence of 0.1–2.4% of all ECs [31]. SCNEC shows similar histology to that of the small cell carcinoma of the lung [32]. According to reports, more than three-quarters (>75%) of esophageal NENs are SCNECs and occur in Eastern nations. SCNEC is generally observed in the middle region of the esophagus with large tumors that contain primitive tumor cells. (b) About 1% of NENs are esophageal LCNECs, which are primarily (>90%) reported in Western nations. Less than 1% of esophageal NENs are esophageal neuroendocrine tumors, which are very rare.

(B) *Staging of* ESCC*:* According to AJCC staging, stage 0 refers to cancer that is still in its early stages (carcinoma in situ or intramucosal carcinoma, Tis), which has not spread to surrounding lymph nodes or distant organs. Stage IA and IB: the cancer has spread to the lamina propria, muscularis mucosa, and muscularis propria. Stage IIA: the cancer has spread up to the muscularis propria or the adventitia; it might be in grade 2–3, located in the upper or middle region of the esophagus. Stage IIB: the cancer has spread to the adventitia, might spread to nearby 1–2 lymph nodes, tissues, or organs (T3 or T1–2/N1). Stage IIIA: the cancer has spread to the muscularis propria (T4a) and also to 6 of the surrounding lymph nodes (N1–N2) but not to the distant organs. Stage IIIB: the cancer has spread to either the muscularis propria or the adventitia and may have spread to 6 nearby lymph nodes. Stage IVA: the cancer has spread to the pleura, the pericardium, or the diaphragm or the trachea, the aorta, the spine, or other crucial structures along with 6 nearby lymph nodes. Stage IVB: the cancer has spread to distant organs such as the liver and lung (M1a) or a distant set of lymph nodes (M1b) or to a distant part of the peritoneum (M1c) [33].

3.2.1 Stages of EAC

Stage 0 refers to cancer that is still in its early stages (carcinoma in situ or intramucosal carcinoma, Tis), which has not spread to lymph nodes or distant organs. Stage IA and IB: the cancer has spread to the lamina propria, muscularis mucosa, submucosa, or the muscularis propria (T1–2) and is grade 1–2, located in any region of the esophagus. Stage IIA: the cancer has spread up to the muscularis propria and might be in grade 3, located in the lower esophagus or gastroesophageal junction. Stage IIB: the cancer has spread to the lamina propria, muscularis mucosa, or the submucosa along with 2 nearby lymph nodes (T1–2/N1) or the adventitia (T3). Stage IIIA: the cancer has spread to the muscularis propria (T4a) and also to 6 of the surrounding lymph nodes (N1–N2) but not to the distant organs. Stage IIIB: the cancer has spread to either the muscularis propria or the adventitia (T3) and may have spread to 6 of the nearby lymph nodes (N2). Stage IVA: the cancer has spread to the pleura, the pericardium, or to the trachea, the aorta, the spine, or other crucial structures along with six surrounding lymph nodes. Stage IVB: the cancer has spread to distant organs such as the liver and lung (M1a) or a distant set of lymph nodes (M1b) or to a distant part of the peritoneum (M1c) [34].

3.3 Pathophysiology

The esophagus is a muscular tube with approximately 18–26 cm in length in adults that extends from the sixth cervical vertebra to the eleventh thoracic vertebra, spanning three anatomical regions [35]. The esophagus has two sphincters; one is located in the upper region at the opening of the esophagus and the other esophageal sphincter is located in the lower region at the ending of the esophagus [36]. The three anatomical regions of the esophagus are cervical, thoracic, and abdominal [37]. The wall of the esophagus consists of four layers: (1) mucosa, (2) submucosa, (3) muscularis propria, and (4) adventitia (Fig. 3.2) [36]. (1) The mucosa lines the esophageal lumen and is the innermost layer. It consists of stratified squamous epithelium followed by the lamina propria (a thin layer of connective tissue) and muscularis mucosa (irregularly arranged smooth muscles) [36]. (2) The submucosa mostly consists of blood vessels, small mucous glands, and connective tissue along with a nerve plexus, which is known as the submucosal or Meissner's plexus [36]. (3) The muscularis propria consists of two different types of layers: an outer longitudinal layer whose contractions cause shortening of the esophagus and an inner circular layer whose contractions cause an increase in luminal pressure, both of which can be striated or smooth muscle [36]. Striated muscles are seen in the proximal region of the esophagus and smooth muscles are seen in the distal region of the esophagus, while the transition zone (between the proximal and distal region ends) consists of both striated and smooth muscles [36]. (4) The outermost layer of the esophagus is adventitia, which connects the esophagus to other surrounding external structures [36]. The submucosal layer of the esophagus contains glands that secrete water, bicarbonate, mucins, epidermal growth factor, and prostaglandins [38]. These secretions are involved in peristalsis along with mucosal clearance and salivary secretion [38]. Generally, EC arises from epithelial cells of the esophagus, but ESCC occurs in the upper two-thirds of the esophagus and EAC arises from glandular cells that are present in the junction of the esophagus and stomach [39]. However, a few rare types, such as neuroendocrine neoplasm carcinomas, develop from the neuroendocrine cells in the esophagus [29].

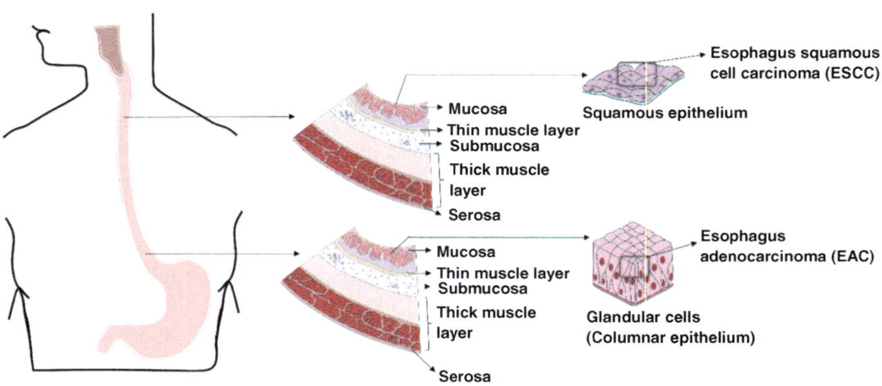

Fig. 3.2 Pathophysiology of ECs along with cell of origin of the main subtypes

3.3.1 Genetics

According to TCGA, ESCC is associated with genetic mutations such as *TP53* (91%), *MLL2* (17%), *NFE2L2* (14%), and amplifications such as *SOX2/T63* (48%) and *FGFR1* (12%) [15]. EGFR is overexpressed in approximately 76% of ESCC cases, followed by CCND1 (46%), CDK4/CDK6 (24%), and MDM2 (6%) [40]. *ALHD2* mutations also play a role in EC pathogenesis [41]. Interestingly, mutations in *ADAM29* and *FAM135B* genes were identified as associated with ESCC [42]. ESCC was shown to be associated with alterations in *ASH1L*, *CREBBP*, *EP300*, *MLL2*, *MLL3*, *SETD1*, *PBRM1*, and *ARID1A* genes [42]. Tylosis, an autosomal condition driven by a missense mutation in the *RHBDF2* gene that results in the activation of EGFR signaling, is associated with ESCC [30]. Mutations in genes such as *FANCD1* and *FANCD2* that are associated with Fanconi anemia, can also result in ESCC [30].

Gastroesophageal reflux disorder (Barrett's esophagus), along with other cancer-causing stimuli, creates genetic and epigenetic changes in the epithelial layer of the esophagus, leading to EAC. The most frequently dysregulated pathways in EACs are the phosphatidylinositol-3-kinase (PI3K) pathway (24%), the TGF-beta pathway (18%), and the WNT/β-catenin pathway [43]. Mutations in *CCNE1* (19% of cases), *cyclin E* (17%) [40], and *MGST1* [44] are associated with EAC. Point mutations in the driver genes *CDK2NA*, *ARID1A*, and *TP53* are significantly altered in EAC. The most frequent copy number alterations in EAC have been found to be in *ERBB2*, *EGFR*, *KRAS*, *FGFR2*, *CCND1*, *CDK6*, *MYC*, *GATA4*, and *GATA6* genes [15]. Esophageal small cell carcinoma is associated with high levels of alterations in genes such as *Syn* with 95.2%, *CD56* with 76.2%, *TTF-1* with 71.4%, *NSE* with 61.9%, *CgA* with 61.9%, *CK* with 57.1%, *EMA* with 61.9%, and *S100* with 19.0% [32].

3.4 Treatment

Successful therapy is challenging due to the organ's peculiar anatomy and the fact that tumor-related symptoms often manifest later in the course of the disease [26]. Treatment strategies for EC include: (a) Endoscopic treatment, (b) Surgical treatment, and (c) Neoadjuvant and adjuvant chemotherapy. (a) *Endoscopic treatment:* Endoscopic mucosal resection (EMR) and endoscopic submucosal dissection (ESD) are two effective treatment options for mucosal cancers. In Western countries, superficial esophageal malignancies such as Barrett's carcinoma are also treated with photodynamic therapy. Endoscopic magnetic resonance imaging (EMR) is one of the endoscopic treatments used to treat esophageal neoplasia. Makuuchi et al. reported a 4.8% complication rate during the removal of esophageal mucosal tumors in a series of 650 patients using EMR (complications: stricture 1.6%, bleeding 3.1%, and perforation 0.7%). In the more recent ESD treatment protocol, a larger portion of the damaged mucosa can be safely removed in one piece, utilizing a variety of endoscopic electrosurgical blades. According to the Japan Esophageal Society, the 5-year overall survival (OS) rate after endoscopic therapy was 83.9%. ESD is typically used for larger lesions, and EMR is recommended for smaller malignancies. ESD is currently, however, also utilized for smaller lesions as a result of the low frequency of problems with the procedure, which is becoming more well-recognized. (b) *Surgical treatment:* Esophagectomy followed by reconstructive surgery is the most efficient course of treatment for patients in whom there is no sign of invasion to the nearby organs or distant metastases. Disappointingly, surgery alone has shown poor 5-year survival rates of 15–40% [26]. There are several surgical options; the decision is made based on the size and location of the primary tumor as well as the therapeutic techniques. (c) *Neoadjuvant and adjuvant chemotherapy:* Two large randomized studies on operable EAC or ESCC examined neoadjuvant treatment with cisplatin and 5-fluorouracil and showed conflicting results [45]. For EC, docetaxel and cisplatin are considered as first-line treatments. Chemotherapy had a response rate of 40% in patients with ESCC and 20% in individuals with EAC, resulting in a 31.3% overall response rate for docetaxel and cisplatin [46]. The median time between progressions was 18.6 weeks for progression-free survival (PFS) and 29.6 weeks for OS [46]. Additionally, first-line treatments for EC include the use of oxaliplatin and capecitabine. The overall response rate with oxaliplatin and capecitabine was 39%, the median OS was 8 months, with a 1-year survival rate of 26% [47]. Docetaxel, 5-fluorouracil, and cisplatin (DFC) were studied as a second-line therapy for patients with postoperative metastatic EC and were found to be promising in patients who are resistant to cisplatin-based chemotherapy [48].

3.5 Conclusion

EC is one of the most common cancers with a significant mortality rate. The incidence of EC is reported to be higher in men than in women. Members with a family history of hiatal hernia, Fanconi anemia, and Tylosis are at a higher risk of developing EC. ECs are predominantly of two subtypes: ESCC and EAC. The incidence of ESCC has been higher than that of EAC in the past; however, in recent years, the incidence of EAC is increasingly reported. GERD and Barrett's esophagus are associated with an increased risk of developing EAC by fivefold and sevenfold, respectively. Early diagnosis of EC reduces the mortality rate and improves the overall survival of the patients. ESCC is associated with mutations in genes such as *TP53*, *MLL2*, and *NFE2L2*, and amplifications of genes such as *SOX2* and *FGFR1*. Treatment strategies for EC comprise endoscopic treatment, surgical treatment, and neoadjuvant and adjuvant chemotherapy. Surgical treatment/esophagectomy is the most effective method for treating patients with no indication of metastasis, followed by chemotherapy with docetaxel and cisplatin or a combination of docetaxel, 5-fluorouracil, and cisplatin.

References

1. Sung H, Ferlay J, Siegel RL, Laversanne M, Soerjomataram I, Jemal A, Bray F. Global cancer statistics 2020: GLOBOCAN estimates of incidence and mortality worldwide for 36 cancers in 185 countries. CA Cancer J Clin. 2021;71(3):209–49.
2. Uhlenhopp DJ, Then EO, Sunkara T, Gaduputi V. Epidemiology of esophageal cancer: update in global trends, etiology and risk factors. Clin J Gastroenterol. 2020;13(6):1010–21.
3. Crew KD, Neugut AI. Epidemiology of upper gastrointestinal malignancies. In: Seminars in oncology, vol. 31. WB Saunders; 2004. p. 450–64.
4. Hongo M, Nagasaki Y, Shoji T. Epidemiology of esophageal cancer: orient to occident. Effects of chronology, geography and ethnicity. J Gastroenterol Hepatol. 2009;24(5):729–35.
5. Bray F, Ferlay J, Soerjomataram I, Siegel RL, Torre LA, Jemal A. Global cancer statistics 2018: GLOBOCAN estimates of incidence and mortality worldwide for 36 cancers in 185 countries. CA Cancer J Clin. 2018;68(6):394–424.
6. Blot WJ, Devesa SS, Fraumeni JF. Continuing climb in rates of esophageal adenocarcinoma: an update. JAMA. 1993;270(11):1320.
7. Brown LM, Hoover RN, Greenberg RS, Schoenberg JB, Schwartz AG, Swanson GM, Liff JM, Silverman DT, Hayes RB, Pottern LM. Are racial differences in squamous cell esophageal cancer explained by alcohol and tobacco use? JNCI J Natl Cancer Inst. 1994;86(17):1340–5.
8. Jiang X, Tseng CC, Bernstein L, Wu AH. Family history of cancer and gastroesophageal disorders and risk of esophageal and gastric adenocarcinomas: a case–control study. BMC Cancer. 2014;14:60.
9. Rosenberg PS, Greene MH, Alter BP. Cancer incidence in persons with Fanconi anemia. Blood. 2003;101(3):822–6.
10. Blaydon DC, Etheridge SL, Risk JM, Hennies HC, Gay LJ, Carroll R, Plagnol V, McRonald FE, Stevens HP, Spurr NK, Bishop DT. RHBDF2 mutations are associated with tylosis, a familial esophageal cancer syndrome. Am J Hum Genet. 2012;90(2):340–6.
11. De Pergola G, Silvestris F. Obesity as a major risk factor for cancer. J Obes. 2013;2013:1.
12. Hampel H, Abraham NS, El-Serag HB. Meta-analysis: obesity and the risk for gastroesophageal reflux disease and its complications. Ann Intern Med. 2005;143(3):199–211.
13. Corley DA, Kubo A, Zhao W. Abdominal obesity and the risk of esophageal and gastric cardia carcinomas. Cancer Epidemiol Biomark Prev. 2008;17(2):352–8.
14. Thrift AP, Pandeya N, Smith KJ, Green AC, Hayward NK, Webb PM, Whiteman DC. *Helicobacter pylori* infection and the risks of Barrett's oesophagus: a population-based case–control study. Int J Cancer. 2012;130(10):2407–16.
15. Smyth EC, Lagergren J, Fitzgerald RC, Lordick F, Shah MA, Lagergren P, Cunningham D. Oesophageal cancer. Nat Rev Dis Primers. 2017;3(1):1–21.
16. Kambhampati S, Xu Y, Meltzer S. Risk factors for progression of Barrett's esophagus to high-grade dysplasia and esophageal carcinoma: 456. Am Coll Gastroenterol. 2016;111:S205–6.
17. Rubenstein JH, Taylor JB. Meta-analysis: the association of oesophageal adenocarcinoma with symptoms of gastro-oesophageal reflux. Aliment Pharmacol Ther. 2010;32(10):1222–7.
18. Kubo A, Levin TR, Block G, Rumore GJ, Quesenberry CP Jr, Buffler P, Corley DA. Dietary patterns and the risk of Barrett's esophagus. Am J Epidemiol. 2008;167(7):839–46.
19. Hvid-Jensen F, Pedersen L, Drewes AM, Sørensen HT, Funch-Jensen P. Incidence of adenocarcinoma among patients with Barrett's esophagus. N Engl J Med. 2011;365(15):1375–83.
20. Zendehdel K, Nyrén O, Edberg A, Ye W. Risk of esophageal adenocarcinoma in achalasia patients, a retrospective cohort study in Sweden. Am Coll Gastroenterol ACG. 2011;106(1):57–61.
21. Stiff G, Alwafi A, Rees BI, Lari J. Corrosive injuries of the oesophagus and stomach: experience in management at a regional paediatric centre. Ann R Coll Surg Engl. 1996;78(2):119.
22. Lee CH, Lee JM, Wu DC, Hsu HK, Kao EL, Huang HL, Wang TN, Huang MC, Wu MT. Independent and combined effects of alcohol intake, tobacco smoking and betel quid chewing on the risk of esophageal cancer in Taiwan. Int J Cancer. 2005;113(3):475–82.

23. Enzinger PC, Mayer RJ. Esophageal cancer. N Engl J Med. 2003;349(23):2241–52.
24. Alsop BR, Sharma P. Esophageal cancer. Gastroenterol Clin. 2016;45(3):399–412.
25. Arnal MJ, Arenas ÁF, Arbeloa ÁL. Esophageal cancer: risk factors, screening and endoscopic treatment in Western and eastern countries. World J Gastroenterol WJG. 2015;21(26):7933.
26. Schweigert M, Dubecz A, Stein HJ. Oesophageal cancer—an overview. Nat Rev Gastroenterol Hepatol. 2013;10(4):230–44.
27. Napier KJ, Scheerer M, Misra S. Esophageal cancer: a review of epidemiology, pathogenesis, staging workup and treatment modalities. World J Gastrointest Oncol. 2014;6(5):112.
28. Yang W, Han Y, Zhao X, Duan L, Zhou W, Wang X, Shi G, Che Y, Zhang Y, Liu J, Zhang H. Advances in prognostic biomarkers for esophageal cancer. Expert Rev Mol Diagn. 2019;19(2):109–19.
29. Lam AK. Updates on World Health Organization classification and staging of esophageal tumors: implications for future clinical practice. Hum Pathol. 2021;108:100–12.
30. Ohashi S, Miyamoto SI, Kikuchi O, Goto T, Amanuma Y, Muto M. Recent advances from basic and clinical studies of esophageal squamous cell carcinoma. Gastroenterology. 2015;149(7):1700–15.
31. Jeene PM, Geijsen ED, Muijs CT, Rozema T, Aleman BM, Muller K, Baas JM, Nuyttens JJ, Wouterse S, Braam PM, Oppedijk V. Small cell carcinoma of the esophagus: a nationwide analysis of treatment and outcome at patient level in locoregional disease. Am J Clin Oncol. 2019;42(6):534.
32. Yun JP, Zhang MF, Hou JH, Tian QH, Fu J, Liang XM, Wu QL, Rong TH. Primary small cell carcinoma of the esophagus: clinicopathological and immunohistochemical features of 21 cases. BMC Cancer. 2007;7:1–8.
33. Hong SJ, Kim TJ, Nam KB, Lee IS, Yang HC, Cho S, Kim K, Jheon S, Lee KW. New TNM staging system for esophageal cancer: what chest radiologists need to know. Radiographics. 2014;34(6):1722–40.
34. Rice TW, Ishwaran H, Ferguson MK, Blackstone EH, Goldstraw P. Cancer of the esophagus and esophagogastric junction: an eighth edition staging primer. J Thorac Oncol. 2017;12(1):36–42.
35. Patti MG, Gantert W, Way LW. Surgery of the esophagus: anatomy and physiology. Surg Clin. 1997;77(5):959–70.
36. Bajwa SA, Toro F, Kasi A. Physiology, esophagus. In: StatPearls [Internet]. 8th ed. StatPearls Publishing; 2022.
37. Fielding JW, Hallissey MT, Lamb PJ, Griffin SM. The anatomy and physiology of the oesophagus. In: Upper gastrointestinal surgery. Springer; 2005. p. 1–5.
38. Yazaki E, Sifrim D. Anatomy and physiology of the esophageal body. Dis Esophagus. 2012;25(4):292–8.
39. Mao WM, Zheng WH, Ling ZQ. Epidemiologic risk factors for esophageal cancer development. Asian Pac J Cancer Prev. 2011;12(10):2461–6.
40. Huang FL, Yu SJ. Esophageal cancer: risk factors, genetic association, and treatment. Asian J Surg. 2018;41(3):210–5.
41. Lewis SJ, Davey Smith G. Alcohol, ALDH2, and esophageal cancer: a meta-analysis which illustrates the potentials and limitations of a Mendelian randomization approach. Cancer Epidemiol Biomark Prev. 2005;14(8):1967–71.
42. Song Y, Li L, Ou Y, Gao Z, Li E, Li X, Zhang W, Wang J, Xu L, Zhou Y, Ma X. Identification of genomic alterations in oesophageal squamous cell cancer. Nature. 2014;509(7498):91–5.
43. Gokulan RC, Garcia-Buitrago MT, Zaika AI. From genetics to signaling pathways: molecular pathogenesis of esophageal adenocarcinoma. Biochim Biophys Acta (BBA) Rev Cancer. 2019;1872(1):37–48.
44. Buas MF, He Q, Johnson LG, Onstad L, Levine DM, Thrift AP, Gharahkhani P, Palles C, Lagergren J, Fitzgerald RC, Ye W. Germline variation in inflammation-related pathways and risk of Barrett's oesophagus and oesophageal adenocarcinoma. Gut. 2017;66(10):1739–47.
45. Kato H, Nakajima M. Treatments for esophageal cancer: a review. Gen Thorac Cardiovasc Surg. 2013;61:330–5.

46. Laack E, Andritzky B, Dürk H, Burkholder I, Edler L, Schuch G, Boeters I, Görn M, Lipp R, Horst H, Popp J. Docetaxel and cisplatin as first-line treatment for patients with metastatic esophageal cancer: a pilot study. Oncol Res Treat. 2005;28(12):647–50.
47. van Meerten E, Eskens FA, Van Gameren EC, Doorn L, van der Gaast A. First-line treatment with oxaliplatin and capecitabine in patients with advanced or metastatic oesophageal cancer: a phase II study. Br J Cancer. 2007;96(9):1348–52.
48. Tanaka T, Fujita H, Sueyoshi S, Tanaka Y, Sasahara H, Mori N, Nagano T, Yamana H, Shirouzu K. Second-line combination chemotherapy with docetaxel for cisplatin-pretreated refractory metastatic esophageal cancer: a preliminary report of initial experience. Chemotherapy. 2007;53(6):449–53.

Stomach Cancer

4

Meghana Korikani, Mohammed Qudrathulla Khan Quadri, Ravikanth Vishnubhotla, Smita C. Pawar, and Rama Krishna Kancha

4.1 Introduction

4.1.1 Epidemiology

Globally, stomach (gastric) cancer (GC) ranked fifth (5.6%) and fourth (7.7%) in incidence and mortality, respectively, among all cancers in the year 2020 [1]. High incidence and mortality rates were observed in Eastern Asia (656,349 new cases and 435,211 deaths) and South-Central Asia (102,676 new cases and 89,595 deaths) [1]. Males have higher incidence (7.1%) and mortality (9.1%) rates when compared to females (4.0% incidence and 6.0% mortality) [1]. GC was reported in elderly people in a few chosen countries, such as China and Korea, and most cases were detected after 55 years of age [2]. The most significant and well-established risk factor for GC is *H. pylori* infection, which displays variations in incidence and correlates with the incidence of GC worldwide [2]. In developing countries, the prevalence of *H. pylori* infection in adults is 76%, and in affluent countries, it is 58% [2]. Furthermore, the estimated incidence of *H. pylori* in South Africa was 77.6%, followed by China (55.8%), Mexico (52.2%), Australia (24.6%), and Denmark (22.1%) [3]. In the United States, the incidence varied between Mexican Americans (62%), non-Hispanic blacks (53%), and non-Hispanic whites (26%) [2].

M. Korikani · M. Q. K. Quadri · R. K. Kancha (✉)
Molecular Medicine and Therapeutics Laboratory, Centre for Plant Molecular Biology, Osmania University, Hyderabad, Telangana, India
e-mail: ramakancha@osmania.ac.in

R. Vishnubhotla
Department of Genomics and Molecular Biology, Institute of Translational Research, Asian Institute of Gastroenterology, Hyderabad, Telangana, India

S. C. Pawar
Department of Genetics, Osmania University, Hyderabad, India

R. K. Kancha (ed.), *Biomedical Aspects of Solid Cancers*,
https://doi.org/10.1007/978-981-97-1802-3_4

4.1.2 Risk Factors

Chronic infection with *Helicobacter pylori* is considered to be the leading cause of noncardiac GC [4]. It increases the risk of distal GC as well as intestinal GC by up to 3–6-fold [5]. The incidence of GC and the geographic variance of *H. pylori* infection are reasonably correlated. Age is associated with an increased risk of GC; between the ages of 60 and 80 years, more than 80% of cases were reported [2]. The development of GC is significantly influenced by dietary factors. Fruits and vegetables can help prevent the development of GC. On the other hand, charbroiled and broiled animal meats and salt-preserved foods accelerate the development of GC [6]. Obesity is a risk factor for gastric carcinoma of the cardiac region [7]. Tobacco smoking is one of the strongest risk factors for GC [8]. Among nondrinkers, smokers have an 80% higher risk of developing GC than nonsmokers [8]. Among smokers, heavy drinkers are at a higher risk (80%) of GC [8]. Epstein-Barr virus (EBV) infection is also associated with an increased risk of GC [9]. EBV is found in 7–16% of gastric adenocarcinomas [10]. Family history is also a risk factor [11]: GCs are mostly sporadic while about 10% show familial aggregation [8]. Less than 3% of all stomach carcinomas are familial and have a Mendelian inheritance pattern [8]. Hereditary diffuse GC (HDGC), the most well-known familial GC, is caused by pathogenic variants in the *CDH1* gene [12]. Some studies have found iodine prophylaxis to be a protective factor against GC [13]. Also, the consumption of hookah and opium can lead to GC [14].

4.1.3 Diagnosis

The most widely used technique to diagnose GC is the upper gastrointestinal endoscopy followed by a biopsy [15]. Other techniques include laparoscopy, a procedure in which a small camera fixed to the end of a tube (laparoscope) is inserted into the body through a small cut in the abdominal region [16]. Common biomarkers for GC are CEA and CA19–9 [17]. Overexpression of HER2, EGFR, VEGFA, NOTCH1, p-mTOR (47–60%), MMP1, MMP7 (32–70%), and loss of expression of CDH1 (69%), TP53, and PTEN are associated with intestinal GC [5]. Overexpression of p-mTOR (58–64%), MMP1, MMP7 (62–90%), MET, TGFB1, SHH/PTCH1/SMO, HER3, FGFR2, PIK3CA and loss of expression of CDH1 (89%), TP53, PTEN were observed in diffuse GC [5].

4.2 Classification

(1) According to Lauren classification, the histological subtypes of GC are (a) intestinal, (b) diffuse, and (c) indeterminate type (Fig. 4.1) [8]. The intestinal type is the most prevalent, followed by the diffuse type and the indeterminate type. Intestinal metaplasia and substantial atrophic gastritis are associated with an increased risk of intestinal subtype malignancies and intestinal tumors from gland-like structures.

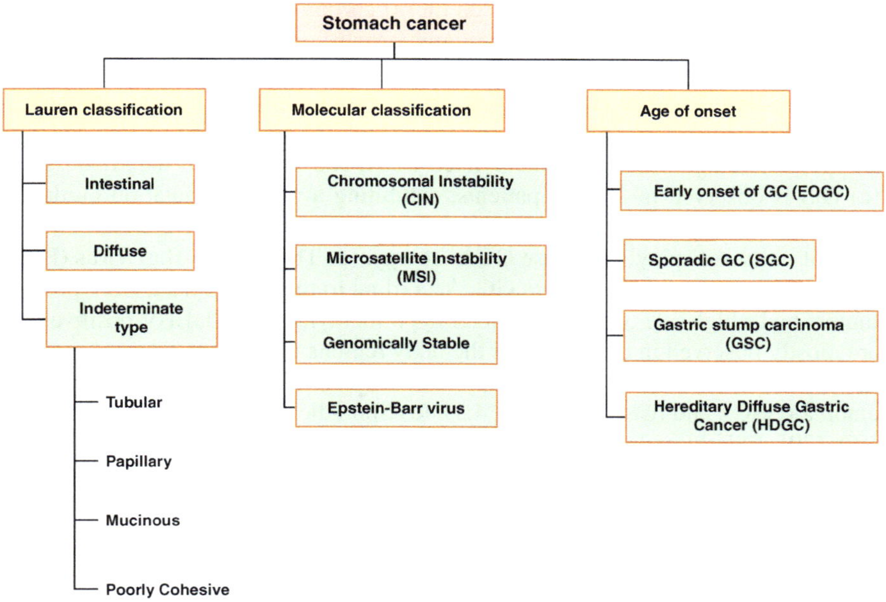

Fig. 4.1 Overview of different types of classification for gastric cancer

Helicobacter pylori infection causes intestinal metaplasia and substantial atrophic gastritis, which ultimately leads to intestinal GC. Diffuse GC is resistant to treatment and has a poor prognosis, which is also characterized by poor differentiation [18]. According to the WHO, GC has four histologic groups: (a) tubular, (b) papillary, (c) mucinous, and (d) poorly cohesive (including signet ring cell carcinoma), which frequently coexists with less dominant components of other histologic patterns (Fig. 4.1) [19]. (a) Early gastric carcinoma's most frequent histologic form is tubular adenocarcinoma. It frequently contains intraluminal mucus, nuclear debris, and inflammatory debris, and it frequently forms grossly polypoid or fungating masses. Histologically, it also shows irregularly distended, fused, or branched tubules of varied diameters. (b) Papillary adenocarcinoma often affects older individuals, develops in the proximal stomach, frequently involves more lymph nodes, and is accompanied by metastasis to the liver. According to histology, it is distinguished by epithelial projections scaffolded by a central fibrovascular core. (c) The presence of mucinous adenocarcinoma is observed in 10% of all stomach carcinomas. According to histology, the tumor is characterized by extracellular mucinous pools that make up at least 50% of the tumor's overall volume. Due to uneven cell clusters and glandular architecture, the tumor cells may occasionally create sporadic signet ring cells that are floating in mucinous pools. (d) A combination of signet ring cells and nonsignet ring cells can be seen in signet ring cell carcinomas and other poorly cohesive carcinomas. Morphologically resembling histiocytes, lymphocytes, or plasma cells are indicative of poorly cohesive nonsignet ring tumor cells [19].

(2) Molecular classification is based on (a) chromosomal instability (CIN), (b) microsatellite instability (MSI), (c) genomic instability (GiS), and (d) Epstein-Barr virus infection (EBV) (Fig. 4.1). (a) CIN accounts for 50% of the incidence of GC, exhibiting significant somatic copy number alterations and correlating with the histology of intestinal GC. (b) MSI accounts for 22% of tumors and is associated with a hypermutated genome, hypermethylated DNA, and silencing of the *MLH1* gene. (c) GiS is observed in 20% of patients, exhibiting a minimal mutation burden as well as somatic copy number alterations. GiS is a more aggressive condition with 73% of tumors displaying diffuse GC histology. (d) The Epstein-Barr virus (EBV) is detected in 9% of patients with GC. According to the TCGA data, EBV-positive tumors had a high rate of DNA promoter hypermethylation [18]. EBV-positive GCs are mostly observed in the fundus or the body regions of the stomach.

(3) GC is also classified into (a) sporadic GC, (b) EOGC, (c) gastric stump carcinoma (GSC), and (d) HDGC (Fig. 4.1). (a) Sporadic GC accounts for 80% of all GCs [20]. Elderly males are more likely to develop sporadic GC; people over the age of 45 are more susceptible [21]. (b) EOGC accounts for 10% of all GCs [20, 22]. This type of cancer is more frequent in women aged less than 45 years [22]. (c) Peptic ulcer disease (PUD), which accounts for 7% of all GC cases, is the most common cause of GSC [23]. Men are more prone to GSC than women [23]. (d) HDGC accounts for only 3% of all GCs and is linked to *CDH1* gene mutations [24, 25].

4.2.1 Staging

The TNM approach was used to categorize GC. Stage 0 indicates cancer that is still in its early stages and has not progressed past the stomach mucosa (also known as carcinoma in situ or intramucosal carcinoma, Tis). Stage IA: Although the cancer has penetrated the lamina propria (T1) through the mucosa, it has not yet spread to the adjacent lymph nodes (N0). If the cancer is in stage IB, it has either spread to the muscularis propria (T2) and there are no surrounding lymph nodes, or it has spread to the lamina propria (T1) and one to two neighboring lymph nodes. When cancer has advanced from the mucosa to the stomach's lamina propria (T1), 3–6 lymph nodes (N2), the muscularis propria (T2), 1–2 surrounding lymph nodes (N1), the subserosa (T3), and no surrounding lymph nodes, it is referred to as stage IIA (N0). In stage IIB, the cancer has spread from the mucosa, but not to any lymph nodes, to the lamina propria (T1), 7–15 nearby lymph nodes (N3a), muscularis propria (T2), 3–6 lymph nodes (N2), subserosa (T3), 1–2 lymph nodes, or serosa (T4). In stage IIIA, the cancer has advanced through the mucosa into the muscularis propria (T2), 7–15 nearby lymph nodes (N3a), or the subserosa (T3), 3–6 nearby lymph nodes (N2), or the serosa (T4a), and 1–2 nearby lymph nodes (N1). Stage IIIB refers to cancer that has spread into the lamina propria (T1) or muscularis propria (T2) and to more than 16 nearby lymph nodes (N3b), to the subserosa (T3) or serosa (T4a), and to 7–15 lymph nodes (N3a), or through the stomach wall to the surrounding area (T4b), and to 3–6 nearby lymph nodes (N2). In stage IIIC, the cancer has spread to the stomach's subserosa (T3) or serosa (T4a/b) and to more than 16 (N3a/b) adjacent lymph nodes. In stage IV, the cancer has spread to a distant portion of the peritoneum or to distant organs such as the liver and the lung (M1).

4.3 Pathophysiology

The wall of the stomach consists of four layers: (a) mucosa, (b) submucosa, (c) muscularis externa, and (d) serosa (Fig. 4.2). (a) *Mucosa* is the innermost layer of the stomach and consists of three parts: surface epithelium, lamina propria, and muscularis mucosae. Surface epithelium is made up of different types of cells: parietal cells, chief cells, and enteroendocrine cells. Invagination of the stomach's surface epithelium into the lamina propria results in the formation of gastric pits and glands that increase the surface area of the epithelium (Fig. 4.2). The four main cell types that line the gastric glands and carry out different functions are the foveolar cells, parietal cells, chief cells, and neuroendocrine cells. (b) *Submucosa* is the second inner layer in the wall of the stomach. It consists of blood vessels, small mucous glands, and connective tissue, along with the nerve plexus. (c) *Muscularis externa* is the third layer that is just below the submucosa, which contains three sublayers of smooth muscles: oblique layer, circular layer, and longitudinal layer. (d) *Serosa* is the outermost layer of the stomach wall. It is made up of squamous epithelium (mesothelium) and a thin layer of connective tissue. Most of GCs are gastric adenocarcinomas that arise from the gastric gland cells of the mucosa of the stomach.

4.3.1 Genetics

In GC, various biological pathways are altered, which include mutations in *TP53* and *BRCA2* genes that are related to genome integrity, *ARID1A* that is involved in chromatin remodeling, *CDH1*, *FAT4*, and *CTNNA1* in cell adhesion, *RHOA* in cytoskeleton and cell motility, and *CTNNB1*, *APC*, and *RNF43* in the Wnt pathway [26]. Frequent mutations in GC were reported in genes *TP53*, *CDH1*, *PTEN*, *ARID1A*, *KRAS*, *B2M*, *MUC3*, *SMAD4*, *PIK3CA*, *RHOA*, *APC*, *ERBB1*, and *HLAB* [20]. Loss

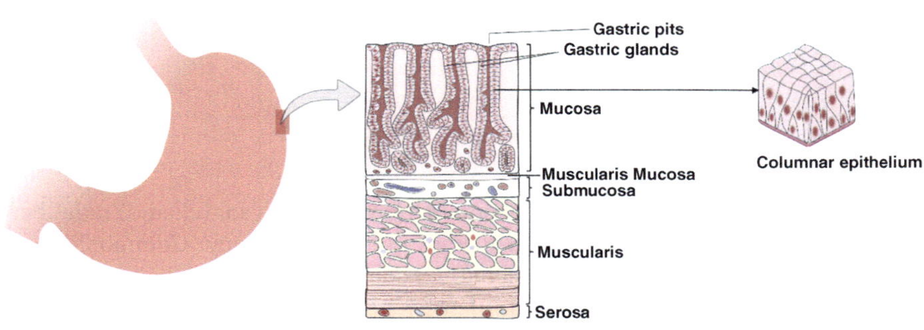

Fig. 4.2 Anatomy and cell of origin of gastric cancer

of heterozygosity (LOH) is a frequent occurrence in GC. Frequent LOH in genes such as *NME1*, *TP53*, and *APC* may have an impact on the assessment of a patient's clinical condition [27]. According to studies on CIN, intestinal GC is associated with increased copy number at the 8q, 17q, and 20q loci as well as with amplified and overexpressed EGF and c-ErbB2, while diffuse GC is characterized by increased copy number at the 12q and 13q loci [27]. MSI-H GCs progress through numerous mutations in genes such as *TGFbRII*, *IGFIIR*, *RIZ*, *TCF4*, *DP2*, *hMSH6*, *hMSH3*, *MED1*, *RAD50*, *BLM*, *ATR*, *MRE11*, *BAX*, *BCL10*, *FAS*, *CASPASE5*, and *APAF1* [28]. The promoter region of genes, namely *CDH1*, *CDKN2A*, *CDKN2B*, and *hMLH1*, are primarily affected by CpG island methylation in GCs, resulting in the downregulation of their expression [29].

Infectious EBV is present in the epithelial cells of GCs in 9% of cases [30]. EBV-positive tumors have an extreme CIMP and lack MSI subtype. All the EBV-positive tumors lacked the MLH1 alterations that are indicative of MSI [20] but display promoter hypermethylation in the CDKN2A region [30] and had mutations in *PIK3CA* (80%), *ARID1A* (55%), and *BCOR* (23%) [18]. Furthermore, amplifications of *JAK2*, *PD-L1*, and *PD-L2* genes were observed in 15% of the EBV-positive tumors [18]. The WHO classifies *H. pylori* as a class I carcinogen and considers it to be the most important environmental risk factor for GC. Interestingly, only 1–2% of individuals infected with the bacteria will develop GC [31]. Chronic inflammation and epigenetic modifications induced by *H. pylori* infection are associated with the promotion of host cell transformation and metastasis [5]. Additionally, oncogenic CagA activates the inflammatory pathway by causing the epithelium to secrete the cytokines IL-8, IL-1, and TNF-27–29 through the NF-kB pathway [5].

Germline variants in the E-cadherin (*CDH1*) gene are found in 30–40% of cases of HDGC, which is an autosomal dominant disorder [32]. Approximately 80% of patients with *CDH1* mutations cause nonsense-mediated decay (NMD) and impair transcript loss [33]. The early onset of GC in *CDH1*-variant carriers may therefore result from this predisposition. Variants in the *RHOA* gene were reported in Asian GC patients resulting in epithelial-mesenchymal transition, similar to that caused by the *CDH1* variants [18]. The most frequent alteration in diffuse-type GC is the loss of E-cadherin function coupled with an overexpression of *EGFR* [34]. According to SNP studies, the *IL-1* gene cluster variants are very significant for GC susceptibility in a variety of ethnic populations, especially in the Caucasian population [35]. TLR polymorphisms have an association with gastrointestinal cancers; especially TLR4 may raise the risk of noncardiac cancer [35].

4.4 Treatment

Treatment for GC includes surgery, chemotherapy, neoadjuvant (chemo) radiotherapy, palliative radiotherapy, targeted therapy, and radiotherapy. Commonly used neoadjuvant chemotherapy for GC includes a combination of epirubicin, cisplatin/oxaliplatin, and 5-FU/capecitabine [36]. Perioperative chemotherapy has shown good results in patients with GC and esophageal-gastric junction cancers [36]. Patients treated with perioperative chemotherapy showed improved overall survival

(OS) and progression-free survival (PFS) in 36% of the patients when compared with operated patients (23%) [36]. Fluoropyrimidine plus oxaliplatin is considered to be the best first-line therapy for GC [37]. Anti-EGFR and anti-VEGF medications may benefit KRAS wild-type patients more than mutant patients. KRAS WT results indicate that anti-EGFR therapeutics may be more successful than anti-VEGF therapy when combined with FOLFIRI or FOLFOX [38]. Irinotecan, docetaxel, and paclitaxel are used as second-line chemotherapy regimens [36]. Radiotherapy is a relatively short and simple treatment option for inoperable GC patients with anemia or for cases with pyloric or cardiac obstruction.

Molecular targeted therapy for GC includes targeting HER2, FGFR2, EGFR, MET, claudin 18.2, and immune-checkpoints. Trastuzumab plus chemotherapy is the first-line therapy for patients with HER2+ gastric cancer. Adding bermarituzumab to the modified FOLFOX6 regimen increases PFS in GCs that overexpress FGFR2b [39]. Patients with MET2+ (moderate)/3+ (strong) gastric or gastroesophageal tumors were treated with onartuzumab in combination with m-FOLFOX6 in the MET gastric trial, which demonstrated a trend towards prolonged overall survival. Clinical trials comparing the antiangiogenic effects of ramucirumab in combination with paclitaxel to paclitaxel alone and as monotherapy versus placebo revealed a significant improvement in OS [39]. Adding zolbetuximab to first-line treatment improved PFS and OS in patients with CLDN18.2-positive GC [39]. Nivolumab was approved for usage in patients with gastric and gastroesophageal cancers in several Asian countries after a trial showed that it increased overall survival when used as a third-line or later-line treatment in Asian patients with gastric and gastroesophageal junction cancers when compared to the placebo [36].

4.5 Conclusion

GC is a heterogeneous disease affecting many individuals; *H. pylori* infection is the most significant risk factor, with age, dietary factors, tobacco smoking, and obesity being additional risk factors. A wide range of novel therapeutics is now being investigated to improve the dismal survival statistics of advanced-stage GC. The combination of neoadjuvant treatment and perioperative chemotherapy is an emerging and most promising strategy to increase the survival rate of patients, with radiation therapy still being the most ideal therapeutic option for advanced-stage GC. In conjunction with chemotherapy, molecular targeted treatment will further provide substantial benefit to the OS of GC patients. More extensive and rigorous efforts in research are still prerequisites to uncover effective treatment regimens for this terminal disease.

References

1. Sung H, Ferlay J, Siegel RL, Laversanne M, Soerjomataram I, Jemal A, Bray F. Global cancer statistics 2020: GLOBOCAN estimates of incidence and mortality worldwide for 36 cancers in 185 countries. CA Cancer J Clin. 2021;71(3):209–49.
2. Ilic M, Ilic I. Epidemiology of stomach cancer. World J Gastroenterol. 2022;28(12):1187.

3. Hooi JK, Lai WY, Ng WK, Suen MM, Underwood FE, Tanyingoh D, Malfertheiner P, Graham DY, Wong VW, Wu JC, Chan FK. Global prevalence of *Helicobacter pylori* infection: systematic review and meta-analysis. Gastroenterology. 2017;153(2):420–9.
4. Plummer M, Franceschi S, Vignat J, Forman D, de Martel C. Global burden of gastric cancer attributable to *Helicobacter pylori*. Int J Cancer. 2015;136(2):487–90.
5. Wadhwa R, Song S, Lee JS, Yao Y, Wei Q, Ajani JA. Gastric cancer—molecular and clinical dimensions. Nat Rev Clin Oncol. 2013;10(11):643–55.
6. Kim J, Cho YA, Choi WJ, Jeong SH. Gene–diet interactions in gastric cancer risk: a systematic review. World J Gastroenterol WJG. 2014;20(28):9600.
7. Poorolajal J, Moradi L, Mohammadi Y, Cheraghi Z, Gohari-Ensaf F. Risk factors for stomach cancer: a systematic review and meta-analysis. Epidemiol Health. 2020;42:e2020004.
8. Machlowska J, Baj J, Sitarz M, Maciejewski R, Sitarz R. Gastric cancer: epidemiology, risk factors, classification, genomic characteristics and treatment strategies. Int J Mol Sci. 2020;21(11):4012.
9. Naseem M, Barzi A, Brezden-Masley C, Puccini A, Berger MD, Tokunaga R, Battaglin F, Soni S, McSkane M, Zhang W, Lenz HJ. Outlooks on Epstein-Barr virus associated gastric cancer. Cancer Treat Rev. 2018;66:15–22.
10. Asakawa Y, Okabe A, Fukuyo M, Li W, Ikeda E, Mano Y, Funata S, Namba H, Fujii T, Kita K, Matsusaka K. Epstein-Barr virus-positive gastric cancer involves enhancer activation through activating transcription factor 3. Cancer Sci. 2020;111(5):1818–28.
11. Yaghoobi M, Bijarchi R, Narod SA. Family history and the risk of gastric cancer. Br J Cancer. 2010;102(2):237–42.
12. Pinheiro H, Oliveira C, Seruca R, Carneiro F. Hereditary diffuse gastric cancer—pathophysiology and clinical management. Best Pract Res Clin Gastroenterol. 2014;28(6):1055–68.
13. Gołkowski F, Szybiński Z, Rachtan J, Sokołowski A, Buziak-Bereza M, Trofimiuk M, Hubalewska-Dydejczyk A, Przybylik-Mazurek E, Huszno B. Iodine prophylaxis—the protective factor against stomach cancer in iodine deficient areas. Eur J Nutr. 2007;46:251–6.
14. Sadjadi A, Derakhshan MH, Yazdanbod A, Boreiri M, Parsaeian M, Babaei M, Alimohammadian M, Samadi F, Etemadi A, Pourfarzi F, Ahmadi E. Neglected role of hookah and opium in gastric carcinogenesis: a cohort study on risk factors and attributable fractions. Int J Cancer. 2014;134(1):181–8.
15. Kim B, Cho SJ. Endoscopic screening and surveillance for gastric cancer. Gastrointest Endosc Clin. 2021;31(3):489–501.
16. Hara K, Ryu S, Okamoto A, Kitagawa T, Marukuchi R, Ito R, Nakabayashi Y. Intraoperative tumor identification during laparoscopic distal gastrectomy: a novel fluorescent clip marking versus metal clip marking and intraoperative gastroscope. J Gastrointest Surg. 2022;26(6):1132–9.
17. Matsuoka T, Yashiro M. Biomarkers of gastric cancer: current topics and future perspective. World J Gastroenterol. 2018;24(26):2818.
18. Sanjeevaiah A, Cheedella N, Hester C, Porembka MR. Gastric cancer: recent molecular classification advances, racial disparity, and management implications. J Oncol Pract. 2018;14(4):217–24.
19. Hu B, El Hajj N, Sittler S, Lammert N, Barnes R, Meloni-Ehrig A. Gastric cancer: classification, histology and application of molecular pathology. J Gastrointest Oncol. 2012;3(3):251.
20. Skierucha M, Milne AN, Offerhaus GJ, Polkowski WP, Maciejewski R, Sitarz R. Molecular alterations in gastric cancer with special reference to the early-onset subtype. World J Gastroenterol. 2016;22(8):2460.
21. Forman D, Burley VJ. Gastric cancer: global pattern of the disease and an overview of environmental risk factors. Best Pract Res Clin Gastroenterol. 2006;20(4):633–49.
22. Milne AN, Offerhaus GJ. Early-onset gastric cancer: learning lessons from the young. World J Gastrointest Oncol. 2010;2(2):59.
23. Sinning C, Schaefer N, Standop J, Hirner A, Wolff M. Gastric stump carcinoma—epidemiology and current concepts in pathogenesis and treatment. Eur J Surg Oncol (EJSO). 2007;33(2):133–9.

24. Fitzgerald RC, Hardwick R, Huntsman D, Carneiro F, Guilford P, Blair V, Chung DC, Norton J, Ragunath K, Van Krieken JH, Dwerryhouse S. Hereditary diffuse gastric cancer: updated consensus guidelines for clinical management and directions for future research. J Med Genet. 2010;47(7):436–44.
25. Luo W, Fedda F, Lynch P, Tan D. CDH1 gene and hereditary diffuse gastric cancer syndrome: molecular and histological alterations and implications for diagnosis and treatment. Front Pharmacol. 2018;9:1421.
26. Lin Y, Wu Z, Guo W, Li J. Gene mutations in gastric cancer: a review of recent next-generation sequencing studies. Tumour Biol. 2015;36:7385–94.
27. McLean MH, El-Omar EM. Genetics of gastric cancer. Nat Rev Gastroenterol Hepatol. 2014;11(11):664–74.
28. Ottini L, Falchetti M, Lupi R, Rizzolo P, Agnese V, Colucci G, Bazan V, Russo A. Patterns of genomic instability in gastric cancer: clinical implications and perspectives. Ann Oncol. 2006;17(7):vii97–vii102.
29. Zheng L, Wang L, Ajani J, Xie K. Molecular basis of gastric cancer development and progression. Gastric Cancer. 2004;7:61–77.
30. Cancer Genome Atlas Research Network. Comprehensive molecular characterization of gastric adenocarcinoma. Nature. 2014;513(7517):202.
31. Tan P, Yeoh KG. Genetics and molecular pathogenesis of gastric adenocarcinoma. Gastroenterology. 2015;149(5):1153–62.
32. Carneiro F, Oliveira C, Suriano G, Seruca R. Molecular pathology of familial gastric cancer, with an emphasis on hereditary diffuse gastric cancer. J Clin Pathol. 2008;61(1):25–30.
33. Oliveira C, Seruca R, Carneiro F. Genetics, pathology, and clinics of familial gastric cancer. Int J Surg Pathol. 2006;14(1):21–33.
34. Bremm A, Walch A, Fuchs M, Mages J, Duyster J, Keller G, Hermannstädter C, Becker KF, Rauser S, Langer R, von Weyhern CH. Enhanced activation of epidermal growth factor receptor caused by tumor-derived E-cadherin mutations. Cancer Res. 2008;68(3):707–14.
35. Camargo MC, Mera R, Correa P, Peek RM Jr, Fontham ET, Goodman KJ, Piazuelo MB, Sicinschi L, Zabaleta J, Schneider BG. Interleukin-1β and interleukin-1 receptor antagonist gene polymorphisms and gastric cancer: a meta-analysis. Cancer Epidemiol Biomark Prev. 2006;15(9):1674–87.
36. Sitarz R, Skierucha M, Mielko J, Offerhaus GJ, Maciejewski R, Polkowski WP. Gastric cancer: epidemiology, prevention, classification, and treatment. Cancer Manag Res. 2018;10:239.
37. Cheng J, Cai M, Shuai X, Gao J, Wang G, Tao K. First-line systemic therapy for advanced gastric cancer: a systematic review and network meta-analysis. Ther Adv Med Oncol. 2019;11:1758835919877726.
38. Kanagavel D, Fedyanin M, Tryakin A, Tjulandin S. Second-line treatment of metastatic gastric cancer: current options and future directions. World J Gastroenterol. 2015;21(41):11621.
39. Nakamura Y, Kawazoe A, Lordick F, Janjigian YY, Shitara K. Biomarker-targeted therapies for advanced-stage gastric and gastro-oesophageal junction cancers: an emerging paradigm. Nat Rev Clin Oncol. 2021;18(8):473–87.

Colorectal Cancer

5

Meghana Korikani, Vijaya Lakshmi Bodiga,
Ravikanth Vishnubhotla, and Rama Krishna Kancha

5.1 Introduction

5.1.1 Epidemiology

Among all cancers, colorectal (bowel) cancer (CRC) ranks third (10%) in incidence and second in mortality (9.4%) [1]. In transitional countries, the incidence rate is roughly four times higher compared to that of transitioning countries [1]. Europe has the highest prevalence rates of colon cancer, followed by Australia/New Zealand and Northern America [1]. Hungary and Norway rank first among men and women, respectively [1]. Rectal cancer is more prevalent in East Asia. Colon and rectal cancers are uncommon in the majority of African and South-Central Asian nations [1]. Hungary (51.2 cases/100,000 persons) has the highest age-standardized annual incidence rates while Gambia has the lowest (1.1 cases/100,000 persons) [2]. In the UK, CRC is the third most common cause of cancer-related deaths in both males (9100 new cases) and females (7600 new cases). Survival rates are 78.3% for one or more years, 58.4% for 5 years or more, and 52.9% for 10 years or more. If diagnosed early, the survival rates are 98% for 1 year or more, 92% for 5 years or more, and 10% for the latest stage.

M. Korikani · R. K. Kancha (✉)
Molecular Medicine and Therapeutics Laboratory, Centre for Plant Molecular Biology, Osmania University, Hyderabad, Telangana, India
e-mail: ramakancha@osmania.ac.in

V. L. Bodiga
Institute of Genetics, Osmania University, Hyderabad, India

R. Vishnubhotla (✉)
Department of Genomics and Molecular Biology, Institute of Translational Research, Asian Institute of Gastroenterology, Hyderabad, Telangana, India

R. K. Kancha (ed.), *Biomedical Aspects of Solid Cancers*,
https://doi.org/10.1007/978-981-97-1802-3_5

5.1.2 Risk Factors

Risk factors for colorectal cancers vary by anatomical site [2]. Smoking increases the risk of developing rectal and proximal colon cancers but not distal colon cancer [3]. Excess adiposity and physical inactivity increase the risk of CRC, strongly for colon cancer rather than rectal cancer [4, 5]. Dietary patterns, consumption of processed meat, and alcohol are other important risk factors [2]. More than 90% of colorectal cancer diagnoses occur in elderly persons over 50 years of age, indicating age as an important risk factor [6]. An increased risk of colorectal cancer occurs in individuals with inherited cancer syndromes (5–7%) and those with a family history of cancer. Hereditary colorectal cancer syndromes are classified into two types: nonpolyposis (HNPCC) and polyposis. Two syndromes that can cause nonpolyposis colorectal cancer are Lynch syndrome and familial colorectal cancer [7]. In contrast, hereditary polyposis syndrome includes familial adenomatous polyposis (FAP) [2]. MUTYH-associated polyposis (MAP) is one of the genetic risks [8]. According to a colonic microbiota study, the risk of developing colorectal cancer may be increased by infection with specific bacterial species like *Fusobacterium nucleatum* [7]. Infection with *Streptococcus bovis* (*S. bovis*) may also increase the risk for CRC [9].

5.1.3 Diagnosis and Biomarkers

Colonoscopy is an invasive procedure to examine the large intestine through an endoscope [10]. It is widely used in the United States, but Poland is the only European country that uses colonoscopy as the only screening procedure for individuals aged between 55 and 66 years [11]. Barium enema is a procedure in which liquid barium is sent into the rectum through a small tube, and an X-ray is taken to identify changes or tumors in the large intestine [10]. Flexible sigmoidoscopy is an examination to detect changes in the lower part of the large intestine by inserting a flexible sigmoidoscope through the rectum [10]. In the UK, a 33% decrease in CRC incidence and a 43% decrease in fatality were observed with sigmoidoscopy [12]. The progression of cancer is associated with high levels of the serum antigen marker CEA, and levels fall after resection of the tumor [10]. The second most extensively studied serum antigen marker for gastrointestinal tumors is the CA19–9 antigen. An increase in the levels of CA19–9 is observed between different tumor stages: 0% for stage I and up to 67% for stage IV [13]. Emerging biomarkers for CRC include protein markers such as nuclear matrix proteins, CCSA-2, CCSA-3, CCSA-4, matrix metalloproteinase 9, S100A8 and S100A9, DNA markers such as *TMEFF2*, *NGFR*, *SEPT9107*, *SEPT9108*, *SEPT914*, *APC*, *KRAS*, *p53142*; *APC*, *MLH1*, and *HLTF143*, and RNA markers such as CDA, MGC20553, BANK1, BCNP1, and MS4A1 [10].

5.2 Classification

Different classifications were proposed based on (1) the anatomic site, (2) genetics, (3) types of polyps, and (4) staging (Fig. 5.1). (1) Based on the anatomic site where the tumor arises, CRC is divided into three subtypes, according to three sections of the colorectum: (a) the proximal colon includes the cecum, ascending colon, hepatic flexure, and transverse colon regions, (b) the distal colon includes splenic flexure, descending colon, and sigmoid colon regions, and (c) the rectum [3].

(2) Colorectal cancer encompasses three major genetic and epigenetic alterations (Fig. 5.1). They are: (a) chromosomal instability (CIN), (b) CpG island methylator phenotype (CIMP), and (c) microsatellite instability (MSI) (Fig. 5.1) [14]. The anomalies in chromosomal copy number and structure are the characteristic features of CIN. Hypermethylation of CpG islands in the promoter regions and consequent silencing of tumor suppressor genes (*MLH1*, *MINT1*, *MINT2*, and *MINT3*) are referred to as the CIMP [15]. MSI is defined by modifications in the length of the microsatellite resulting from mutations in the DNA mismatch-repair genes (*MLH1*) [2]. CpG island hypermethylation is a process that inactivates DNA mismatch repair genes and results in high levels of MSI. Here, MSI is not mutually exclusive with CIMP. Around 70% of MSI-high colorectal tumors are also CIMP-high [2].

(3) Based on the types of polyps, CRCs are grouped into two classes: (a) adenomatous polyps (85–90%) and (b) serrated polyps (10–15%) (Fig. 5.1) [2]. The adenoma-carcinoma pathway accounts for around 70–90% of all CRCs, while the serrated neoplasia pathway accounts for approximately 10–20% of CRCs [7]. (a) There are two pathways that lead to adenomatous polyps: (1) adenoma-carcinoma pathway in which inactivating variant(s) in the *APC* gene lead to the development of adenoma and (2) activating variant(s) in the *KRAS* oncogene and inactivating variant(s) in the *TP53* tumor suppressor lead to CRC [2]. (b) Serrated polyps are caused due to the serrated pathway in which the oncogene *BRAF* is mutated leading to the activation of the MAPK pathway and consequently resulting in hyperplastic

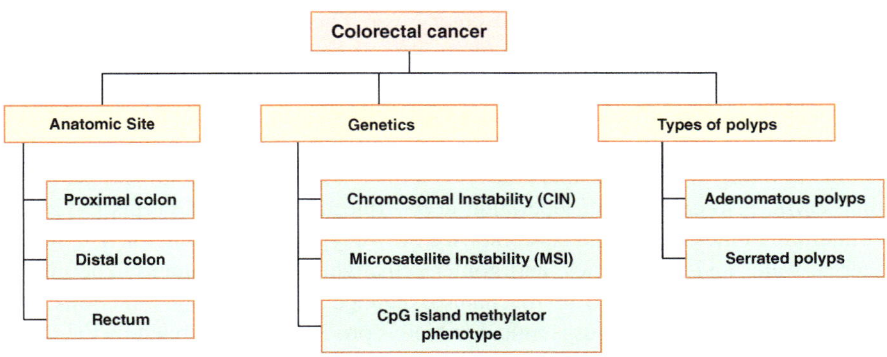

Fig. 5.1 Classification of colorectal cancer

polyp or serrated polyps [2]. The adenoma–carcinoma pathway is associated with the development of the CIN-positive CRC, while the serrated neoplasia pathway is associated with CIMP resulting in MSI-positive CRC subtypes [2, 7].

(4) CRC is classified based on the TNM system in which T stands for the tumor's size, N for the cancer's invasion to adjacent lymph nodes, and M for the cancer's invasion to distant regions (other organs such as the liver or lungs). According to AJCC staging, stage 0 (carcinoma in situ or intramucosal carcinoma, Tis): the cancer that is still in its early stages and has not spread beyond the mucosa of the colon or rectum. Stage I: the tumor has entered the submucosa through the muscularis mucosa (T1) and may have spread into the muscularis propria as well (T2). Stage IIA: the cancer has spread only up to the outermost layers of the colon or rectum. Stage IIB: the cancer has spread through the colon or rectum wall but has not spread to other nearby lymph nodes, tissues, or organs (T4a). Stage IIC: the tumor invades colon or rectum wall and has spread to other nearby tissues or organs. (T4b). Stage IIIA: the cancer has spread through the mucosa into the submucosa (T1) or the muscularis propria (T2) or the visceral peritoneum and also to one to three of the surrounding lymph nodes (N1–N2a). Stage IIIB: the cancer has spread from the mucosa into the submucosa or muscularis propria and may have spread to four to seven nearby lymph nodes. Stage IIIC: the cancer has spread to the outermost layers of the colon or rectum (T3) or through the visceral peritoneum (T4a) and has spread to 1 (N1 or N2) to 7 (N2b) surrounding lymph nodes. Stages IVA, IVB, and IVC indicate that the cancer has metastasized to distant organs such as the liver and lungs (M1a), distant lymph nodes (M1b), or distant peritoneum (M1c).

5.3 Pathophysiology

One-fifth of the gastrointestinal (GI) tract's length of about 5 feet is made up of the large intestine. It is divided into four sections: cecum, colon, rectum, and anal canal. The mucosa, submucosa, muscular layer, and serosa are the four layers that make up the large intestine (Fig. 5.2). The inner circular layer and the outer longitudinal layer of smooth muscle constitute the muscular layer. The wall of the large intestine is lined with a simple columnar epithelium [16]. It has invaginations (the intestinal glands) rather than evaginations that are observed in the small intestine (villi). Both the small and large intestines contain goblet cells, which produce mucin to create mucus in water. However, goblet cells are more prominent in the large intestine. The epithelial lining of the small intestine and colon contains a gland known as an intestinal crypt, also called the Lieberkühn crypt. Intestinal villi and crypts cover the epithelium of the colon, which is composed of two types of cells: enterocytes, which secrete water and electrolytes, and goblet cells, which secrete mucus. The mucus layer protects the intestine from mechanical damage and pathogenic infections. The primary component of mucus is mucin, which is produced and secreted by the intestinal goblet cells. CRC displays altered mucin expression and atypical glycosylation contributing to impaired mucus function. Mucus has a dual function in CRC, preventing the development of cancer at its earliest stages but also accelerating tumor

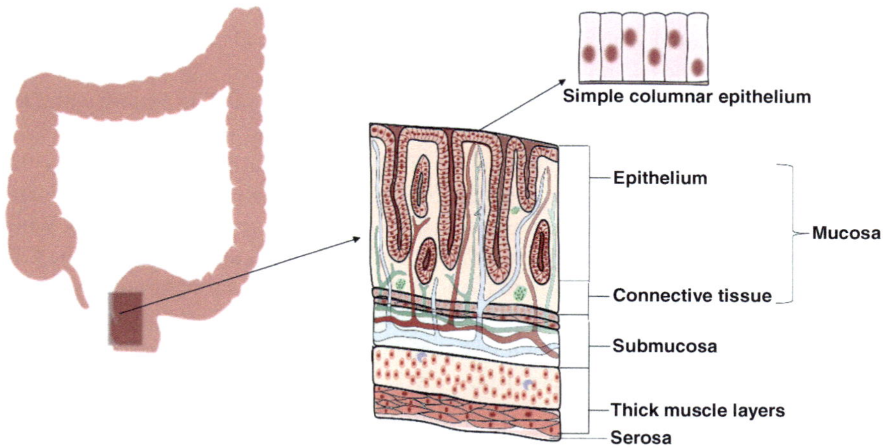

Fig. 5.2 Anatomy and pathophysiology of colorectal cancer

growth and cancer progression at late stages by aiding in immune evasion, tumor cell invasion, and reducing anticancer drug efficacy [17, 18]. New epithelium develops at this location because the cells there are constantly being worn down by the passage of food. The basal region of the crypt, which lies farthest from the intestinal lumen, contains multipotent stem cells. Most colorectal tumors are assumed to be driven by stem cells or stem-cell-like cells. These cancer stem cells are located at the base of the colonic crypts and are essential for the development of tumors [19]. Most cancers are primarily caused by polyps. Over the course of 10–15 years, this procedure starts with an abnormal crypt, evolves into a polyp (a neoplastic precursor lesion), and ultimately results in colorectal cancer [7].

5.3.1 Genetics

Sequential progression of CRC from adenoma to carcinoma is a result of a series of genetic and epigenetic events that align with clinical pathological alterations [20]. Oncogenes that are altered in colorectal cancer include *KRAS*, *EGFR*, *ERBB2*, *TGFA*, and *TGFB1*, and tumor suppressor genes include *APC*, *TP53*, *CDKN1B*, as well as LOH 18q and deletion 5q allele [21]. The *TP53* gene is mutated in about 50% of all sporadic colorectal cancers [21]. Initially, the loss of the *APC* gene (regulates cellular differentiation) in the normal epithelium of the colon or rectum leads to the formation of early adenomas [22]. This early adenoma transforms into intermediate adenoma due to mutations in the *KRAS* gene, which promotes the growth of an adenoma [22]. Loss of 18q with the *SMAD4* gene leads to late adenoma where cell apoptosis is suppressed, and cell proliferation is enhanced [22]. Finally, mutations in *TP53*, *TGFBR2*, *IGF2R*, and *BAX* genes result in carcinoma [20]. African-Americans and women (51–62%) are more likely to develop proximal sporadic colon tumors and exhibit a pattern with high levels of CIMP and MSI and are more frequently associated with mutated *KRAS* and *BRAF* [23]. Distal colorectal tumors have a better prognosis and exhibit CIN [23].

CRC can be caused by adenomatous or serrated polyps. (a) The majority of CRC cases (70–90%) follow the traditional adenoma–carcinoma–metastasis model [23]. These phenotypic changes are connected to the accumulating genetic events that make up "*APC-KRAS-TP53*," known as the Vogelstein model. Inactivating variants or deletions in the *APC* gene are associated with the emergence of adenoma, while inactivating variants or deletions in *TP53* and dsDNA breakage that drives the CIN are associated with adenocarcinoma, and *KRAS* activating variants are associated with invasive/metastatic disease [23]. (b) About 10% of CRCs are caused by the serrated neoplasia pathway, which can result in one of two progression presentations: (1) microvesicular hyperplastic polyps can progress to traditional serrated adenomas, which can further progress to MSS carcinomas, or (2) goblet cell-rich hyperplastic polyps can progress to sessile serrated adenomas, which can then progress to either MSI or microsatellite stable (MSS) carcinomas. These serrated neoplasms frequently have activating mutations in *BRAF* or *KRAS* genes, elevated CIMP, and hypermutation rates, while *APC* mutations are less common [23].

Colorectal cancer is caused due to various pathways such as chromosomal instability, microsatellite instability, and aberrant DNA methylation. CIN is associated with the loss of heterozygosity, which makes it susceptible to a second hit. CIN in CRC is a result of loss of tumor suppressor genes such as *APC*, *TP53*, and *SMAD4*, as well as an oncogenic *KRAS*. Despite the fact that CIN is present in the majority of colorectal tumors, only a few genes have been identified that cause this phenotype, and there is no known general mechanism to explain how these genes operate [21]. The primary diver gene of CIN carcinogenesis is *APC* [24]. The succeeding driver gene mutations have been observed in *KRAS*, *SMAD4*, and *TP53* [25]. The canonical Wnt and MAPK pathways are clinically relevant in CIN [24]. (1) The canonical Wnt pathway is involved in cell proliferation and differentiation. According to TCGA, 94% of all CRC tumors exhibit alterations in the Wnt signaling pathway. Inactivating variants in APC and CTNNB1 genes, which are part of the Wnt signaling pathway, are seen in 80% of the tumors [26]. Germline variants in the *APC* gene result in FAP (Familial adenomatous polyposis), an autosomal dominant disorder [21]. Additionally, variants in the *SOX9* gene, deletions in *TCF7L2*, and overexpression of the frizzled receptor were observed alterations in the Wnt signaling pathway [26]. (2) *KRAS* is highly mutated in 30–50% of all CRCs [27]. Phosphatidylinositol 3-kinase (*PI3K*) is mutated in 20% of the cases with CRC [24].

CRCs can be caused by the MSI pathway, which results from alterations in mismatch repair (MMR) genes. The loss of function of the MMR genes *MLH1*, *MSH2*, *MSH3*, *MSH6*, and *PMS2* that are caused by hypermutation, promotes the growth of CRC. Germline variants in MMR genes result in Lynch syndrome [25]. Hypermethylation of the MSH2 promoter is caused by the germline deletion of its direct upstream gene in a few Lynch syndrome individuals. MSH2 controls the identification of mismatches and initiates DNA repair by forming heterodimers with MSH6 or MSH3 [28]. Around 10–15% of all sporadic colon cancer cases are caused due to hypermethylation of the *MLH1* gene, resulting in gene silencing [25]. In CRC, hypoxia, inflammation, and cellular stress lead to the loss of function of the *MSH3* gene [29]. CRC exhibits elevated levels of IL-6 that activate STAT-3 as well as MMP-9, which degrades type IV collagen leading to metastasis [30, 31]. Moreover, persistent inflammatory conditions such as inflammatory bowel disease enhance the risk of CRC. Changes in the microbiome may be one explanation, resulting in an increase in inflammatory and pro-tumorigenic cytokines [32].

5.4 Treatment

Treatment for CRC includes laparoscopy, surgery, radiotherapy (rectal cancers), and systematic treatment/chemotherapy. In randomized trials and population studies, laparoscopy is the gold standard of treatment for colon cancer in many parts of the world [7]. Rectal cancer surgery is more difficult due to the accessibility and delicate structure of the pelvis [33]. Preoperative radiation, which is based on the clinical stage and surgical quality, reduces risks to an absolute minimum. For metastatic CRC, chemotherapy is usually a combination of different drugs such as fluoropyrimidines, oxaliplatin [34], and irinotecan [35]. Patients with metastatic CRC often receive multiple courses of therapy based on their conditions [7]. Rectal cancer adjuvant therapy has not been as successful with other medications that work well in metastatic circumstances (such as biologics and irinotecan). Adjuvant chemotherapy usually lasted 6 months in the past. The IDEA alliance discovered that limiting adjuvant chemotherapy to 3 months could reduce toxicity such as neuropathy without compromising the effectiveness of treatment for at least low-risk stage III colon cancers [36].

First-line treatments with FOLFIRI and FOLFOX have been demonstrated to be successful in some populations when combined with anti-EGFR or anti-VEGF antibodies for patients with metastatic colorectal cancer [37]. Additional evidence indicates that FOLFIRI or FOLFOX treatment combined with anti-VEGF and anti-EGFR therapies may be more detrimental to KRAS mutant patients [37]. When combined with first-line fluorouracil, folinic acid, and irinotecan (FOLFIRI), both cetuximab and bevacizumab can improve outcomes in patients with metastatic colorectal cancer [38]. In a trial, the FOLFIRI plus cetuximab group had an objective response of 62% as compared to the FOLFIRI plus bevacizumab group (58%). However, the median overall survival was 28.7 months in the cetuximab group as compared to 25 months for the bevacizumab group [38]. Immunotherapy for CRC includes three FDA-approved immune checkpoint inhibitors (ICI): Pembrolizumab, Nivolumab, and Ipilimumab [39]. ICI treatment efficiency in CRC patients can be influenced by the microsatellite instability (MSI) status, which is categorized into three groups: microsatellite instability-high (MSI-H), microsatellite instability-low (MSI-L), and microsatellite stable (MSS) [39]. BAT25, BAT26, D5S346, D2S123, and D17S250 are the five MSI markers that are used to assess MSI status using immunohistochemical labeling and polymerase chain reaction [39]. If two or more of these 5 markers are positive in the tumor it is classified as MSI-H, and if only one of these 5 markers is positive, it is classified as MSI-L [40]. ICIs are more potent on metastatic CRC individuals with MSI high tumors. When nivolumab and ipilimumab were combined, the disease control rate for CRC patients with MSI-H tumors was 80%, which was significantly higher than the rate for patients with microsatellite stable tumors [41].

5.5 Conclusion

Colon cancer is still one of the leading causes of cancer death worldwide. Though it was considered the disease of Western countries, the prevalence of CRC is increasing elsewhere in the present decade due to changes in lifestyle and diet patterns. Early diagnosis helps increase the survival rate. The onset, progression, and metastasis of CRC are influenced by genetic and epigenetic factors. The genetic factors involved in CRC are chromosomal instability, microsatellite instability, and aberrant DNA methylation in different regions of the colon and rectum. Altered microbiota and a high density of certain bacteria are identified as biomarkers for early diagnosis of CRC. Altered expression of mucin and changes in glycation pattern are also causative factors for immune evasion and tumor cell invasion. Recent developments have identified that the combination of chemo/radiotherapies and targeted therapy has good efficacy in treating CRCs. As the gastrointestinal tract is the primary organ that is directly exposed to the diet, a controlled and planned diet can prevent the onset of the disease.

References

1. Sung H, Ferlay J, Siegel RL, Laversanne M, Soerjomataram I, Jemal A, Bray F. Global cancer statistics 2020: GLOBOCAN estimates of incidence and mortality worldwide for 36 cancers in 185 countries. CA Cancer J Clin. 2021;71(3):209–49.
2. Keum N, Giovannucci E. Global burden of colorectal cancer: emerging trends, risk factors and prevention strategies. Nat Rev Gastroenterol Hepatol. 2019;16(12):713–32.
3. Murphy N, Ward HA, Jenab M, Rothwell JA, Boutron-Ruault MC, Carbonnel F, Kvaskoff M, Kaaks R, Kühn T, Boeing H, Aleksandrova K. Heterogeneity of colorectal cancer risk factors by anatomical subsite in 10 European countries: a multinational cohort study. Clin Gastroenterol Hepatol. 2019;17(7):1323–31.
4. Dong Y, Zhou J, Zhu Y, Luo L, He T, Hu H, Liu H, Zhang Y, Luo D, Xu S, Xu L. Abdominal obesity and colorectal cancer risk: systematic review and meta-analysis of prospective studies. Biosci Rep. 2017;37(6):BSR20170945.
5. de Rezende LF, de Sá TH, Markozannes G, Rey-López JP, Lee IM, Tsilidis KK, Ioannidis JP, Eluf-Neto J. Physical activity and cancer: an umbrella review of the literature including 22 major anatomical sites and 770,000 cancer cases. Br J Sports Med. 2018;52(13):826–33.
6. Haggar FA, Boushey RP. Colorectal cancer epidemiology: incidence, mortality, survival, and risk factors. Clin Colon Rectal Surg. 2009;22(04):191–7.
7. Dekker E, Tanis PJ, Vleugels JLA, Kasi PM, Wallace MB. Colorectal cancer. Lancet. 2019;394(10207):1467–80.
8. Yu H, Hemminki K. Genetic epidemiology of colorectal cancer and associated cancers. Mutagenesis. 2020;35(3):207–19.

9. Wong SH, Yu J. Gut microbiota in colorectal cancer: mechanisms of action and clinical applications. Nat Rev Gastroenterol Hepatol. 2019;16(11):690–704.
10. Pawa N, Arulampalam T, Norton JD. Screening for colorectal cancer: established and emerging modalities. Nat Rev Gastroenterol Hepatol. 2011;8(12):711–22.
11. Regula J, Rupinski M, Kraszewska E, Polkowski M, Pachlewski J, Orlowska J, Nowacki MP, Butruk E. Colonoscopy in colorectal-cancer screening for detection of advanced neoplasia. N Engl J Med. 2006;355(18):1863–72.
12. Atkin WS, Edwards R, Kralj-Hans I, Wooldrage K, Hart AR, Northover JM, Parkin DM, Wardle J, Duffy SW, Cuzick J. Once-only flexible sigmoidoscopy screening in prevention of colorectal cancer: a multicentre randomised controlled trial. Lancet. 2010;375(9726):1624–33.
13. Hundt S, Haug U, Brenner H. Blood markers for early detection of colorectal cancer: a systematic review. Cancer Epidemiol Biomark Prev. 2007;16(10):1935–53.
14. Ogino S, Goel A. Molecular classification and correlates in colorectal cancer. J Mol Diagn. 2008;10(1):13–27.
15. Mojarad EN, Kuppen PJ, Aghdaei HA, Zali MR. The CpG island methylator phenotype (CIMP) in colorectal cancer. Gastroenterol Hepatol Bed Bench. 2013;6(3):120.
16. Azzouz LL, Sharma S. Physiology, large intestine. In: StatPearls [internet]. Treasure Island (FL): StatPearls Publishing; 2021.
17. Kufe DW. Mucins in cancer: function, prognosis and therapy. Nat Rev Cancer. 2009;9(12):874–85.
18. Jonckheere N, Skrypek N, Van Seuningen I. Mucins and tumor resistance to chemotherapeutic drugs. Biochim Biophys Acta (BBA) Rev Cancer. 2014;1846(1):142–51.
19. Medema JP. Cancer stem cells: the challenges ahead. Nat Cell Biol. 2013;15(4):338–44.
20. Luo XJ, Zhao Q, Liu J, Zheng JB, Qiu MZ, Ju HQ, Xu RH. Novel genetic and epigenetic biomarkers of prognostic and predictive significance in stage II/III colorectal cancer. Mol Ther. 2021;29(2):587–96.
21. Munteanu I, Mastalier B. Genetics of colorectal cancer. J Med Life. 2014;7(4):507.
22. Vogelstein B, Papadopoulos N, Velculescu VE, Zhou S, Diaz LA Jr, Kinzler KW. Cancer genome landscapes. Science. 2013;339(6127):1546–58.
23. Li J, Ma X, Chakravarti D, Shalapour S, DePinho RA. Genetic and biological hallmarks of colorectal cancer. Genes Dev. 2021;35(11–12):787–820.
24. Pino MS, Chung DC. The chromosomal instability pathway in colon cancer. Gastroenterology. 2010;138(6):2059–72.
25. Fischer J, Walker LC, Robinson BA, Frizelle FA, Church JM, Eglinton TW. Clinical implications of the genetics of sporadic colorectal cancer. ANZ J Surg. 2019;89(10):1224–9.
26. Palma S, Zwenger AO, Croce MV, Abba MC, Lacunza E. From molecular biology to clinical trials: toward personalized colorectal cancer therapy. Clin Colorectal Cancer. 2016;15(2):104–15.
27. Santini D, Loupakis F, Vincenzi B, Floriani I, Stasi I, Canestrari E, Rulli E, Maltese PE, Andreoni F, Masi G, Graziano F. High concordance of KRAS status between primary colorectal tumors and related metastatic sites: implications for clinical practice. Oncologist. 2008;13(12):1270–5.
28. Chen W, Swanson BJ, Frankel WL. Molecular genetics of microsatellite-unstable colorectal cancer for pathologists. Diagn Pathol. 2017;12(1):1–2.
29. Bellizzi AM, Frankel WL. Colorectal cancer due to deficiency in DNA mismatch repair function: a review. Adv Anat Pathol. 2009;16(6):405–17.
30. Grivennikov SI, Greten FR, Karin M. Immunity, inflammation, and cancer. Cell. 2010;140(6):883–99.
31. Zeng ZS, Huang Y, Cohen AM, Guillem JG. Prediction of colorectal cancer relapse and survival via tissue RNA levels of matrix metalloproteinase-9. J Clin Oncol. 1996;14(12):3133–40.
32. Wang X, Yang Y, Huycke MM. Microbiome-driven carcinogenesis in colorectal cancer: models and mechanisms. Free Radic Biol Med. 2017;105:3–15.
33. Ma B, Gao P, Song Y, Zhang C, Zhang C, Wang L, Liu H, Wang Z. Transanal total mesorectal excision (taTME) for rectal cancer: a systematic review and meta-analysis of oncological and

perioperative outcomes compared with laparoscopic total mesorectal excision. BMC Cancer. 2016;16(1):1–3.
34. Haller DG, Tabernero J, Maroun J, De Braud F, Price T, Van Cutsem E, Hill M, Gilberg F, Rittweger K, Schmoll HJ. Capecitabine plus oxaliplatin compared with fluorouracil and folinic acid as adjuvant therapy for stage III colon cancer. J Clin Oncol. 2011;29(11):1465–71.
35. Van Cutsem E, Labianca R, Bodoky G, Barone C, Aranda E, Nordlinger B, Topham C, Tabernero J, André T, Sobrero AF, Mini E. Randomized phase III trial comparing biweekly infusional fluorouracil/leucovorin alone or with irinotecan in the adjuvant treatment of stage III colon cancer: PETACC-3. J Clin Oncol. 2009;27(19):3117–25.
36. Grothey A, Sobrero AF, Shields AF, Yoshino T, Paul J, Taieb J, Souglakos J, Shi Q, Kerr R, Labianca R, Meyerhardt JA. Duration of adjuvant chemotherapy for stage III colon cancer. N Engl J Med. 2018;378(13):1177–88.
37. Ridouane Y, Lopes G, Ku G, Masud H, Haaland B. Targeted first-line therapies for advanced colorectal cancer: a Bayesian meta-analysis. Oncotarget. 2017;8(39):66458.
38. Heinemann V, von Weikersthal LF, Decker T, Kiani A, Vehling-Kaiser U, Al-Batran SE, Heintges T, Lerchenmüller C, Kahl C, Seipelt G, Kullmann F. FOLFIRI plus cetuximab versus FOLFIRI plus bevacizumab as first-line treatment for patients with metastatic colorectal cancer (FIRE-3): a randomised, open-label, phase 3 trial. Lancet Oncol. 2014;15(10):1065–75.
39. Johdi NA, Sukor NF. Colorectal cancer immunotherapy: options and strategies. Front Immunol. 2020;11:1624.
40. Kawakami H, Zaanan A, Sinicrope FA. Microsatellite instability testing and its role in the management of colorectal cancer. Curr Treat Options Oncol. 2015;16:1–5.
41. Overman MJ, Lonardi S, Wong KY, Lenz HJ, Gelsomino F, Aglietta M, Morse MA, Van Cutsem E, McDermott R, Hill A, Sawyer MB. Durable clinical benefit with nivolumab plus ipilimumab in DNA mismatch repair-deficient/microsatellite instability-high metastatic colorectal cancer. J Clin Oncol. 2018;36(8):773–9.

Liver Cancer

6

Sai Sandeep Annamaraju, Sai Charitha Mullaguri, Sharat Putta, Ravikanth Vishnubhotla, and Rama Krishna Kancha

6.1 Introduction

Epidemiology: Worldwide, liver cancer ranks sixth in incidence with 905,677 new diagnoses, accounting for 4.7% of all cancer cases, and third in terms of mortality with 830,180 deaths, accounting for 8.3% of all deaths due to cancer [1]. An 18% 5-year survival rate of LC makes it the second most lethal cancer [2]. The death rate due to liver cancer has increased from 7.2 to 10.3 deaths per 100,000 during the period 2000 to 2016 [2]. An incidence of greater than one million cases was estimated to occur by the end of 2025 [3], and more than one million deaths were projected to occur by the end of 2030 [2]. The reported incidence is highest in Eastern Asia (491,687 cases) followed by South-Eastern Asia (99,265 cases) and South-Central Asia (54,698 cases). Similarly, the mortality was highest in Eastern Asia (449,534 deaths) followed by South-Eastern Asia (95,668 deaths) and South-Central Asia (52,769 deaths).

Based on statistics from the GLOBOCAN factsheet for the year 2020, the global incidence was significantly higher in males (632,320 cases with a cumulative risk of 1.65) compared to females (273,357 cases with a cumulative risk of 0.60). Similarly, the global mortality rates were also higher in males (577,522 deaths, cumulative risk 1.49) than in females (252,658 deaths, cumulative risk 0.55). The higher incidence and mortality rates in males than in females were seen in all regions except Central

S. S. Annamaraju · S. C. Mullaguri · R. K. Kancha (✉)
Molecular Medicine and Therapeutics Laboratory, CPMB, Osmania University, Hyderabad, India
e-mail: ramakancha@osmania.ac.in

S. Putta
Krishna Institute of Medical Sciences, Secunderabad, Telangana, India

R. Vishnubhotla
Department of Genomics and Molecular Biology, Institute of Translational Research, Asian Institute of Gastroenterology, Hyderabad, Telangana, India

R. K. Kancha (ed.), *Biomedical Aspects of Solid Cancers*,
https://doi.org/10.1007/978-981-97-1802-3_6

America, where higher rates of incidence (5895 males; 5924 females) and mortality (5584 males; 5647 females) were observed in females. Globally, a total of 534,000 cases and 485,000 deaths were reported in the year 2019 [4]. The majority (75–85% of reported cases) of liver cancers are hepatocellular carcinomas (HCC) [1]. The mean/median age at diagnosis of HCC is 69, 65, 62, 59, 52, and 45 years in Japan, Europe, North America, South Korea, China, and Africa, respectively [5]. Taiwan and Japan have significantly higher median survival (≥60 months) for patients with HCC, which is due to better surveillance and treatment strategies [5]. The least median survival (2.5 months) for patients with HCC was observed in sub-Saharan Africa [5].

Risk factors: Almost all diseases or conditions that cause chronic liver injury eventually lead to cirrhosis of the liver, where there is extensive scarring and remodeling of the liver. Nearly 90% of all HCC develops in patients with chronic liver disease or cirrhosis [3]. Cirrhosis causes an increased risk of the occurrence of HCC, with a yearly incidence of 2–4% [2]. Conditions that can cause HCC in the absence of or before the development of cirrhosis include chronic hepatitis B virus (HBV) and hepatitis C virus (HCV) infections, nonalcoholic steatohepatitis (NASH), aflatoxin-contaminated foods, and excess alcohol intake [6]. Globally, HBV infections are responsible for almost half of the HCC cases, about 60% in Asia and Africa, while 20% in the Western world [3]. In patients with cirrhosis caused by HBV and HCV infection, the annual incidence of HCC was observed to be 2–5% [5]. In HBV endemic regions, HBV-associated HCC occurs even in the absence of cirrhosis, accounting for nearly 50% of reported cases [5]. Chronic HBV infection is endemic to Eastern Asian and most African countries, whereas the prevalence of HCV is high in North America (USA), Europe, and Japan [7, 8]. The risk due to HCV infection is significantly reduced due to patients undergoing treatment with antiviral drugs to obtain a sustained virological response [6, 8]. HBV/HDV (hepatitis D virus) coinfection increases the risk of HCC when compared to HBV infection alone [3]. A male-to-female ratio of 3.1:2 might be due to the cumulative effect of risk factors in males and differences in sex hormones [3]. Exposure to aflatoxins (a mycotoxin) and aristolochic acid (a mutagenic compound) are also major risk factors [5]. Aflatoxin is endemic to Western Africa, where >90% of the general population are exposed to it [5]. Nearly 20–30% of patients with nonalcoholic fatty liver disease (NAFLD) develop into NASH [6]. Around 15–20% of HCC cases reported in Western countries were due to NASH [3].

Diagnosis: Ultrasonography and the levels of serum α-fetoprotein (AFP) are used for surveillance of HCC in high-risk populations [9]. Except for early detection, HCC of any stage can be detected by ultrasonography with a sensitivity of 84% [9]. For early detection, the sensitivities of ultrasonography without AFP and ultrasonography in combination with AFP were 45% and 63%, respectively [10]. Contrast-enhanced multiphasic CT or MRI are typically used for further evaluation/diagnosis of a focal lesion identified on ultrasound. Arterial phase hyperenhancement (APHE) followed by portal venous or delayed phase washout are imaging diagnostic techniques for HCC [11]. Biopsy is not recommended for diagnostic purposes in patients with typical imaging features, particularly where liver resection or transplantation are being considered. However, histological diagnosis may be required in patients without cirrhosis and/or patients with inconclusive imaging data [2]. Among blood-based surveillance tests, the GALAD score is used for the detection of NASH with or without cirrhosis [9]. The GALAD score was found to be superior over ultrasonography [9]. The GALAD score includes two demographic risk factors (gender and age) and three tumor markers (AFP L3%, AFP, des-γ carboxyprothrombin) [9]. To confirm the diagnosis, immunohistochemical analysis of HSP-70, glypican-3, glutamine synthase, and clathrin heavy chains can be performed [11].

6.2 Classification

HCCs can be classified based on (i) molecular markers, (ii) immune status, and (iii) staging. (i) Based on molecular features of surgically removed tumors, HCC can be broadly classified into (a) proliferation class and (b) nonproliferation class, with each class accounting for 50% of reported cases (Fig. 6.1) [12, 13]. The proliferation class is distinguished by the expression of molecular signals related to cell division and nonproliferation by features related to normal liver physiology [14]. (a) The proliferation class has HBV-related etiology with a poor prognosis [13]. This class was presented with aggressive clinical behavior that includes high serum AFP, poor cell differentiation, high-grade tumors, high vascular invasion, TP53 inactivation, *FGF19/CCND1* amplifications, chromosomal instability, and activation of oncogenic pathways [12, 14]. The proliferation class is further classified into the first group (S1) and second group (S2) (Fig. 6.1) [15]. The first group (S1 or WNT-associated TGF beta group), which accounts for 20% of HCC cases, is associated with noncanonical activation of WNT signaling and an immune-exhausted tumor microenvironment [15]. The second group (S2 or progenitor cell group), which accounts for 25–30% of HCC cases, is associated with high expression of *EPCAM*, *CK19*, *IGF2*, and a 36 CpG signature (a DNA hypermethylation signature) [13, 14]. (b) The nonproliferation class has HCV and alcohol-related etiologies and has comparatively better clinical outcomes [2]. This class is characterized by cells with low

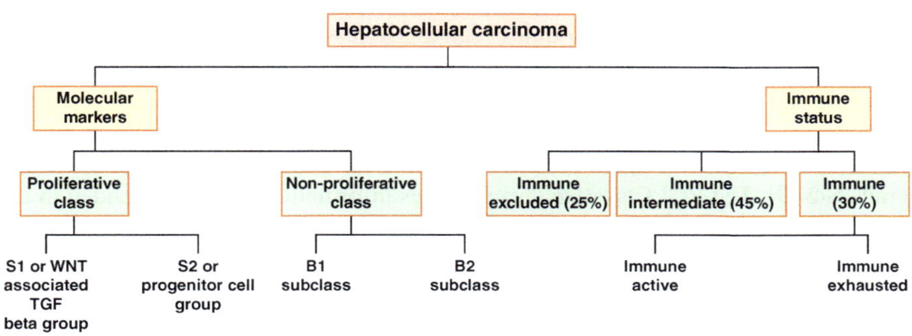

Fig. 6.1 Classification of hepatocellular carcinoma based on molecular markers and immune status of tumor

tumor grade (well-differentiated tumors), less vascular invasion, chromosomal stability, and gene expression resembling that of normal hepatocytes [2, 12]. The nonproliferation class is diverse and can be categorized into (b1) first and (b2) second subclasses (Fig. 6.1) [3, 13]. The b1 subclass possesses mutations in *TERT* promotor and canonical activation of WNT signaling due to variants in *CTNNB1* while retaining normal liver function [12, 15]. The b2 subclass is characterized by IFN-gamma signaling [3].

(ii) Based on infiltration of immune cells, HCC tumors are classified into (a) immune (immune-active and immune-exhausted), (b) immune-intermediate, and (c) immune-excluded classes (Fig. 6.1) [3, 13, 16]. (a) About 30% of HCCs are categorized under the immune class, which is characterized by the presence of high immune cell infiltration, overexpression of PD1/PDL1, presence of granzyme B and perforin 1, activation of IFN gamma signaling, and absence of *CTNNB1* variants [16]. Based on T cell response, the immune class is further classified into (a1) active immune (active $CD4^+$ helper T cells and $CD8^+$ cytotoxic T cell response and expression of adaptive response genes) and (a2) exhaustive immune (TGF beta regulated genes are activated leading to immunosuppression) (Fig. 6.1) [16]. The active immune class accounts for 65%, and the exhausted immune class accounts for 35% of the immune class [16]. The exhaustive immune class overlaps with the proliferation class [13]. (b) The immune intermediate class accounts for 45% of HCCs. (c) About 25% of the HCCs are categorized under the immune-excluded class, which is characterized by fewer B cells, T cells, and increased T regulatory cells in the tumor microenvironment [13]. This class harbors variants in the *CTNNB1* gene and high chromosomal aberrations [13]. The immune-excluded class overlaps with the first subclass of the nonproliferative class (*CTNNB1* mutated subclass) [13]. While immune-excluded tumors are resistant to immune checkpoint inhibitors (ICIs), immune-active class responds to ICIs [3].

(iii) The Barcelona Clinic Liver Cancer (BCLC) staging system classifies HCC into five stages based on the extent of disease (size of tumor), liver function (considering Child-Pugh score), and liver performance status (based on Eastern Cooperative Oncology Group (ECOG) performance status) [17]. The five stages of HCC are: (a) BCLC stage 0 (very early stage), which includes patients with a single nodule of <2 cm, Child-Pugh class A, and ECOG grade 0 [17], (b) BCLC stage A includes patients with a single or ≤ 3 nodules with a size less than 3 cm, Child-Pugh class A-B, and ECOG grade 0 [7], (c) BCLC stage B includes patients with multinodular tumor, Child-Pugh class A-B, and ECOG grade 0 [9], (d) BCLC stage C includes patients with portal invasion (N1, M1), Child-Pugh class A-B, and ECOG grade 1–2 [7, 11], and (e) BCLC stage D includes patients with Child-Pugh class C and ECOG grade > 2 [9]. The BCLC system also provides information on recommended treatment strategies and estimated overall survival (OS) based on the stage at which a patient is diagnosed [18, 19].

6.3 Pathophysiology

Liver is the largest solid organ in the human body and weighs approximately 1.2 to 1.5 kg in a full-grown adult. It is usually reddish-brown in color and positioned in the upper right quadrant of the abdominal cavity, underneath the diaphragm (Fig. 6.2). The liver consists of hepatic lobules, which are hexagonal in shape and supported by thin connective tissue. Each hepatic lobule is made up of many hepatic cells (hepatocytes) (Fig. 6.2). Parenchymal cells, including hepatocytes and cholangiocytes, and nonparenchymal cells that include Kupffer cells, fibroblasts, stellate cells and endothelial cells, are the components of the liver [20]. Hepatocytes account for nearly 60–80% of the total liver mass [20]. Hepatocytes have significant cell plasticity (ability to proliferate in response to cell injury) [3]. They can dedifferentiate to form precursor cells (which have properties similar to progenitor cells) [3, 21]. Either mature hepatocytes or liver stem cells were thought to be the cells of origin for HCC (Fig. 6.2) [3]. Progenitor cells (hepatoblasts) can also lead to a subgroup of HCC by malignant transformation with both cholangiocytic (cholangiocarcinoma, CCA) and hepatocytic (HCC) differentiation (classical HCC-CCA or cHCC-CCA) [21]. The mixed cHCC-CCA accounts for an incidence between 1.0 and 14.2% of the primary liver cancers [22]. HCCs can be formed from two types of precursors, (a) cirrhosis and (b) HCAs (hepatocellular adenomas) [21]. (a) The majority of HCCs (90%) are caused due to cirrhosis/chronic hepatitis [23]. Carcinogenesis occurs through multiple steps that include small monoclonal dysplastic foci (size less than 1 mm), dysplastic nodules (size greater than 1 mm), early HCC (nearly 2 mm), progressed HCC (nearly 2 cm), and advanced HCC (greater than 2 cm) [23, 24]. Dysplastic foci and dysplastic nodules are premalignant in

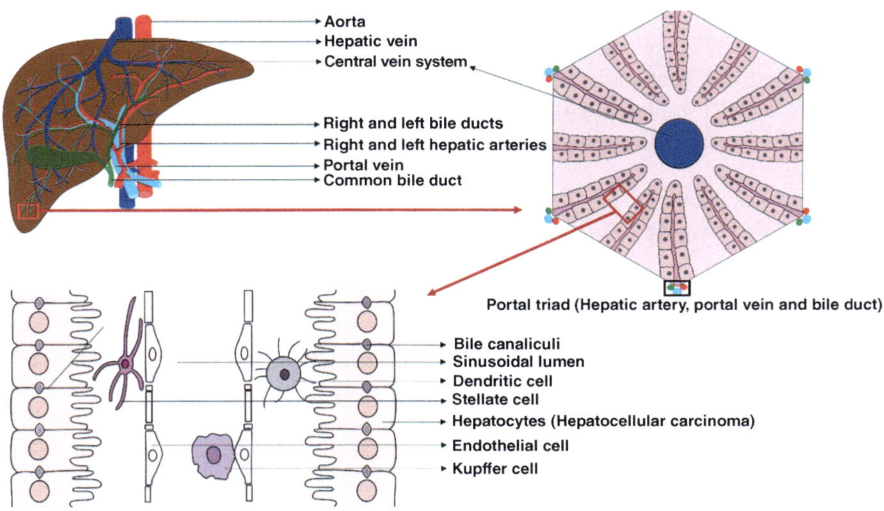

Fig. 6.2 Pathophysiology of hepatocellular cancer. The basic anatomy of the liver along with the portal triad and the different types of cells present in the liver were shown

nature, while early HCCs and progressed HCCs are considered as malignant lesions [23]. Dysplastic nodules differ from normal liver parenchyma tissue by color, size, and texture [25]. Based on cellular atypia, the dysplastic nodules are classified into low-grade (LGDN) and high-grade dysplastic nodules (HGDN) [24]. LGDN and HGDN are associated with a 9% and 32% risk for transformation into HCC, respectively [21]. LGDN have low cellular atypia, slightly increased cell density and nucleo-cytoplasmic ratio, while HGDN have comparatively higher cellular atypia, increased cell density, high nucleo-cytoplasmic ratio, and nuclear hyperchromasia (darker nucleus) [24, 25]. LGDN, HGDN, and early HCCs are hypovascular or isovascular, while progressed HCCs are hypervascular in nature [25].

Telomerase reactivation leading to the lengthening of telomeres is a major event in the pathogenesis of cirrhosis and the initiation of tumors [14]. The telomerase gene is reactivated in more than 90% of HCC cases, which include mutations in the *TERT* promoter (54–60%), insertions in the *TERT* promoter (10–15%), and *TERT* amplifications (5–6%) [14]. *TERT* promoter mutation acts as a gatekeeper mutation in the initiation of the tumor [21]. *TERT* promoter mutations were observed in 6% of LGDN, 19% of HGDN, 61% of the early HCCs, and 41% of established HCCs [26]. The relatively stable mutations in the *TERT* promoter between early and advanced HCC indicate that it is a gatekeeper gene and it does not have any role in the progression of HCC [21]. Further, the absence of *TP53* and *CTNNB1* variants in dysplastic nodules plays a role in tumor progression rather than in tumor initiation [21].

(b) Rarely, in patients without CLD (chronic liver disease), HCC can also develop from benign HCAs [14]. Nearly 3% of HCAs are transformed into HCCs [27]. HCA occurs in the normal liver due to monoclonal proliferation of hepatocytes [14]. HCA is associated with female predominance, accounting for 85% of cases, and oral contraception usage was noted in 87% of individuals (with a median usage of 13 years) [14, 27]. The median age at diagnosis for HCA is 38 years [27]. HCAs can be classified into four molecular groups: *HNF1A* mutated group (30–40% of total HCA), *CTNNB1* mutated group (10–15%), inflammatory group (40–50%), and sonic hedgehog mutated group (5%) [28].

6.4 Treatment

Initial stages (stage 0-A): Surgical resection, liver transplantation, or local ablation are potential curative treatment options (preferred in the same order) for early-stage patients (stage 0-A). These options can provide a median OS of nearly 5 years [29]. Resectability of the liver is an option only for a small number of patients who are clinically presented with either single nodules, normal liver function, and absence of cirrhosis, or "child-pugh A" patients with well-compensated cirrhosis [30]. Patients undergoing surgical resection have high 5-year survival rates (nearly 70%) [30]. However, complete cure with surgery is not always possible as there is a 50–70% of 5-year recurrence rate [31]. Patients with recurrence can be considered for liver transplantation [29]. The 5-year and 10-year survival rates in patients who underwent transplantation were 70% and 50%, respectively [3]. The long-term outcomes due to transplantation are better than resection; however, the role of transplantation has been limited due to organ shortage [3]. Radio frequency ablation was considered to be superior to PEI (percutaneous ethanol injection) in terms of providing OS benefit [32].

Intermediate stage patients (stage B): By the time patients are diagnosed, more than half of them have reached the intermediate or advanced stages [33]. For patients diagnosed with intermediate-stage cancer (stage B), TACE (transarterial chemoembolization) is adopted as the standard treatment strategy [34]. TACE embolizes (blocks the abnormal blood vessel that contains tumor) the tumor and introduces chemotherapeutic or radioactive particles into the arterial system supporting the tumor [35]. A median survival duration of less than 20 months has been reported when TACE is performed in real-life cohorts, which include patients with portal vein invasion, a large tumor burden, and declining liver function [34]. TACE is the only method that has exhibited a survival benefit over the best supportive care for HCC patients who cannot be treated with resection, transplantation, or ablation [35]. Nevertheless, most of the patients (50%) will eventually undergo treatment with systemic therapy [3].

The advanced stage patients (stage C): The advanced-stage patients, including patients with portal invasion and extrahepatic spread but preserved liver function, should be considered for systemic therapy [36]. The first-line regimens include sorafenib, lenvatinib, and a combination of atezolizumab and bevacizumab [3, 37]. Sorafenib is the standard of care treatment for a long time for advanced HCC [34]. Survival is significantly higher with sorafenib treatment (10.7 months) when compared to the placebo (7.9 months) [38]. Similarly, survival was comparable for lenvatinib (13.6 months) and sorafenib (12.3 months) [39]. The atezolizumab and bevacizumab combination (12-month OS: 67.2%) has superior survival outcomes than the standard sorafenib treatment (12-month OS: 54.6%) [36, 40]. Based on a meta-analysis, the atezolizumab plus bevacizumab combination showed superior OS and progression-free survival (PFS) compared to lenvatinib and nivolumab [41]. The second-line systemic therapies for HCC include regorafenib, ramucirumab, and cabozantinib [37]. Regorafenib treatment also showed higher OS (10.6 months) when compared to the placebo (7.8 months) [42, 43]. Another kinase inhibitor, cabozantinib, resulted in a median OS of 10.2 months as compared to 8.0 months with placebo [44]. Ramucirumab inhibits VEGFR2, and the median OS is 8.5 months as compared to 7.3 months with the placebo group [45]. For refractory patients with AFP levels of 400 ng/mL, ramucirumab is an additional treatment option [41]. Based on phase Ib/II data, the anti-PD1 drug pembrolizumab might be a potential treatment option in patients with advanced HCC who progressed after sorafenib treatment [46]. Pembrolizumab provided a median OS of 12.9 months [47]. Nivolumab, an anti-PD1 drug which is currently in phase-II trials, showed an objective response rate (ORR) of 14% with a median OS of 15.6 months [3] and is currently used in the second-line setting [47]. The anti-CTLA4 antibody ipilimumab plus nivolumab is currently in phase I trials [48]. This combination showed a high ORR and proved to exhibit clinical benefits in patients already treated with sorafenib

[48]. The lenvatinib plus pembrolizumab showed an OS of 22 months and was approved in the first-line setting [47].

6.5 Conclusion

HCC is one of the prime causes of cancer-related deaths across the world [49]. Cirrhosis of the liver, viral hepatitis, and alcohol constitute the major risk factors for HCC, whilst NASH is emerging as the most important risk worldwide [50, 51]. The developmental pathophysiology of HCC involves the interplay of genetics, viral and nonviral risk factors, the microenvironment, and immune cells. Despite advances in management, mortality from liver cancer remains high, with a 5-year survival of 18% [52]. Prognosis is critically dependent on the stage of the disease, with early diagnosis offering the best chance for a cure. Detection at an early stage is possible only through dedicated screening of high-risk populations using ultrasound [53]. Early-stage HCC is responsive to curative treatments. A major concern in the management of HCC is the lack of effective therapies for intermediate and advanced-stage HCC. In this regard, immune checkpoint inhibitors have provided a significant step forward in recent years by prolonging survival in advanced unresectable HCC [40]. In addition to advances in treatment modalities, HCC burden can be reduced by HBV vaccination, eradication of viral hepatitis C, modifying lifestyle, and improving early diagnostic techniques.

References

1. Sung H, Ferlay J, Siegel RL, Laversanne M, Soerjomataram I, Jemal A, Bray F. Global cancer statistics 2020: GLOBOCAN estimates of incidence and mortality worldwide for 36 cancers in 185 countries. CA Cancer J Clin. 2021;71(3):209–49.
2. Villanueva A. Hepatocellular carcinoma. N Engl J Med. 2019;380:1450–62.
3. Llovet JM, Kelley RK, Villanueva A, Singal AG, Pikarsky E, Roayaie S, Lencioni R, Koike K, Zucman-Rossi J, Finn RS. Hepatocellular carcinoma. Nat Rev Dis Primers. 2021;7:6.
4. Kocarnik JM, Compton K, Dean FE, Fu W, Gaw BL, Harvey JD, Henrikson HJ, Lu D, Pennini A, Xu R, Ababneh E. Cancer incidence, mortality, years of life lost, years lived with disability, and disability-adjusted life years for 29 cancer groups from 2010 to 2019: a systematic analysis for the global burden of disease study 2019. JAMA Oncol. 2022;8(3):420–44.
5. Yang JD, Hainaut P, Gores GJ, Amadou A, Plymoth A, Roberts LR. A global view of hepatocellular carcinoma: trends, risk, prevention and management. Nat Rev Gastroenterol Hepatol. 2019;16(10):589–604.
6. Kulik L, El-Serag HB. Epidemiology and management of hepatocellular carcinoma. Gastroenterology. 2019;156(2):477–91.
7. Forner A, Reig M, Bruix J. Hepatocellular carcinoma. Lancet. 2018;391(10127):1301–14.
8. Shiani A, Narayanan S, Pena L, Friedman M. The role of diagnosis and treatment of underlying liver disease for the prognosis of primary liver cancer. Cancer Control. 2017;24(3):1073274817729240.
9. Yang JD, Heimbach JK. New advances in the diagnosis and management of hepatocellular carcinoma. BMJ. 2020;371:m3544.

10. Tzartzeva K, Obi J, Rich NE, Parikh ND, Marrero JA, Yopp A, Waljee AK, Singal AG. Surveillance imaging and alpha fetoprotein for early detection of hepatocellular carcinoma in patients with cirrhosis: a meta-analysis. Gastroenterology. 2018;154(6):1706–18.
11. Bruix J, Reig M, Sherman M. Evidence-based diagnosis, staging, and treatment of patients with hepatocellular carcinoma. Gastroenterology. 2016;150(4):835–53.
12. Calderaro J, Ziol M, Paradis V, Zucman-Rossi J. Molecular and histological correlations in liver cancer. J Hepatol. 2019;71(3):616–30.
13. Llovet JM, Montal R, Sia D, Finn RS. Molecular therapies and precision medicine for hepatocellular carcinoma. Nat Rev Clin Oncol. 2018;15(10):599–616.
14. Zucman-Rossi J, Villanueva A, Nault JC, Llovet JM. Genetic landscape and biomarkers of hepatocellular carcinoma. Gastroenterology. 2015;149(5):1226–39.
15. Hoshida Y, Toffanin S, Lachenmayer A, Villanueva A, Minguez B, Llovet JM. Molecular classification and novel targets in hepatocellular carcinoma: recent advancements. In Seminars in liver disease 2010 (Vol. 30, 01, pp. 035–051). Thieme Medical Publishers.
16. Sia D, Jiao Y, Martinez-Quetglas I, Kuchuk O, Villacorta-Martin C, de Moura MC, Putra J, Camprecios G, Bassaganyas L, Akers N, Losic B. Identification of an immune-specific class of hepatocellular carcinoma, based on molecular features. Gastroenterology. 2017;153(3):812–26.
17. Tellapuri S, Sutphin PD, Beg MS, Singal AG, Kalva SP. Staging systems of hepatocellular carcinoma: a review. Indian J Gastroenterol. 2018;37:481–91.
18. Ayuso C, Rimola J, Vilana R, Burrel M, Darnell A, García-Criado Á, Bianchi L, Belmonte E, Caparroz C, Barrufet M, Bruix J. Diagnosis and staging of hepatocellular carcinoma (HCC): current guidelines. Eur J Radiol. 2018;101:72–81.
19. Bruix J, da Fonseca LG, Reig M. Insights into the success and failure of systemic therapy for hepatocellular carcinoma. Nat Rev Gastroenterol Hepatol. 2019;16(10):617–30.
20. Sia D, Villanueva A, Friedman SL, Llovet JM. Liver cancer cell of origin, molecular class, and effects on patient prognosis. Gastroenterology. 2017;152(4):745–61.
21. Craig AJ, Von Felden J, Garcia-Lezana T, Sarcognato S, Villanueva A. Tumour evolution in hepatocellular carcinoma. Nat Rev Gastroenterol Hepatol. 2020;17(3):139–52.
22. Beaufrère A, Calderaro J, Paradis V. Combined hepatocellular-cholangiocarcinoma: an update. J Hepatol. 2021;74(5):1212–24.
23. Di Tommaso L, Sangiovanni A, Borzio M, Park YN, Farinati F, Roncalli M. Advanced precancerous lesions in the liver. Best Pract Res Clin Gastroenterol. 2013;27(2):269–84.
24. Park YN. Update on precursor and early lesions of hepatocellular carcinomas. Arch Pathol Lab Med. 2011;135(6):704–15.
25. Roskams T, Kojiro M. Pathology of early hepatocellular carcinoma: conventional and molecular diagnosis. In Seminars in liver disease 2010 (Vol. 30, 01, pp. 017–025). Thieme Medical Publishers.
26. Nault JC, Ningarhari M, Rebouissou S, Zucman-Rossi J. The role of telomeres and telomerase in cirrhosis and liver cancer. Nat Rev Gastroenterol Hepatol. 2019;16(9):544–58.
27. Nault JC, Couchy G, Balabaud C, Morcrette G, Caruso S, Blanc JF, Bacq Y, Calderaro J, Paradis V, Ramos J, Scoazec JY. Molecular classification of hepatocellular adenoma associates with risk factors, bleeding, and malignant transformation. Gastroenterology. 2017;152(4):880–94.
28. Nault JC, Bioulac-Sage P, Zucman-Rossi J. Hepatocellular benign tumors—from molecular classification to personalized clinical care. Gastroenterology. 2013;144(5):888–902.
29. Galle PR, Forner A, Llovet JM, Mazzaferro V, Piscaglia F, Raoul JL, Schirmacher P, Vilgrain V. EASL clinical practice guidelines: management of hepatocellular carcinoma. J Hepatol. 2018;69(1):182–236.
30. Raza A, Sood GK. Hepatocellular carcinoma review: current treatment, and evidence-based medicine. World J Gastroenterol. 2014;20(15):4115–27.
31. Sugawara Y, Hibi T. Surgical treatment of hepatocellular carcinoma. Biosci Trends. 2021;15(3):138–41.
32. Tian G, Yang S, Yuan J, Threapleton D, Zhao Q, Chen F, Cao H, Jiang TA, Li L. Comparative efficacy of treatment strategies for hepatocellular carcinoma: systematic review and network meta-analysis. BMJ Open. 2018;8(10):e021269.

33. Chen Z, Xie H, Hu M, Huang T, Hu Y, Sang N, Zhao Y. Recent progress in treatment of hepatocellular carcinoma. Am J Cancer Res. 2020;10(9):2993.
34. Vogel A, Cervantes A, Chau I, Daniele B, Llovet JM, Meyer T, Nault JC, Neumann U, Ricke J, Sangro B, Schirmacher P. Correction to:"hepatocellular carcinoma: ESMO clinical practice guidelines for diagnosis, treatment and follow-up". Ann Oncol. 2019;30(5):871–3.
35. Viveiros P, Riaz A, Lewandowski RJ, Mahalingam D. Current state of liver-directed therapies and combinatory approaches with systemic therapy in hepatocellular carcinoma (HCC). Cancers. 2019;11(8):1085.
36. Reig M, Forner A, Rimola J, Ferrer-Fàbrega J, Burrel M, Garcia-Criado Á, Kelley RK, Galle PR, Mazzaferro V, Salem R, Sangro B. BCLC strategy for prognosis prediction and treatment recommendation: the 2022 update. J Hepatol. 2022;76(3):681–93.
37. Huang A, Yang XR, Chung WY, Dennison AR, Zhou J. Targeted therapy for hepatocellular carcinoma. Signal Transduct Target Ther. 2020;5(1):146.
38. Llovet JM, Ricci S, Mazzaferro V, Hilgard P, Gane E, Blanc JF, De Oliveira AC, Santoro A, Raoul JL, Forner A, Schwartz M. Sorafenib in advanced hepatocellular carcinoma. N Engl J Med. 2008;359(4):378–90.
39. Kudo M, Finn RS, Qin S, Han KH, Ikeda K, Piscaglia F, Baron A, Park JW, Han G, Jassem J, Blanc JF. Lenvatinib versus sorafenib in first-line treatment of patients with unresectable hepatocellular carcinoma: a randomised phase 3 non-inferiority trial. Lancet. 2018;391(10126):1163–73.
40. Finn RS, Qin S, Ikeda M, Galle PR, Ducreux M, Kim TY, Kudo M, Breder V, Merle P, Kaseb AO, Li D. Atezolizumab plus bevacizumab in unresectable hepatocellular carcinoma. N Engl J Med. 2020;382(20):1894–905.
41. Sonbol MB, Riaz IB, Naqvi SA, Almquist DR, Mina S, Almasri J, Shah S, Almader-Douglas D, Junior PL, Mahipal A, Wee W. Systemic therapy and sequencing options in advanced hepatocellular carcinoma: a systematic review and network meta-analysis. JAMA Oncol. 2020;6(12):e204930.
42. Ettrich TJ, Seufferlein T. Regorafenib. Recent Results Cancer Res. 2018;211:45–56.
43. Granito A, Forgione A, Marinelli S, Renzulli M, Ielasi L, Sansone V, Benevento F, Piscaglia F, Tovoli F. Experience with regorafenib in the treatment of hepatocellular carcinoma. Ther Adv Gastroenterol. 2021;14:17562848211016959.
44. Abou-Alfa GK, Meyer T, Cheng AL, El-Khoueiry AB, Rimassa L, Ryoo BY, Cicin I, Merle P, Chen Y, Park JW, Blanc JF. Cabozantinib in patients with advanced and progressing hepatocellular carcinoma. N Engl J Med. 2018;379(1):54–63.
45. Zhu AX, Kang YK, Yen CJ, Finn RS, Galle PR, Llovet JM, Assenat E, Brandi G, Pracht M, Lim HY, Rau KM. Ramucirumab after sorafenib in patients with advanced hepatocellular carcinoma and increased α-fetoprotein concentrations (REACH-2): a randomised, double-blind, placebo-controlled, phase 3 trial. Lancet Oncol. 2019;20(2):282–96.
46. Zhu AX, Finn RS, Edeline J, Cattan S, Ogasawara S, Palmer D, Verslype C, Zagonel V, Fartoux L, Vogel A, Sarker D. Pembrolizumab in patients with advanced hepatocellular carcinoma previously treated with sorafenib (KEYNOTE-224): a non-randomised, open-label phase 2 trial. Lancet Oncol. 2018;19(7):940–52.
47. Luo XY, Wu KM, He XX. Advances in drug development for hepatocellular carcinoma: clinical trials and potential therapeutic targets. J Exp Clin Cancer Res. 2021;40(1):172.
48. Yau T, Kang YK, Kim TY, El-Khoueiry AB, Santoro A, Sangro B, Melero I, Kudo M, Hou MM, Matilla A, Tovoli F. Efficacy and safety of nivolumab plus ipilimumab in patients with advanced hepatocellular carcinoma previously treated with sorafenib: the CheckMate 040 randomized clinical trial. JAMA Oncol. 2020;6(11):e204564.
49. Llovet JM, Castet F, Heikenwalder M, Maini MK, Mazzaferro V, Pinato DJ, Pikarsky E, Zhu AX, Finn RS. Immunotherapies for hepatocellular carcinoma. Nat Rev Clin Oncol. 2022;19(3):151–72.
50. Estes C, Razavi H, Loomba R, Younossi Z, Sanyal AJ. Modeling the epidemic of nonalcoholic fatty liver disease demonstrates an exponential increase in burden of disease. Hepatology. 2018;67(1):123–33.

51. Prabhakar T, Kaushal K, Prasad M, Gupta E, Sood A, Jain AK, Shukla A, Goel A, Duseja A, Saraya A, Shah S. Etiologic fractions in patients of hepatocellular carcinoma in India with and without a background of cirrhosis: a multi-centric study. Hepatol Int. 2023;17(3):745–52.
52. Jemal A, Ward EM, Johnson CJ, Cronin KA, Ma J, Ryerson AB, Mariotto A, Lake AJ, Wilson R, Sherman RL, Anderson RN. Annual report to the nation on the status of cancer, 1975–2014, featuring survival. JNCI J Natl Cancer Inst. 2017;109(9):djx030.
53. Heimbach JK, Kulik LM, Finn RS, Sirlin CB, Abecassis MM, Roberts LR, Zhu AX, Murad MH, Marrero JA. AASLD guidelines for the treatment of hepatocellular carcinoma. Hepatology. 2018;67(1):358–80.

7 Pancreatic Cancer

Sai Sandeep Annamaraju, Sai Charitha Mullaguri,
Sharat Putta, Ravikanth Vishnubhotla,
and Rama Krishna Kancha

7.1 Introduction

Epidemiology and risk factors: Worldwide, pancreatic cancer ranks fourteenth in incidence with 495,773 new cases, accounting for 2.6% of all cancers, and seventh in mortality with 466,003 deaths, accounting for 4.7% of all cancers [1]. The 5-year and 1-year survival rates are about 9% and 24%, respectively [2, 3]. According to GLOBOCAN, the incidence and mortality in 2020 were higher in Eastern Asia with 181,450 new cases and 173,212 deaths, followed by Northern America (62,643 new cases; 53,277 deaths) and South America (28,030 new cases; 27,118 deaths). The highest age-standardized incidence and death rates were observed in Western Europe (8.6 cases/100,000; 7.8 deaths/100,000). The incidence was higher in males (262,865 new cases; cumulative risk 0.66) when compared to females (232,908 new cases; cumulative risk 0.45). Similarly, mortality in pancreatic cancer was higher in males (246,840 deaths; cumulative risk 0.62) when compared to females (219,163 deaths; cumulative risk 0.41) [1]. However, in South America, the incidence and mortality were slightly higher in females (14,264 new cases; 13,772 deaths) than in males (13,766 new cases; 13,346 deaths). The majority of pancreatic cancers are pancreatic ductal adenocarcinomas (PDACs) [4]. Interestingly, mortality rates in stomach, colorectal, and liver cancers were decreasing due to advances in treatment strategies,

S. S. Annamaraju · S. C. Mullaguri · R. K. Kancha (✉)
Molecular Medicine and Therapeutics Laboratory, Centre for Plant Molecular Biology,
Osmania University, Hyderabad, India
e-mail: ramakancha@osmania.ac.in

S. Putta
Krishna Institute of Medical Sciences, Secunderabad, Telangana, India

R. Vishnubhotla
Department of Genomics and Molecular Biology, Institute of Translational Research, Asian Institute of Gastroenterology, Hyderabad, Telangana, India

R. K. Kancha (ed.), *Biomedical Aspects of Solid Cancers*,
https://doi.org/10.1007/978-981-97-1802-3_7

whereas mortality rates in PDACs still remain high [3]. Reasons for persistent high mortality from PDAC include advanced disease at presentation, lack of optimal screening modalities, poorly defined "risk population," and advanced age at presentation. The percentage of stage-specific diagnoses is 20% at the resectable stage (stage I-II), 30% at the intermediate stage (stage III), and 50% at the metastatic stage (stage IV) [5]. The average survival period for patients diagnosed with metastatic PDACs is less than 1 year [6]. Smoking, chronic diabetes mellitus, nonhereditary chronic pancreatitis, obesity, intraductal papillary mucinous neoplasms (IPMNs), and some of the genetic syndromes are the major risk factors [7]. IPMNs are mucus-producing papillary epithelial neoplasms, which can develop into invasive PDACs [3, 8]. Hereditary pancreatitis is characterized by *PRSS1* and *SPINK1* gene variants [3, 8, 9].

Diagnosis: Majority (60–70%) of pancreatic cancers arise from either the pancreatic head or neck and are characterized by biliary obstruction, weight loss, painless jaundice, cholangitis, and main pancreatic duct obstruction [10]. Other less common subtypes that arise from the pancreatic body and pancreatic tail are characterized by epigastric pain and/or back pain [10]. Multidetector CT angiography is the common imaging technique used for detection [11]. Pancreatic malignancies are less dense when compared to pancreatic parenchyma, and the dual-phase has a crucial role in proper visualization of the vasculature [12]. MRCP (magnetic resonance cholangiopancreatography) is an alternative technique that further evaluates lesions in the liver and biliary tract to detect metastasis [10]. Additionally, endoscopic ultrasound can also be used to detect nearby lymph nodes [13]. Serum biomarkers such as CA 19–9 have higher sensitivity (79–81%) and specificity (82–90%) in the diagnosis of pancreatic cancer [10, 14].

7.2 Classification

Pancreatic cancers are classified based on (i) histology, (ii) molecular profiling, and (iii) staging. (i) Based on histology, pancreatic cancers are classified into (a) ductal carcinomas/exocrine pancreatic cancers and (b) nonductal cancers (Fig. 7.1) [15]. (a) Ductal carcinomas: PDACs account for >90% of exocrine pancreatic cancers among ductal carcinomas (Fig. 7.1) [4, 15]. There are certain subtypes of ductal carcinoma that are highly related to PDACs but classified as different types, including adeno-squamous carcinoma, osteoclastic giant cell carcinoma, and a few rare subtypes (Fig. 7.1) [16]. Adeno-squamous carcinoma (with >15% of squamous cell component) is an uncommon subtype with both glandular and squamous cell differentiation, accounting for 1–4% of exocrine pancreatic cancers [15, 16]. Osteoclastic giant cell carcinoma accounts for 1.4% of pancreatic cancer cases [16]. Other subtypes of ductal carcinomas include colloid carcinoma (1–3% of exocrine pancreatic cancers) and medullary carcinoma [16]. (b) Nonductal cancers: These are rare and account for 5% of total pancreatic malignant neoplasms (Fig. 7.1) [16]. These cancers include pancreatic neuroendocrine neoplasms (PanNENs), acinar cell carcinomas, pancreatoblastomas, and solid pseudo-papillary neoplasms (SPNs) (Fig. 7.1) [15].

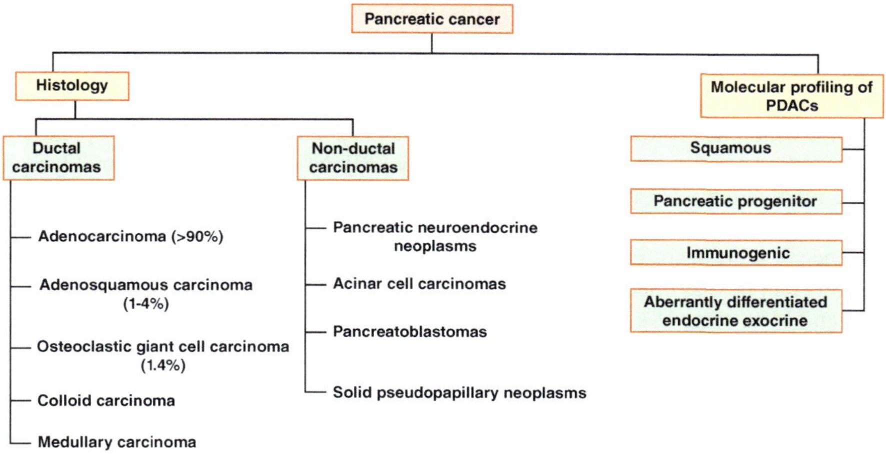

Fig. 7.1 Classification of pancreatic cancer based on histology and pancreatic ductal adenocarcinoma based on the molecular profiling of tumors

(ii) Based on molecular analysis of 456 surgically resected PDAC samples, Bailey et al. classified PDACs into four molecular subtypes that are associated with different survival rates and histopathology [17, 18]. The subtypes include (a) squamous, (b) pancreatic progenitor, (c) immunogenic, and (d) Aberrantly Differentiated Endocrine Exocrine (ADEX) (Fig. 7.1) [17]. (a) Squamous subtype: It is the largest subtype (31% of total incidence) and is characterized by poor prognosis [19]. Characteristic features of the squamous subtype include variants in *TP53* and *KDM6A*, inflammation, autophagy, activation of *MYC,* hypoxia, and alterations in TGFβ and WNT signaling cascades [19]. This subtype is referred to as squamous, as many of the genes mutated in this subtype are highly expressed in C2 squamous-like classes of bladder, head and neck, breast, and lung cancers [18]. (b) Pancreatic progenitor subtype: It accounts for 19% of incidence and contains differentially expressed transcription factors [18]. Additionally, transcriptional networks involved in the oxidation of fatty acids, steroid hormones, drug metabolism, glycosylation (involved in mucin production), and the occurrence of IPMNs are characteristic features of this subtype [17]. This subtype has an overall survival (OS) of 23.7 months [19]. (c) Immunogenic subtype: It has an incidence of 29% and OS of 25.6 months [19]. It is characterized by features similar to that of the pancreatic progenitor subtype and additionally includes up-regulation of CTLA4 and PD1 proteins and differentially expressed genes involved in various immune functions [17]. (d) ADEX subtype: It accounts for 21% of incidence and has an OS of 30 months [19]. It includes differentially expressed genes involved in exocrine activity (*MIST* and *NR5A2*) and the development of insulin-producing beta cells (*MODY*, *INS*, *NEUROD1*, and *NKX2–2*) [17].

(iii) *Staging:* The TNM staging system by AJCC is the most commonly used staging protocol for pancreatic cancer [12]. TNM indicates tumor diameter, the number of regional lymph nodes, and the extent of metastasis, respectively [12]. T1 specifies a tumor with a diameter of 2 cm or less, which is restricted within the pancreas [20]. T2 indicates a tumor with a maximum diameter of >2 cm and ≤ 4 cm that is present within the pancreas [21]. T3 refers to a tumor with a diameter of >4 cm, which has spread beyond the pancreas [21]. T4 refers to a tumor spreading to the celiac axis or superior mesenteric artery [20]. N0 specifies no regional lymph node involvement, N1 refers to the involvement of 1–3 regional lymph nodes, and N2 refers to the involvement of 4 or more lymph nodes [21]. M0 indicates the absence of metastasis, and M1 specifies metastasis to distant organs [20]. Pancreatic cancers can be classified into four stages: stage IA (T1, N0, and M0), stage IB (T2, N0, and M0), stage IIA (T3, N0, and M0), stage IIB (T1-T3, N1, and M0), stage III (T1-T3, N2, M0 or T4, any N, and M0) and stage IV (any T, any N, and M1) [20].

7.3 Pathophysiology

Anatomy: The pancreas lies posterior to the stomach and is a heterocrine gland comprising both exocrine and endocrine functions. The exocrine part accounts for 98% of the pancreas, within which the endocrine part is embedded. Various digestive enzymes are produced by the exocrine pancreas and are secreted into the duodenum. The endocrine part (islets) produces hormones that are released directly into the blood. The pancreas is surrounded and incompletely lobulated by loose connective tissue. Each lobule (acini) is made up of spherical clusters of pyramidal acinar cells that secrete digestive enzymes. Intralobular ducts originate from each acinus, which unite to form interlobular ducts; interlobular ducts further merge to eventually form the main pancreatic duct (Fig. 7.2). The pancreas consists of four anatomical segments, including the head, uncinate process, body, and tail (Fig. 7.2). The head and uncinate are located slightly toward the right of the midline within the "C" loop formed by the medial duodenal wall. The body lies posterior to the stomach, and the tail continues into the hilum of the spleen. The majority of PDACs occur in the pancreatic head (60–70%), while about 30% occur in the body and tail [22].

Cell of origin: The major cell types in the pancreas include acinar cells (exocrine), ductal cells (epithelial cells), and α, β, δ, and ε cells (endocrine cells) (Fig. 7.2) [4]. Pancreatic stem cells are multipotent; they can differentiate into both endocrine and exocrine cells. Interestingly, mature cells of the pancreas have the ability to de-differentiate [23]. Mature acinar cells have significant plasticity [24]. In response to certain macro and micro environmental stimuli, these cells can de-differentiate into a progenitor phenotype (expressing ductal markers) through acinar to ductal metaplasia (ADM) [4, 24]. ADM was frequently found in injured pancreatic tissue, closely associated with PDACs [23].

PDACs develop by accumulating a series of stepwise mutations from normal mucosa to distinct precursor lesions, eventually leading to malignancy [14]. The majority of PDACs arise from precursor lesions referred to as PanINs (pancreatic intraepithelial neoplasms), while a minor proportion of the PDACs (4%) arise from cystic neoplasms such as IPMNs (intraductal papillary mucinous neoplasms) and

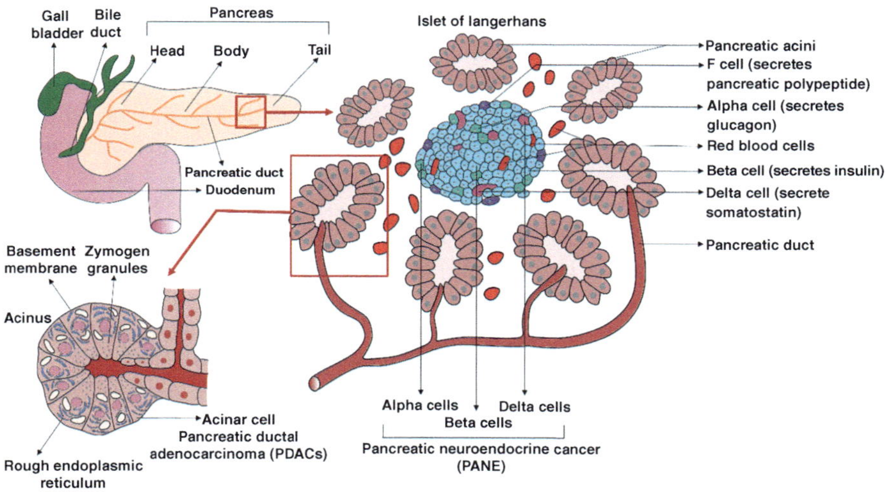

Fig. 7.2 Pathophysiology of pancreatic cancer. Basic anatomy of pancreas and the cell of origin of major subtypes of pancreatic cancer were shown

MCNs (mucinous cystic neoplasms) [16, 25]. PDACs mostly occur as solitary lesions, though some exist as multifocal lesions [22].

PanINs: PanINs arise from pancreatic ducts and are less than 5 mm in size. The majority of the PanINs arise from *KRAS*-driven acinar cells [23]. PanINs are microscopic, flat or papillary, noninvasive, epithelial microscopic precursor lesions with varying degrees of atypia and mucin production [26]. PanINs may play a role in localized pancreatitis; the subsequent epithelial injury and repair process might contribute to the development of malignancies [14]. Based on cytological atypia, PanINs are classified into two types, namely low-grade (PanIN1A/1B, PanIN2) and high-grade (PanIN3) lesions [27]. It is estimated that it will take around 11.3 and 12.3 years for men and women, respectively, to progress from PanIN3 to PDAC [28]. *KRAS* plays an important role in the silencing of various acinar cell housekeeping genes and up-regulation of homeobox genes such as *PDX1* and *SOX9* [24]. Point mutations in *KRAS* (particularly in codon 12) were identified in nearly 90% of grade 1 and grade 2 PanINs [7]. In addition to activating mutations, the *KRAS* gene also harbors amplifications resulting in higher tumor-promoting potential. Further, overexpression of *AKT2* and *PI3K* was observed, leading to increased tumor survival [4]. The process of acinar-to-ductal metaplasia was mediated by hyperactivity of the *KRAS* (demonstrated by in vitro mouse acinar cells that transdifferentiate into duct-like cells) [24]. ADM generally was a reversible process leading to repopulation of the pancreas; however, when oncogenic *KRAS* gene or growth factor signaling was altered, ADM becomes irreversible [24]. Transformation into PanINs was considered as the initial step [4]. In PanIN2 and PanIN3, mutational inactivation in *SMAD4*, *TP53*, and *CDKN2A* takes place, indicating that *KRAS* mutations have a crucial role in tumor initiation, while *SMAD4*, *TP53*, and *CDKN2A* mutations were acting as rate-limiting steps in the progression into PDAC [7]. Additionally, germline variants in *BRCA1/2*, *PALB2*, and *ATM*, as well as somatic variants in the DNA mismatch repair genes, were also observed in a subset of tumors [4]. Alterations in epigenetic regulatory circuits that include loss of function variants in the SWI/SNF complex were found in 10–15% of pancreatic cancer patients [7].

IPMNs: These were the most common type of cystic neoplasms [13]. IPMNs are visible epithelial neoplasms (>1 cm in size) that are rarely flat, predominantly papillary, noninvasive, occurring in the main pancreatic ducts [26]. The average age at diagnosis is 60–70 years [29]. Though the majority of IPMNs are asymptomatic, nearly 25% of IPMNs progress to invasive cancers [7]. The incidence of PDAC can vary according to the type of ducts from which they arise [14]. IPMNs can be classified into main duct (15–21%), branch duct (41–64%), and mixed type (22–38%) [13]. IPMNs found in the main pancreatic ducts have a higher malignancy than those found in the branch pancreatic ducts [7]. Studies demonstrated that malignant cells are present in 70% of main duct IPMNs when compared to 25% in the branch duct resected IPMNs [14]. The characteristic cytological features include the presence of thick extracellular mucin, groups of mucinous glandular epithelial cells, papillary clusters, single cells with varying degrees of cytological atypia, and cyst debris [29]. Mutations in IPMNs include *KRAS* (40–65%), *GNAS* (40–85%), and *RNF43* (50%) [7]. IPMNs were also classified based on the degree of dysplasia into low grade and high grade [26, 30]. They account for 40% of the total cystic neoplasms [31].

MCN: MCNs are mucin-producing epithelial neoplasms that contain ovarian-type stroma [31]. They account for 23% of the total resected pancreatic tumors [32]. MCNs often occur in the pancreatic body or tail and are significantly more common in females than in males (20:1) [29]. They usually affect patients at 40–50 years of age [31]. These neoplasms do not connect with the ductal system of the pancreas and are not present as multiple cysts [29, 30]. One-third of the MCNs can lead to invasive carcinoma [30]. Like other epithelial tumors, activating mutations in the *KRAS* are early genetic alterations while *TP53* and *SMAD4* act as late events; MCNs do not have any subtype specific genetic alterations [29].

7.4 Treatment

Surgery: Fewer than 20% of patients have localized tumors that are resectable at diagnosis, whilst about 85% of patients have locally advanced or metastasized cancers [33, 34]. The survival of patients with surgical resection is 20.1–28.0 months [35]. For pancreatic cancers in the head, a pancreaticoduodenectomy (Whipple procedure) is performed, which involves the resection of the pancreatic head, duodenum, gallbladder, and common bile duct [35, 36]. Pancreaticoduodenectomy is classified into two types based on gastric antrum removal (classic Whipple procedure) or preservation (pyloric-preserving Whipple procedure) [36]. There is no significant difference between classic and pyloric-preserving Whipple procedures in terms of long-term survival and complications; however, the operating time, blood loss, and potential bile reflux are less in the pyloric-preserving Whipple procedure [36]. For the treatment of pancreatic tail cancers, distal pancreatectomy with splenectomy is performed [34, 37]. The aim of the resection is to remove the tumor in its entirety, with the margins of the resected specimen being free of microscopic disease (R_0). R_0 resection results in long-term survival among patients without node involvement [35]. After the resection, treatment with adjuvant therapy can improve OS and disease-free survival rates [38].

Adjuvant therapy: The current standard treatment for patients who undergo surgery is a 6-month adjuvant therapy with mFOLFIRINOX in patients who are fit enough, or 6 months of treatment with gemcitabine plus capecitabine combination [38]. The PRODIGE-24 study provided an OS of 54.4 months (3-year survival of more than 60%) with mFOLFIRINOX when compared to 35.0 months with gemcitabine monotherapy [39]. Despite this obvious survival benefit, the usage was limited to fewer patients due to the high toxicity associated with mFOLFIRINOX [33]. The ESPAC-4 study showed a survival advantage upon treatment with gemcitabine plus capecitabine combination (28 months) when compared to gemcitabine alone (25.5 months) [40]. Less fit patients who are older than 70 years with ECOG performance status of 2, or patients who exhibit contraindication to FOLFIRINOX can benefit from gemcitabine plus capecitabine combination [33].

Systemic therapy: For metastatic disease, FOLFIRINOX or gemcitabine plus nab-paclitaxel combination were recommended as first-line treatment regimens [39, 41]. These drugs showed significant improvement when compared to gemcitabine monotherapy [42, 43]. The PRODIGE4/ACCORD11 study revealed that when compared to gemcitabine monotherapy, FOLFIRINOX had superior outcomes with 11.1 months, 48.4%, and 6.4 months of OS, 1-year survival, and progression-free survival (PFS) with FOLFIRINOX as compared to 6.8 months, 20.6%, and 3.3 months with gemcitabine monotherapy [39, 44]. However, FOLFIRINOX was associated with increased toxicity profiles (hazard ratio-0.57), with a higher occurrence of neutropenia, thrombocytopenia, diarrhea, sensory neuropathy, and liver enzyme derangement [45]. The MPACT study confirmed that the usage of gemcitabine plus nab-paclitaxel has better survival (8.5 months) than the gemcitabine monotherapy (6.7 months) [41]. Various gemcitabine-based therapies that include gemcitabine alone or with either capecitabine or erlotinib were also recommended as first-line therapies [38]. PDAC with mutations in *BRCA 1/2* were sensitive to platinum-based agents, and patients with germline *BRCA1* mutations can benefit from olaparib as maintenance therapy [46].

Appropriate second-line treatment regimen is selected based on the first-line treatment and patient criteria [42]. The nanoliposomal-irinotecan, 5-FU, and folinic acid combination was a new second-line regimen that was suitable only for those patients who are progressing on gemcitabine-based therapy [33]. Currently, mFOLFOX6 as well as a combination of nanoliposomal-irinotecan, 5-FU, and folinic acid are the two second-line regimens [38, 47]. There is supportive evidence for the usage of gemcitabine plus nab-paclitaxel combination after treatment with FOLFIRINOX [48]. The mFOLFIRINOX reported the longest median OS of

14.4 months in a phase I/II trial [49]. A median overall response rate (ORR) of 13 months was observed with mFOLFIRINOX among patients who were unresponsive to gemcitabine plus nab-paclitaxel combination; hence mFOLFIRINOX can be considered as second-line treatment in these patients with good performance status [43]. Second-line therapy with gemcitabine was recommended for those who received prior mFOLFIRINOX [43]. Entrectinib, a TRK inhibitor, is currently in phase II trials [50]. As a second-line setting, the FDA approved larotrectinib for patients with *NTRK* gene fusions and pembrolizumab for patients with mismatch repair deficiency (MRD) [47]. Drugs in phase-I trials, such as ulixertinib (in combination with nab-paclitaxel plus gemcitabine) and KO-947 (alone), were used to inhibit ERK1/2 [50]. Ulixertinib was approved in the first-line setting and KO-947 was approved as the second-line setting [50].

7.5 Conclusion

Worldwide, the burden of pancreatic cancer has increased drastically over the past few decades [51]. The 5-year survival, however, remains dismally low at 10%. This is consequent to the fact that 90% of tumors are detected at a late stage, with the cancer being either unresectable or associated with systemic metastases at diagnosis [52]. In contrast, 5-year survival in resectable disease is significantly better, underscoring the need for early detection. Surveillance can, however, be offered to the subgroup of patients with inherited mutations, with an objective to detect and treat early-stage disease. Surgical removal of the tumor represents the only curative option and is typically feasible in early-stage disease [10]. Advanced disease, which is unresectable and/or metastatic, is treated with FOLFIRINOX or gemcitabine plus albumin-bound (nab) paclitaxel. Future strategies to reduce the burden of the disease should include smoking and alcohol cessation, obesity prevention, in addition to screening high-risk individuals for early disease. Advances in genomics, stromal therapies, and immunotherapies, whilst making best use of conventional therapies including chemotherapy and radiotherapy, can facilitate tailor-made treatments for individual patients [53].

References

1. Sung H, Ferlay J, Siegel RL, Laversanne M, Soerjomataram I, Jemal A, Bray F. Global cancer statistics 2020: GLOBOCAN estimates of incidence and mortality worldwide for 36 cancers in 185 countries. CA Cancer J Clin. 2021;71(3):209–49.
2. Bradley SD, Talukder AH, Lai I, Davis R, Alvarez H, Tiriac H, Zhang M, Chiu Y, Melendez B, Jackson KR, Katailiha A. Vestigial-like 1 is a shared targetable cancer-placenta antigen expressed by pancreatic and basal-like breast cancers. Nat Commun. 2020;11(1):5332.
3. Ushio J, Kanno A, Ikeda E, Ando K, Nagai H, Miwata T, Kawasaki Y, Tada Y, Yokoyama K, Numao N, Tamada K. Pancreatic ductal adenocarcinoma: epidemiology and risk factors. Diagnostics. 2021;11(3):562.

4. Orth M, Metzger P, Gerum S, Mayerle J, Schneider G, Belka C, Schnurr M, Lauber K. Pancreatic ductal adenocarcinoma: biological hallmarks, current status, and future perspectives of combined modality treatment approaches. Radiat Oncol. 2019;14(1):1–20.
5. Loveday BP, Lipton L, Thomson BN. Pancreatic cancer: an update on diagnosis and management. Aust J Gen Pract. 2019;48(12):826–31.
6. Hayashi A, Hong J, Iacobuzio-Donahue CA. The pancreatic cancer genome revisited. Nat Rev Gastroenterol Hepatol. 2021;18(7):469–81.
7. Ryan DP, Hong TS, Bardeesy N. Pancreatic adenocarcinoma. N Engl J Med. 2014;371(11):1039–49.
8. Klein AP. Pancreatic cancer epidemiology: understanding the role of lifestyle and inherited risk factors. Nat Rev Gastroenterol Hepatol. 2021;18(7):493–502.
9. Matsubayashi H, Takaori K, Morizane C, Maguchi H, Mizuma M, Takahashi H, Wada K, Hosoi H, Yachida S, Suzuki M, Usui R. Familial pancreatic cancer: concept, management and issues. World J Gastroenterol. 2017;23(6):935.
10. Mizrahi JD, Surana R, Valle JW, Shroff RT. Pancreatic cancer. Lancet. 2020;395(10242): 2008–20.
11. Zhang L, Sanagapalli S, Stoita A. Challenges in diagnosis of pancreatic cancer. World J Gastroenterol. 2018;24(19):2047.
12. Chu LC, Goggins MG, Fishman EK. Diagnosis and detection of pancreatic cancer. Cancer J. 2017;23(6):333–42.
13. Singhi AD, Koay EJ, Chari ST, Maitra A, Singhi AD, Koay EJ, Chari ST, Maitra A. Early detection of pancreatic cancer: opportunities and challenges. Gastroenterology. 2019;156(7):2024–40.
14. McGuigan A, Kelly P, Turkington RC, Jones C, Coleman HG, McCain RS. Pancreatic cancer: A review of clinical diagnosis, epidemiology, treatment and outcomes. World J Gastroenterol. 2018;24(43):4846.
15. Collisson EA, Bailey P, Chang DK, Biankin AV. Molecular subtypes of pancreatic cancer. Nat Rev Gastroenterol Hepatol. 2019;16(4):207–20.
16. Mostafa ME, Erbarut-Seven I, Pehlivanoglu B, Adsay V. Pathologic classification of" pancreatic cancers": current concepts and challenges. Chin Clin Oncol. 2017;6(6):59.
17. Du Y, Zhao B, Liu Z, Ren X, Zhao W, Li Z, You L, Zhao Y. Molecular subtyping of pancreatic cancer: translating genomics and transcriptomics into the clinic. J Cancer. 2017;8(4):513.
18. Bailey P, Chang DK, Nones K, Johns AL, Patch AM, Gingras MC, Miller DK, Christ AN, Bruxner TJ, Quinn MC, Nourse C, Australian Pancreatic Cancer Genome I, Munzy DM, Fisher WE, Karim SA, Eshleman JR, Hruban RH, Pilarsky C, Morton JP, Sansom OJ, Scarpa A, Musgrove EA, Bailey UM, Hofmann O, Sutherland RL, Wheeler DA, Gill AJ, Gibbs RA, Pearson JV, Waddell N, Biankin AV, Grimmond SM. Genomic analyses identify molecular subtypes of pancreatic cancer. Nature. 2016;531(7592):47–52.
19. Torres C, Grippo PJ. Pancreatic cancer subtypes: a roadmap for precision medicine. Ann Med. 2018;50(4):277–87.
20. Van Roessel S, Kasumova GG, Verheij J, Najarian RM, Maggino L, De Pastena M, Malleo G, Marchegiani G, Salvia R, Ng SC, De Geus SW. International validation of the eighth edition of the American Joint Committee on Cancer (AJCC) TNM staging system in patients with resected pancreatic cancer. JAMA Surg. 2018;153(12):e183617.
21. Liao X, Zhang D. The 8th edition American joint committee on cancer staging for hepato-pancreato-biliary cancer: a review and update. Arch Pathol Lab Med. 2021 May 1;145(5):543–53.
22. Luchini C, Capelli P, Scarpa A. Pancreatic ductal adenocarcinoma and its variants. Surg Pathol Clin. 2016;9(4):547–60.
23. Yamaguchi J, Yokoyama Y, Kokuryo T, Ebata T, Nagino M. Cells of origin of pancreatic neoplasms. Surg Today. 2018;48:9–17.
24. Storz P. Acinar cell plasticity and development of pancreatic ductal adenocarcinoma. Nat Rev Gastroenterol Hepatol. 2017;14(5):296–304.

25. Hruban RH, Adsay NV, Albores-Saavedra J, Compton C, Garrett ES, Goodman SN, Kern SE, Klimstra DS, Klöppel G, Longnecker DS, Lüttges J. Pancreatic intraepithelial neoplasia: a new nomenclature and classification system for pancreatic duct lesions. Am J Surg Pathol. 2001;25(5):579–86.
26. Basturk O, Hong SM, Wood LD, Adsay NV, Albores-Saavedra J, Biankin AV, Brosens LA, Fukushima N, Goggins M, Hruban RH, Kato Y. A revised classification system and recommendations from the Baltimore consensus meeting for neoplastic precursor lesions in the pancreas. Am J Surg Pathol. 2015;39(12):1730.
27. Kim JY, Hong SM. Precursor lesions of pancreatic cancer. Oncol Res Treat. 2018;41(10):603–10.
28. Peters ML, Eckel A, Mueller PP, Tramontano AC, Weaver DT, Lietz A, Hur C, Kong CY, Pandharipande PV. Progression to pancreatic ductal adenocarcinoma from pancreatic intraepithelial neoplasia: results of a simulation model. Pancreatology. 2018;18(8):928–34.
29. Pittman ME, Rao R, Hruban RH. Classification, morphology, molecular pathogenesis, and outcome of premalignant lesions of the pancreas. Arch Pathol Lab Med. 2017;141(12):1606–14.
30. Hruban RH, Takaori K, Canto M, Fishman EK, Campbell K, Brune K, Kern SE, Goggins M. Clinical importance of precursor lesions in the pancreas. J Hepato-Biliary-Pancreat Surg. 2007;14:255–63.
31. Ozcan K, Klimstra DS. A review of mucinous cystic and Intraductal neoplasms of the Pancreatobiliary tract: recent advances. Arch Pathol Lab Med. 2022;146(3):298–311.
32. Distler M, Aust D, Weitz J, Pilarsky C, Grützmann R. Precursor lesions for sporadic pancreatic cancer: PanIN, IPMN, and MCN. Biomed Res Int. 2014;2014:474905.
33. De Dosso S, Siebenhüner AR, Winder T, Meisel A, Fritsch R, Astaras C, Szturz P, Borner M. Treatment landscape of metastatic pancreatic cancer. Cancer Treat Rev. 2021 May;1(96):102180.
34. Kleeff J, Korc M, Apte M, La Vecchia C, Johnson CD, Biankin AV, Neale RE, Tempero M, Tuveson DA, Hruban RH, Neoptolemos JP. Pancreatic cancer (primer). Nat Rev Dis Primers. 2016;2(1):160222.
35. Jeune F, Coriat R, Prat F, Dousset B, Vaillant JC, Gaujoux S. Pancreatic cancer surgical management. Presse Med. 2019;48(3):e147–58.
36. Huettner FJ, Fitzmaurice C, Schwarzer G, Seiler CM, Antes G, Buechler MW, Diener MK. Pylorus-preserving pancreaticoduodenectomy (pp Whipple) versus pancreaticoduodenectomy (classic Whipple) for surgical treatment of periampullary and pancreatic carcinoma. Cochrane Database Syst Rev. 2016;2:CD006053.
37. Torphy RJ, Fujiwara Y, Schulick RD. Pancreatic cancer treatment: better, but a long way to go. Surg Today. 2020;50:1117–25.
38. Springfeld C, Jäger D, Büchler MW, Strobel O, Hackert T, Palmer DH, Neoptolemos JP. Chemotherapy for pancreatic cancer. La Presse Medicale. 2019;48(3):e159–74.
39. Conroy T, Desseigne F, Ychou M, Bouché O, Guimbaud R, Bécouarn Y, Adenis A, Raoul JL, Gourgou-Bourgade S, de la Fouchardière C, Bennouna J. FOLFIRINOX versus gemcitabine for metastatic pancreatic cancer. N Engl J Med. 2011;364(19):1817–25.
40. Neoptolemos JP, Palmer DH, Ghaneh P, Psarelli EE, Valle JW, Halloran CM, Faluyi O, O'Reilly DA, Cunningham D, Wadsley J, Darby S. Comparison of adjuvant gemcitabine and capecitabine with gemcitabine monotherapy in patients with resected pancreatic cancer (ESPAC-4): a multicentre, open-label, randomised, phase 3 trial. Lancet. 2017;389(10073):1011–24.
41. Von Hoff DD, Ervin T, Arena FP, Chiorean EG, Infante J, Moore M, Seay T, Tjulandin SA, Ma WW, Saleh MN, Harris M. Increased survival in pancreatic cancer with nab-paclitaxel plus gemcitabine. N Engl J Med. 2013;369(18):1691–703.
42. Ellenrieder V, König A, Seufferlein T. Current standard and future perspectives in first-and second-line treatment of metastatic pancreatic adenocarcinoma. Digestion. 1960;94(1):44–9.
43. Singh RR, O'Reilly EM. New treatment strategies for metastatic pancreatic ductal adenocarcinoma. Drugs. 2020;80(7):647–69.
44. Cheema AR, O'Reilly EM. Management of metastatic pancreatic adenocarcinoma. Surgical Clinics. 2016;96(6):1391–414.

45. Pokorny AM, Chin VT, Nagrial AM, Yip D, Chantrill LA. Metastatic pancreatic ductal adenocarcinoma: diagnosis and treatment with a view to the future. Intern Med J. 2018;48(6):637–44.
46. Hammel P, Zhang C, Matile J, Colle E, Hadj-Naceur I, Gagaille MP, Bouattour M, Cros J, de Mestier L, Lamuraglia M. PARP inhibition in treatment of pancreatic cancer. Expert Rev Anticancer Ther. 2020;20(11):939–45.
47. Lellouche L, Palmieri LJ, Dermine S, Brezault C, Chaussade S, Coriat R. Systemic therapy in metastatic pancreatic adenocarcinoma: current practice and perspectives. Ther Adv Med Oncol. 2021;13:17588359211018539.
48. Blomstrand H, Batra A, Cheung WY, Elander NO. Real-world evidence on first-and second-line palliative chemotherapy in advanced pancreatic cancer. World J Clin Oncol. 2021;12(9):787.
49. Ramanathan RK, McDonough SL, Philip PA, Hingorani SR, Lacy J, Kortmansky JS, Thumar J, Chiorean EG, Shields AF, Behl D, Mehan PT. Phase IB/II randomized study of FOLFIRINOX plus pegylated recombinant human hyaluronidase versus FOLFIRINOX alone in patients with metastatic pancreatic adenocarcinoma: SWOG S1313. J Clin Oncol. 2019;37(13):1062.
50. Nevala-Plagemann C, Hidalgo M, Garrido-Laguna I. From state-of-the-art treatments to novel therapies for advanced-stage pancreatic cancer. Nat Rev Clin Oncol. 2020;17(2):108–23.
51. Pourshams A, Sepanlou SG, Ikuta KS, Bisignano C, Safiri S, Roshandel G, Sharif M, Khatibian M, Fitzmaurice C, Nixon MR, Abbasi N. The global, regional, and national burden of pancreatic cancer and its attributable risk factors in 195 countries and territories, 1990–2017: a systematic analysis for the global burden of disease study 2017. Lancet Gastroenterol Hepatol. 2019;4(12):934–47.
52. Siegel RL, Miller KD, Fuchs HE, Jemal A. Cancer statistics, 2022. CA Cancer J Clin. 2022;72(1):7–33.
53. Wood LD, Canto MI, Jaffee EM, Simeone DM. Pancreatic cancer: pathogenesis, screening, diagnosis and treatment. Gastroenterology. 2022;163:386.

Biliary Tract Cancers

8

Sai Sandeep Annamaraju, Sai Charitha Mullaguri,
Ravikanth Vishnubhotla, and Rama Krishna Kancha

8.1 Introduction

Epidemiology: Biliary tract cancers (BTCs) are malignancies that include cholangiocarcinoma (CCA) and gallbladder cancer (GBC) [1, 2]. BTCs account for nearly 3% of all cancers [1] with a mortality rate of 3.58 deaths per 100,000 [3]. According to AJCC, the 5-year survival rates were 50%, 30%, 10%, and 0% for patients with stages I, II, III, and IV, respectively [1]. Among the three subtypes of CCAs that were classified based on the anatomic site of origin, perihilar cholangiocarcinoma (PCCA) accounts for 50–60%, distal cholangiocarcinoma (DCCA) constitutes 20–30%, and intrahepatic cholangiocarcinoma (ICCA) accounts for 10–20% of all cases [4]. PCCA and DCCA together constitute extrahepatic cholangiocarcinomas (ECCA) [1, 2]. The 5-year survival rates were 10%, 11%, and 8% for PCCA, DCCA, and ICCA, respectively [4]. Interestingly, the incidence of CCA is as high as 85 cases per 100,000 in Southeast Asia, which can be attributed to liver fluke parasites [2–4].

In the year 2020, GBC ranked 23rd worldwide in incidence (115,949 new cases) and 20th in mortality (84,695 deaths) [5]. According to the GLOBOCAN, the incidence and mortality were high in Eastern Asia (43,628 cases; 33,014 deaths), followed by South-Central Asia (32,026 cases; 24,675 deaths) and South America (7948 cases; 5109 deaths). High age-standardized incidence rates were observed in South-Central Asia (1.7 cases/100,000), followed by Northern Africa (1.5

S. S. Annamaraju · S. C. Mullaguri · R. K. Kancha (✉)
Molecular Medicine and Therapeutics Laboratory, Centre for Plant Molecular Biology, Osmania University, Hyderabad, India
e-mail: ramakancha@osmania.ac.in

R. Vishnubhotla
Department of Genomics and Molecular Biology, Institute of Translational Research, Asian Institute of Gastroenterology, Hyderabad, Telangana, India

R. K. Kancha (ed.), *Biomedical Aspects of Solid Cancers*,
https://doi.org/10.1007/978-981-97-1802-3_8

cases/100,000), Eastern Asia (1.4 cases/100,000), and South America (1.4 cases/100,000). The incidence of GBC was higher in females (74,887 new cases) when compared to males (41,062 new cases) [5]. Similarly, the mortality rate was also higher in females (54,430 deaths) when compared to males (30,265 deaths) [5]. Interestingly, GBC is the only gastrointestinal cancer that has a higher incidence in females than in males [3, 4]. The 5-year survival rate for GBC is around 20% [4].

Risk factors: Major risk factors for CCA include primary sclerosing cholangitis, Lynch syndrome, and biliary duct anomalies (common to both ICCA and ECCA) [1, 3]. *Opisthorchis viverrine* and *Clonorchis sinensis* are liver trematodes that are endemic to North-East Thailand, China, Vietnam, Cambodia, and Laos, and these regions are considered as hotspots for CCA [1]. Additionally, risk factors for ICCA include obesity, diabetes, cirrhosis, hepatitis B and C, and hepatolithiasis [1, 3]. For ECCA, gallstones are considered a major risk factor [1, 3]. Major risk factors for GBC include gallstones, gallbladder polyps, chronic cholecystitis, *Salmonella typhi*, obesity, and diabetes [1]. Cholelithiasis is the major cause of the high prevalence of GBC in India and Chile [3, 4, 6].

Diagnosis and screening: The common imaging techniques in CCA include ultrasonography, CEUS (contrast-enhanced ultrasonography), CT, MRI, and 18FDG-PET (18 fluorodeoxyglucose-positron emission tomography) [7]. (a) ICCA: Dynamic CT or MRI scans with arterial phase enhancement followed by delayed phase washout are generally used to detect hepatocellular carcinoma (HCC), and ICCA can be detected due to enhancement in the peripheral arterial phase followed by delayed phase enhancement [8, 9]. ICCA can be distinguished from HCC due to the absence of cirrhosis [10]. CA19–9 levels higher than 1000 U/ml can also be used for additional conclusions in the detection of ICCA [9]. (b) ECCA: Jaundice due to biliary obstruction is a very common symptom in ECCA; jaundice is less frequent in ICCA [7, 11]. Blood tests to detect biliary obstruction were performed, which include raised WBC, neutrophilia, and elevated C-reactive protein [8]. A combination of CT, MRI, and MRCP is used to detect both PCCA and DCCA [9]. Endoscopic ultrasonography is also widely used in PCCA and DCCA due to the high tumor detection rate [9]. An optimized FISH was used to detect chromosomal aneusomy in CCA with a sensitivity of 93% and a specificity of 100% [9]. (c) GBC: A CT scan might display GBC as an infiltrative malignancy with a mass of cells in the gallbladder, though small lesions might not be observed [8]. Enhanced CT is used for determination of staging as it detects local invasion into the portal vein and hepatic artery, as well as distant metastasis [8].

8.2 Classification

Different classifications were made based on (i) anatomic site, (ii) tumor growth patterns, and (iii) staging. (i) Based on the anatomic site of the origin of the tumor, CCAs were categorized into ICCA and ECCA (Fig. 8.1) [1, 2]. ECCA is the most prevalent subtype in BTCs and was further classified into perihilar cholangiocarcinoma (PCCA) and distal cholangiocarcinoma (DCCA) (Fig. 8.1) [1, 2]. (ii) Based

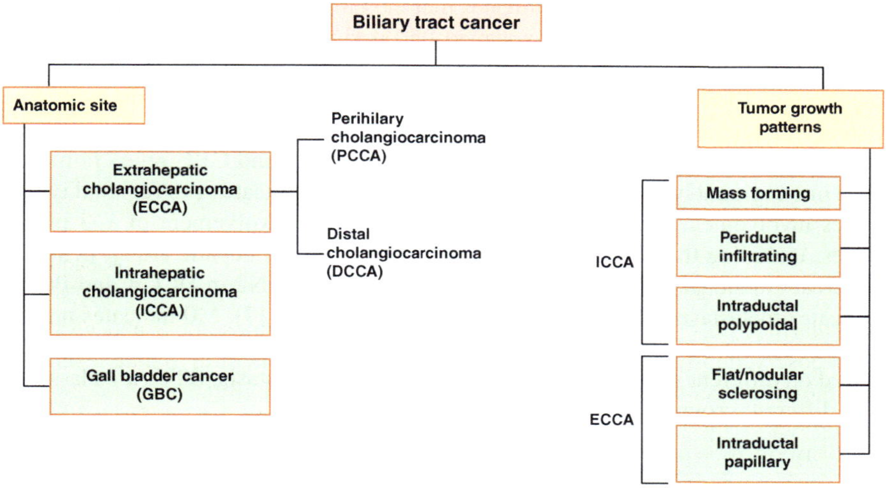

Fig. 8.1 Classification of biliary tract cancers based on site of origin and growth patterns of tumors

on tumor growth patterns, ICCA, PCCA, and DCCA were classified into different growth types (Fig. 8.1). ICCA was classified into mass-forming, periductal infiltrating, and intraductal growth types (Fig. 8.1) [8, 10]. The mass-forming type (78% of ICCA cases) was characterized by a mass located within the liver parenchyma, while periductal infiltrating, corresponding to 16% of ICCA cases, was characterized by longitudinal infiltration along the bile ducts, and intraductal growth type (6% of ICCA cases) was characterized by polypoidal growth in the bile ducts [8, 10]. However, PCCA and DCCA can be flat/nodular sclerosing (73% of ECCA cases) and intraductal papillary type (27% of ECCA cases) (Fig. 8.1) [8]. Two types of precursor lesions, biliary intraepithelial neoplasia (BiINs) and intraductal papillary neoplasms of the bile duct (IPNBs), lead to these growth patterns [8].

(iii) The TNM system by AJCC is the most commonly used staging system for ICCA, PCCA, DCCA, and GBCs [8, 12]. According to AJCC, T_{is} is the carcinoma in situ or high-grade dysplasia [7, 12]. In ICCA, T1 is classified into T1a (a single tumor with a size of 5 cm or less) and T1b (a single tumor with a size of >5 cm) and tumor invasion is absent; T2 refers to a single invaded tumor or multiple tumors with or without invasion, T3 implies tumor extension up to the visceral peritoneum, and T4 in ICCA specifies tumors spreading to local extrahepatic structures [7]. In PCCA, T1 indicates a tumor restricted to the bile duct that extends into the fibrous tissue of the muscle layer, T2 is classified into T2a (tumor infiltrates beyond the bile duct) and T2b (tumor extends to the liver parenchyma), T3 specifies tumor spreading up to the unilateral branches of the portal vein and hepatic artery, and T4 in PCCA refers to tumor invasion into the portal vein, portal vein branches bilaterally with portal vein hepatic artery involvement [7]. In DCCA, T1, T2, and T3 indicate tumor infiltrating the bile duct wall with depths of <5 mm, 5-12 mm, and > 12 mm, respectively, while T4 refers to tumor invasion into the celiac axis and common hepatic artery [7]. In GBC, T1 indicates that the tumor spreads into the lamina propria or muscle layer, T2 specifies spread into peri-muscular connective tissue, T3 indicates perforation into the serosa or direct invasion into the liver or adjacent organs, and T4 refers to the spreading of the tumor into the main portal vein or into two or more hepatic organs [12]. N0 indicates no regional lymph node involvement in ICCA, PCCA, DCCA, and GBC [7, 12]. N1 in ICCA and GBC refers to metastasis into regional lymph nodes, whereas N1 in DCCA indicates 1–3 regional lymph nodes involvement [7, 12]. N1 in PCCA refers to the involvement of 1–3 lymph nodes, including the hilar, cystic duct, common bile duct, hepatic artery, posterior pancreatoduodenal, and portal vein lymph nodes [7, 12]. N2 in DCCA and PCCA indicates metastasis into 4 or more regional lymph nodes [7]. M0 indicates no distant metastasis, and M1 indicates distant metastasis in all four subtypes [7, 12]. Based on different stages of tumor development and metastasis, BTCs are classified into different prognostic stages.

8.3 Pathophysiology

Anatomy: The bile is a dark green to yellowish fluid produced in the liver. It is stored and concentrated in the gallbladder and eventually secreted into the duodenum during digestion. The biliary tract/tree is a ductal system that collects bile from the liver and releases it into the second part of the duodenum (Fig. 8.2). The biliary tree is classified into intrahepatic and extrahepatic biliary tree (Fig. 8.2). The intrahepatic ducts are made up of bile ductules that connect to form segmental ducts, which further merge to form the right and left hepatic ducts (Fig. 8.2). The extrahepatic biliary tree includes extrahepatic segments of the right and left hepatic ducts,

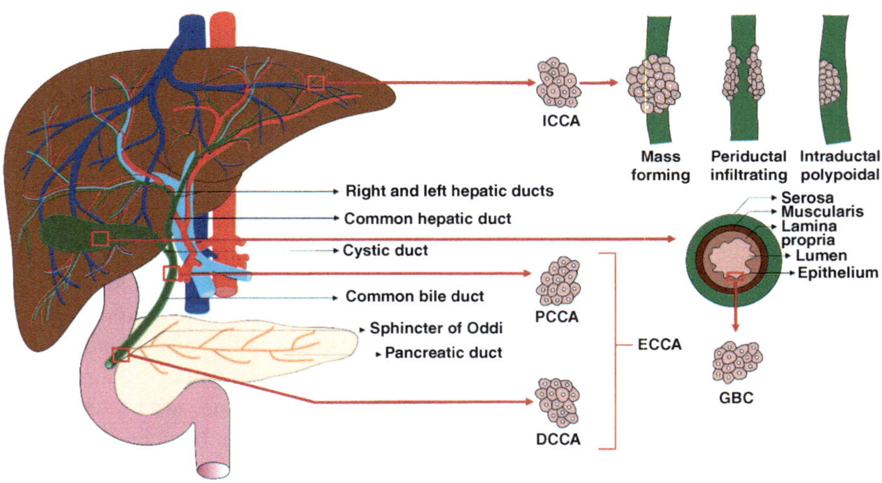

Fig. 8.2 Pathophysiology of biliary tract cancers. The biliary system and the sites of origin of GBC and subtypes of cholangiocarcinoma are shown

common hepatic ducts, and common bile ducts (Fig. 8.2). The gallbladder is a flask-shaped, blind-ending diverticulum that drains into the extrahepatic ducts through the cystic duct (Fig. 8.2).

Cell of origin and histopathology: ICCAs arise either from hepatic stem cells (hepatoblasts) that reside in the canals of Hering of small intrahepatic ducts or from biliary tree stem cells (BTSCs) that reside in the peribiliary glands of large intrahepatic and extrahepatic ducts [13]. Small duct CCAs (small duct ICCAs) or mixed CCAs are derived from hepatoblasts, while the large duct CCAs (large duct ICCAs, PCCAs, and DCCAs) arise from BTSCs [13]. Histologically, PCCA and DCCA have similar appearances to that of the large duct ICCAs [14]. Hepatoblasts form mature hepatocytes and intrahepatic mature cholangiocytes; therefore, they can give rise to variable phenotypes with mixed components (e.g., classical HCC-CCA) [15]. Biliary progenitor cells within the peribiliary glands can form mucin-producing tumors of both intrahepatic (large duct ICCA) and extrahepatic origin (PCCA and DCCA) [16]. Extrahepatic ducts share their origin with the pancreas and are formed before the intrahepatic ducts, eventually merging during embryonic development [4]. Gallbladder cancers are derived from mature cholangiocytes and gallbladder epithelial cells [4].

ICCA: ICCAs originate from the intrahepatic bile ducts that lie close to the second branch of the right and left main hepatic ducts (second-order bile ducts) [8]. WHO has classified ICCA into three types: mass-forming, which contributes to 78%, followed by periductal infiltrating (16%) and intraductal growth type (6%) [8]. The mass-forming type exhibits nodular lesions or masses in the hepatic parenchyma, the periductal type shows carcinoma spreading into portal tracts with narrowing of the affected bile ducts, and the intraductal type is polypoid or papillary growth within the lumen of the dilated bile ducts [17]. Based on anatomical and histologic features, ICCAs can be classified into small duct ICCAs (occur at the peripheral liver) and large duct ICCAs (frequently occur at the perihilar portion of the liver); this classification has clinicopathologic, molecular, and therapeutic significance [14, 18]. The large duct ICCAs consist of mucin-producing columnar cells with papillary architecture and show an infiltrative growth pattern [18]. The tumor cells of the large duct type resemble classic PDACs and have similarities with PCCA in terms of immunohistochemistry and gene expression profiles [16, 19]. Small bile ducts indicate septal and interlobular bile ducts that predominantly exhibit mass-forming growth [4, 17]. The tumor cells of small duct ICCAs are cuboidal with negligible eosinophilic cytoplasm and limited or absence of mucin [16, 19]. The cholangiolar type (small duct ICCA) has comparatively better prognosis and survival rates than the bile duct type (large duct ICCA) [20]. Nearly 45% of the bile duct type (large duct ICCA) contains precancerous lesions such as biliary intraepithelial neoplasms (BilIN) and intraductal papillary neoplasms of bile ducts (IPNBs), whereas the lesions were observed only in 4% of cholangiolar type (small duct ICCAs) [20].

ECCA: PCCA can arise anywhere between second-order ducts and the insertion of the cystic duct [21]. Perihilar bile ducts specify the right and left hepatic ducts, their first branches, and the proximal portion of the extrahepatic bile duct [11, 17].

DCCA originates from the epithelium distal to the cystic duct [8]. Most ECCAs are well to moderately differentiated adenocarcinomas along with abundant fibrous stroma [16]. Histopathologically, most ECCAs are of the pancreatobiliary type [16]. ECCAs are commonly periductal infiltrating tumors, and a few PCCAs are associated with intraductal growth patterns [16].

GBC: GBC arises from the fundus of the gallbladder or from the cystic duct [4, 8]. The pathological outcomes of GBC include intestinal as well as pseudopyloric metaplasia, low-grade, and high-grade dysplasia [22]. Pseudopyloric gland metaplasia is associated with 50% of specimens; however, they do not have any consequential significance for the occurrence of carcinoma, while the goblet cell metaplasia and foveolar metaplasia need closer monitoring [23]. Low-grade and high-grade dysplasia are the primary pathological outcomes of interest; low-grade dysplasia is difficult to define with low clinical significance, while high-grade dysplasia is associated with architectural atypia and is referred to as carcinoma in situ [22].

Precursor lesions: BilINs and IPNBs are the two major precursors to BTC [16]. BilINs are similar to PanINs (pancreatic intraepithelial neoplasia) and are classified into three grades (BilIN1, 2, and 3) [24]. The BilIN1 are flat or micropapillary neoplasms with basal nuclei and mild nuclear abnormalities (mild dysplasia), BilIN2 are associated with moderate dysplasia, and BilIN3 are characterized by severe dysplasia [24, 25]. Both BilIN2 and BilIN3 are pseudopapillary or micropapillary in nature with loss of polarity [25]. IPNBs are rare precursors of the invasive ICCAs and ECCAs [26]. IPNBs are more common in men than in women [16]. The incidence of IPNBs among all bile duct cancers ranges between 7 and 38% [25]. They share histological and clinical features of IPMNs of the pancreas [25].

Genetics: S100P is an immunohistochemical marker, which is expressed in the large duct ICCA and ECCA, but it is negative for small duct ICCA, whereas NCAM and N-cadherins are expressed in the small duct ICCA and are negative for large duct ICCA [18]. Subtype specific genetic alterations are seen in BTC: ICCA (*FGFR2 fusions*, *IDH1/2*, *EPHA2*, and *BAP1*), ECCA (*PRKCA* or *PRKCB* fusions, *ELF3*, and *ARID1B* mutations), and GBC (*EGFR*, *ERBB3*, *PTEN*, *ARID2*, *MLL2*, *MLL3*, and *TERT* promoter mutations) [27]. ECCAs are positive for CK7 and CK19 [16]. ECCAs exhibit overlapping mutations with PDACs that include *KRAS*, *P16/CDKN2A*, *TP53*, and *SMAD4* [16]. Additionally, *ERBB2* mutations were also observed in nearly 20–30% of the ECCAs [28]. In ICCAs, genetic alterations such as *KRAS*, *TP53*, or *MAPK/mTOR* are associated with a poor prognosis compared to *FGFR* genetic alterations [28]. In GBC, mutations in *KRAS*, *TP53*, and *ERBB2* mutations occur at higher frequencies [29].

8.4 Treatment

Surgery: Radical resection is the current treatment option for BTC, but it is possible only in 25–30% of all BTC patients [30]. The 5-year survival rate is only 26% after the resection [30]. Liver resection is the mainstay in the treatment of ICCA, though fewer patients are eligible for resection [31]. Surgical resection in PCCA is carried out by lobectomy with bile duct resection, which is performed in patients who comply with the exclusion criteria, such as the absence of metastatic disease or underlying primary sclerosing cholangitis [9]. Surgical resection in DCCA involves pancreaticoduodenectomy, though for smaller tumors, removal of the extrahepatic biliary tree with lymph nodes is performed [9].

Adjuvant therapy: Though advanced diagnostic techniques and better patient selection have improved the resection rates, the recurrence rate remains very high at 50–60% [32]. Treatment with adjuvant systemic therapy after surgery is associated with better outcomes when compared to observation alone [33]. Management of CCA and GBC involves surgical resection followed by adjuvant therapy with capecitabine [34]. The BILCAP trial (447 patients were included; ICCA-19%, hilar-29%, DCCA-35%, and GBC-17%) revealed that patients treated with capecitabine had a median overall survival (OS) of 51.1 months as compared to 36.4 months in the observation group [35]. Similarly, the median recurrence-free survival (RFS) improved to 24.4 months from 17.5 months [35]. The phase-III ACTICCA-1 trial and a phase-II South Korean trial are both currently randomizing resected patients to cisplatin and gemcitabine combination therapy and capecitabine single agent [36]. Additionally, two independent phase-III trials that include the GEMOX regimen and gemcitabine plus capecitabine combination are currently under evaluation in comparison with capecitabine monotherapy [36].

Systemic therapy: Majority of the BTC patients are diagnosed at advanced stages; in the absence of targetable genetic alterations, these patients will undergo first-line chemotherapy with gemcitabine and cisplatin combination (GC) or gemcitabine and oxaliplatin combination (GEMOX), followed by a second-line therapy with 5-fluorouracil and oxaliplatin/irinotecan [34, 37]. The results of the ABC-02 phase-III clinical trial revealed the superiority of GC when compared to the gemcitabine alone and the median OS was significantly prolonged by 3.6 months (GC: 11.7 months; Gemcitabine alone: 8.1 months), without significant addition of toxicity [38]. However, nearly 40% of the patients in this cohort were associated with gallbladder cancer; therefore, at least for PCCA and DCCA, novel therapies can be considered [9]. When contraindications such as renal insufficiency are observed with cisplatin, it can be replaced with oxaliplatin (GEMOX) [39]. The median progression-free survival (PFS) and the median OS for GEMOX were 3.4 to 6.5 months and 8.3 to 15.4 months, respectively [37]. For elderly patients, the single-agent gemcitabine is still considered [39]. Fluoropyrimidines such as 5-fluorouracil, capecitabine, and S-1 are often used in the second-line setting [39]. Upon progression, FOLFOX may be used if performance status is good and if oxaliplatin was not used as the first-line treatment [33]. Targetable genetic alterations in BTCs include *FGFR2* fusions, *IDH1* mutations, *BRAF*-V600E mutation, *NTRK* fusions, *HER2* amplification, and microsatellite instability [33]. The IDH1 inhibitor ivosidenib showed a median PFS of 2.7 months vs 1.4 months with placebo [33, 40]. Though it was only a minor improvement, the PFS at 6 and 12 months was 32% and 21.9%, respectively [33, 40].

Drugs targeting HER2 showed synergistic antitumor effects in combination with chemotherapy agents [41]. Pemigatinib is a selective inhibitor of FGFR 1–3 and is approved for ICCA patients with *FGFR2* fusions [42]. Based on phase-II data, pemigatinib showed a median PFS and OS of 9.2 and 15 months; infigratinib, an antiangiogenic drug, also received FDA approval very recently [34, 39]. Infigratinib is a nonselective pan-FGFR inhibitor and showed a significant overall response rate (ORR) of 14.8% and a disease control rate of 75.4%, with an estimated PFS of 5.8 months [43, 44]. Dabrafenib, a potent inhibitor of RAF proteins, is currently under evaluation for BTC [33]. Addition of erlotinib to the GEMOX and cediranib significantly improved the response rates; however, these drugs did not show any survival advantage [45]. The single-arm phase-II studies with bevacizumab, sunitinib, and vandetanib exhibited limited efficacy [45]. Larotrectinib, a TRK inhibitor, has shown a positive response to *NTRK* gene fusion-positive malignancies with a response rate of 75% [33].

8.5 Conclusion

Biliary tract cancers, including cholangiocarcinoma and gallbladder cancer, are rare and have poor prognosis. Advanced cytological tests, such as FISH, are useful in diagnosis. The genomic landscape of biliary tract cancers has revealed potential actionable drug targets. Molecular alterations in *FGFR*, *IDH1*, *BRAF*, and *NTRK*, *HER2* amplifications, and microsatellite instability can be targeted. Surgical resection is the main treatment option for localized cancers, while locoregional and systemic therapies are first-line treatment options for advanced and unresectable tumors. Additionally, palliative therapy might improve the quality of life for patients with advanced-stage cancer.

References

1. Valle JW, Lamarca A, Goyal L, Barriuso J, Zhu AX. New horizons for precision medicine in biliary tract CancersPrecision medicine in BTC. Cancer Discov. 2017;7(9):943–62.
2. Turkes F, Carmichael J, Cunningham D, Starling N. Contemporary tailored oncology treatment of biliary tract cancers. Gastroenterol Res Pract. 2019;2019:7698786.
3. Tariq NU, McNamara MG, Valle JW. Biliary tract cancers: current knowledge, clinical candidates and future challenges. Cancer Manag Res. 2019;11:2623–42.
4. Moeini A, Haber PK, Sia D. Cell of origin in biliary tract cancers and clinical implications. JHEP Reports. 2021;3(2):100226.
5. Sung H, Ferlay J, Siegel RL, Laversanne M, Soerjomataram I, Jemal A, Bray F. Global cancer statistics 2020: GLOBOCAN estimates of incidence and mortality worldwide for 36 cancers in 185 countries. CA Cancer J Clin. 2021;71(3):209–49.
6. Kayhanian H, Smyth EC, Braconi C. Emerging molecular targets and therapy for cholangiocarcinoma. World journal of gastrointestinal oncology. 2017;9(7):268.
7. Forner A, Vidili G, Rengo M, Bujanda L, Ponz-Sarvisé M, Lamarca A. Clinical presentation, diagnosis and staging of cholangiocarcinoma. Liver Int. 2019;39:98–107.

8. Valle JW, Kelley RK, Nervi B, Oh DY, Zhu AX. Biliary tract cancer. Lancet. 2021;397(10272):428–44.
9. RizviS K. Cholangiocarcinoma- evolving concepts and therapeutic strategies. NatRev ClinOncol. 2018;15:95.
10. Blechacz B, Komuta M, Roskams T, Gores GJ. Clinical diagnosis and staging of cholangiocarcinoma. Nat Rev Gastroenterol Hepatol. 2011;8(9):512–22.
11. Banales JM, Marin JJ, Lamarca A, Rodrigues PM, Khan SA, Roberts LR, Cardinale V, Carpino G, Andersen JB, Braconi C, Calvisi DF. Cholangiocarcinoma 2020: the next horizon in mechanisms and management. Nat Rev Gastroenterol Hepatol. 2020;17(9):557–88.
12. Shukla SK, Singh G, Shahi KS, Pant P. Staging, treatment, and future approaches of gallbladder carcinoma. J Gastrointest Cancer. 2018;49:9–15.
13. Cardinale V, Carpino G, Reid L, Gaudio E, Alvaro D. Multiple cells of origin in cholangiocarcinoma underlie biological, epidemiological and clinical heterogeneity. World journal of gastrointestinal oncology. 2012;4(5):94.
14. Babushkina EA, Belokopytova LV, Grachev AM, Meko DM, Vaganov EA. Variation of the hydrological regime of Bele-Shira closed basin in southern Siberia and its reflection in the radial growth of Larix sibirica. Reg Environ Chang. 2017;17:1725–37.
15. Raggi C, Invernizzi P, Andersen JB. Impact of microenvironment and stem-like plasticity in cholangiocarcinoma: molecular networks and biological concepts. J Hepatol. 2015;62(1):198–207.
16. Krasinskas AM. Cholangiocarcinoma. Surg Pathol Clin. 2018;11(2):403–29.
17. Nakanuma Y, Kakuda Y. Pathologic classification of cholangiocarcinoma: new concepts. Best Pract Res Clin Gastroenterol. 2015;29(2):277–93.
18. Hayashi A, Misumi K, Shibahara J, Arita J, Sakamoto Y, Hasegawa K, Kokudo N, Fukayama M. Distinct clinicopathologic and genetic features of 2 histologic subtypes of intrahepatic cholangiocarcinoma. Am J Surg Pathol. 2016;40(8):1021–30.
19. Rodrigues PM, Olaizola P, Paiva NA, Olaizola I, Agirre-Lizaso A, Landa A, Bujanda L, Perugorria MJ, Banales JM. Pathogenesis of cholangiocarcinoma. Annu Rev Pathol. 2021;16:433–63.
20. Liau JY, Tsai JH, Yuan RH, Chang CN, Lee HJ, Jeng YM. Morphological subclassification of intrahepatic cholangiocarcinoma: etiological, clinicopathological, and molecular features. Mod Pathol. 2014;27(8):1163–73.
21. Razumilava N, Gores GJ. Classification, diagnosis, and management of cholangiocarcinoma. Clin Gastroenterol Hepatol. 2013;11(1):13–21.
22. Koshiol J, Bellolio E, Vivallo C, Cook P, Roa JC, McGee EE, Losada H, Van Dyke AL, Van De Wyngard V, Prado R, Villaseca M. Distribution of dysplasia and cancer in the gallbladder: an analysis from a high cancer-risk population. Hum Pathol. 2018;82:87–94.
23. Roa JC, Basturk O, Adsay V. Dysplasia and carcinoma of the gallbladder: pathological evaluation, sampling, differential diagnosis and clinical implications. Histopathology. 2021;79(1):2–19.
24. Zen Y, Adsay NV, Bardadin K, Colombari R, Ferrell L, Haga H, Hong SM, Hytiroglou P, Klöppel G, Lauwers GY, Van Leeuwen DJ. Biliary intraepithelial neoplasia: an international interobserver agreement study and proposal for diagnostic criteria. Mod Pathol. 2007;20(6):701–9.
25. Rocha FG, Lee H, Katabi N, DeMatteo RP, Fong Y, D'Angelica MI, Allen PJ, Klimstra DS, Jarnagin WR. Intraductal papillary neoplasm of the bile duct: a biliary equivalent to intraductal papillary mucinous neoplasm of the pancreas? Hepatology. 2012;56(4):1352–60.
26. Schlitter AM, Born D, Bettstetter M, Specht K, Kim-Fuchs C, Riener MO, Jeliazkova P, Sipos B, Siveke JT, Terris B, Zen Y. Intraductal papillary neoplasms of the bile duct: stepwise progression to carcinoma involves common molecular pathways. Mod Pathol. 2014;27(1):73–86.
27. Nakamura H, Arai Y, Totoki Y, Shirota T, Elzawahry A, Kato M, Hama N, Hosoda F, Urushidate T, Ohashi S, Hiraoka N. Genomic spectra of biliary tract cancer. Nat Genet. 2015;47(9):1003–10.

28. Churi CR, Shroff R, Wang Y, Rashid A, Kang HC, Weatherly J, Zuo M, Zinner R, Hong D, Meric-Bernstam F, Janku F. Mutation profiling in cholangiocarcinoma: prognostic and therapeutic implications. PLoS One. 2014;9(12):e115383.
29. Sharma A, Sharma KL, Gupta A, Yadav A, Kumar A. Gallbladder cancer epidemiology, pathogenesis and molecular genetics: recent update. World J Gastroenterol. 2017;23(22):3978.
30. Vogel A, Saborowski A. Cholangiocellular carcinoma. Digestion. 2017;95(3):181–5.
31. Mazzaferro V, Gorgen A, Roayaie S, dit Busset MD, Sapisochin G. Liver resection and transplantation for intrahepatic cholangiocarcinoma. J Hepatol. 2020;72(2):364–77.
32. Zhao DY, Lim KH. Current biologics for treatment of biliary tract cancers. J Gastrointest Oncol. 2017;8(3):430.
33. Sutherland M, Ahmed O, Zaidi A, Ahmed S. Current progress in systemic therapy for biliary tract cancers. J Hepatobiliary Pancreat Sci. 2022;29(10):1094–107.
34. Lamarca A, Edeline J, Goyal L. How I treat biliary tract cancer. ESMO open. 2022;7(1):100378.
35. Primrose JN, Fox RP, Palmer DH, Malik HZ, Prasad R, Mirza D, Anthony A, Corrie P, Falk S, Finch-Jones M, Wasan H. Capecitabine compared with observation in resected biliary tract cancer (BILCAP): a randomised, controlled, multicentre, phase 3 study. Lancet Oncol. 2019;20(5):663–73.
36. Rizzo A, Brandi G. Adjuvant systemic treatment in resected biliary tract cancer: state of the art, controversies, and future directions. Cancer Treat Res Commun. 2021;27:100334.
37. Sasaki T, Isayama H, Nakai Y, Koike K. Current status of chemotherapy for the treatment of advanced biliary tract cancer. Korean J Intern Med. 2013;28(5):515.
38. Valle J, Wasan H, Palmer DH, Cunningham D, Anthoney A, Maraveyas A, Madhusudan S, Iveson T, Hughes S, Pereira SP, Roughton M. Cisplatin plus gemcitabine versus gemcitabine for biliary tract cancer. N Engl J Med. 2010;362(14):1273–81.
39. Vogel A, Saborowski A. Current and future systemic therapies in biliary tract cancer. Visceral Medicine. 2021;37(1):32–8.
40. Marin JJ, Prete MG, Lamarca A, Tavolari S, Landa-Magdalena A, Brandi G, Segatto O, Vogel A, Macias RI, Rodrigues PM, Casta AL. Current and novel therapeutic opportunities for systemic therapy in biliary cancer. Br J Cancer. 2020;123(7):1047–59.
41. Tella SH, Kommalapati A, Borad MJ, Mahipal A. Second-line therapies in advanced biliary tract cancers. Lancet Oncol. 2020;21(1):e29–41.
42. Goyal L, Kongpetch S, Crolley VE, Bridgewater J. Targeting FGFR inhibition in cholangiocarcinoma. Cancer Treat Rev. 2021;95:102170.
43. Xie C, McGrath NA, Monge Bonilla C, Fu J. Systemic treatment options for advanced biliary tract carcinoma. J Gastroenterol. 2020;55:944–57.
44. Zhang W, Zhou H, Wang Y, Zhang Z, Cao G, Song T, Zhang T, Li Q. Systemic treatment of advanced or recurrent biliary tract cancer. Biosci Trends. 2020;14(5):328–41.
45. Kelley RK, Bridgewater J, Gores GJ, Zhu AX. Systemic therapies for intrahepatic cholangiocarcinoma. J Hepatol. 2020;72(2):353–63.

Kidney Cancer

9

Nusrath Banu, Anil Kumar Pasupulati,
Krishna Chaitanya Puligundla, and Rama Krishna Kancha

9.1 Introduction

Epidemiology: Kidney cancer is the 13th most frequent malignancy, with 179,368 deaths, accounting for 1.8% of all cancer-related deaths [1, 2]. In 2020, 431,288 new cases were reported, accounting for 2.2% of all cancer cases [1]. The incidence and mortality rates were highest in Eastern Asia (108,503 cases and 54,658 deaths), followed by Northern America (76,975 cases and 16,791 deaths), and Central and Eastern Europe (49,772 cases and 20,238 deaths) [1]. Further, the global incidence and mortality were more significant in males (271,249 cases, cumulative risk 0.70; 115,600 deaths, cumulative risk 0.28) than in females (160,039 cases, cumulative risk 0.36; 63,768 deaths, cumulative risk 0.12) [1]. The age-standardized incidence rate was highest in North America (12.2 per 100,000), followed by North Europe, Australia, and New Zealand, which showed similar rates (10.3 per 100,000) [1]. The least incidence rate was observed in Central Africa (1.0 per 100,000), followed by Melanesia and South-Central Asia with incidences of 1.2 and 1.4 per 100,000, respectively [1]. In the United States (US), the incidence has increased from 7.1/100,000 in 1975 to 14.9/100,000 in 2016 [3]. However, kidney cancer incidence has plateaued after peaking at 16.0/100,000 in 2008 [3]. In the United States, people with kidney cancer are diagnosed at an average age of 64, with the majority being

N. Banu · R. K. Kancha (✉)
Molecular Medicine and Therapeutics Laboratory, CPMB, Osmania University, Hyderabad, India
e-mail: ramakancha@osmania.ac.in

A. K. Pasupulati
Department of Biochemistry, School of Life Sciences, Hyderabad, India

K. C. Puligundla (✉)
Department of Medical Oncology, MNJ Institute of Oncology and Regional Cancer Centre, Hyderabad, India

R. K. Kancha (ed.), *Biomedical Aspects of Solid Cancers*,
https://doi.org/10.1007/978-981-97-1802-3_9

diagnosed between the ages of 65 and 74 [3]. The age-standardized mortality was 3.6/100,000 in the year 2016 [3]. In the United States, the age-standardized incidence rate was higher for black men (15.6/100,000) than for white men (14.0/100,000) [3].

Among kidney cancers, renal cell carcinoma (RCC) is the most frequent, accounting for 1–3% of all human malignancies [4–6]. RCC is further divided into (a) clear cell carcinoma, which accounts for 75%, and (b) nonclear cell carcinoma, which accounts for 25% of all RCC cases [7, 8]. Wilms tumor (WT), rhabdoid renal tumor, kidney sarcomas, and renal carcinomas are malignant renal tumors that account for 5% of all childhood cancers [9]. WT is more common in children, and its prevalence varies across the globe and by ethnicity [9]. The incidence rate of kidney cancers in children was 8.3 per million; North America and Europe have higher incidence rates (9–10 per million) as compared to the Asian regions (4–5 per million) [9]. Among adults with kidney cancer in the United States, RCC is the deadliest, with a survival rate of 46.8% in 1977 [3]. However, this survival rate has increased significantly to 76% between 2009 and 2015 [3]. Survival varies according to the disease stage at the time of diagnosis: 93% for stage I, 72.5% for stage II/III, and 12% for stage IV [3]. It is predicted that the overall incidence will decrease in most developed countries and increase in most developing countries through 2030 [10].

Risk factors: The risk factors can be categorized as unalterable and alterable factors [3]. Unalterable risk factors include age (above 60), gender (males), and race, with African Americans, Hispanic Americans, and Native Americans being most affected [3, 11]. Alterable risk factors include obesity, alcohol consumption, smoking, occupational exposure (trichloroethylene and aristolochic acid), and drugs (acetaminophen and nonaspirin NSAIDs) [3, 12]. High BMI (overweight/obesity) is one of the major risk factors, accounting for 18.5% of the population burden of kidney cancer, followed by smoking (16.6%) and occupational trichloroethylene exposure (0.1%) [12]. A history of chronic kidney disease, kidney stones, hypertension, and diabetes has also been shown to be additional risk factors for kidney cancer [2, 12]. It is estimated that overweight and obese individuals show an increased risk of 28% and 77%, respectively, when compared to normal individuals; 26% of kidney cancer cases worldwide are caused by high BMI [2, 13]. An increased 25% risk in men and 35% in women was observed for every 5 kg increase in body weight [3]. Regular physical activity reduces RCC risk by 22% [3, 14]. Tobacco smoking is the primary risk factor, with an increased risk associated with increased pack-years [3, 13, 15]. Further, compared to nonsmokers, an increased risk of 15% and 30% is estimated among former and current smokers, respectively, and continued smoking after RCC diagnosis worsens overall survival [2, 3, 16]. Moreover, smoking is the cause of 6% of kidney cancer deaths [2].

Excessive drinking of alcohol is associated with an increased risk, while moderate drinking is associated with a slight protective effect against RCC [2, 12]. Studies have shown that the risk is reduced by 20% among alcohol consumers when compared to nondrinkers or light drinkers because the consumption of alcohol was found to increase insulin sensitivity, indirectly lowering the risk of kidney cancer [2, 12]. Occupational exposure to trichloroethylene increases the risk by 30–40% [2,

12]. A history of hypertension increases the risk by double or triple among whites and blacks, respectively [2]. It was also observed that the highest Hazard Ratio (HR) for RCC-related death in men was 1.18 (95% CI) [17].

Screening and Diagnosis: Diagnosis can involve an MRI, CT scan, X-ray, blood and urine tests, biopsy, and tumor biomarker testing [18]. RCC is often diagnosed during thoracoabdominal imaging prescribed to diagnose abdomen-related issues. MRI is mainly advised for incompletely defined masses or contraindications to CT scans [18]. Renal mass biopsy is becoming more common as an alternative to partial or radical nephrectomy. Evaluation of paraneoplastic disease and metastatic RCC malignancy is done using chest and abdominal imaging [18]. RCC diagnosis by examining the physical triad of gross hematuria, flank pain, and a palpable abdominal mass is associated with advanced disease [18]. Biomarkers such as KIM-1 in plasma and aquaporin (AQP1)/perilipin (PLIN2) in urine offer potential detection methods [19]. The RCC of the clear cell type is often diagnosed at a very advanced stage and therefore has a poor survival rate [18]. One method of diagnosis is to look for heritable disorders associated with the development of RCC. In most cases, molecular genetic testing will unequivocally confirm the diagnosis, especially for well-studied genes like *VHL*, which have a broad spectrum of germline mutations [20]. *FLCN* germline mutation testing is advised for patients with Birt-Hogg Dube (BHD) symptoms such as fibrofolliculomas (FF), pulmonary cysts, or various types of renal malignancies (most notably hybrid-oncocytic RCC) [21].

9.2 Classification

According to the 2016 WHO classification, kidney cancers are classified as (i) renal cell tumors, (ii) metanephric tumors, (iii) nephroblastic and cystic tumors, (iv) mesenchymal tumors, (v) mixed epithelial and stromal tumor family, (vi) neuroendocrine tumors, (vii) miscellaneous tumors, and (viii) metastatic tumors (Fig. 9.1) [22].

Renal cell tumors that develop from the renal tubule epithelium constitute 90% of kidney malignancies. Based on histopathological and genetic findings, RCC is further classified into: (a) clear cell RCC (65–70%), (b) papillary RCC (10–15%), (c) chromophobe RCC (5–7%), (d) clear cell papillary RCC (3–4%), (e) collecting (bellini) duct carcinoma (1%), (f) medullary RCC (1%), (g) MiT family translocation RCC (1%), (h) multilocular cystic renal neoplasm of low malignant potential (< 1%), (i) hereditary leiomyomatosis with RCC (<1%), (j) succinate dehydrogenase deficient RCC (<1%), (k) mucinous tubular and spindle cell carcinoma (<1%), (l) tubulocystic RCC (< 1%), (m) acquired cystic kidney disease-associated RCC (<1%), (n) RCC-unclassified (<1%), (o) oncocytoma (3–7%), and (p) papillary adenoma (7%) (Fig. 9.1) [4, 6]. RCC can be further grouped into malignant tumors and benign tumors. All RCCs are malignant except clear cell papillary RCC and multilocular cystic renal neoplasm of low malignant potential, whereas papillary adenoma and oncocytoma are benign tumors [22, 23]. Some rare entities, not yet well characterized in terms of morphology, immunohistochemistry, or genetic

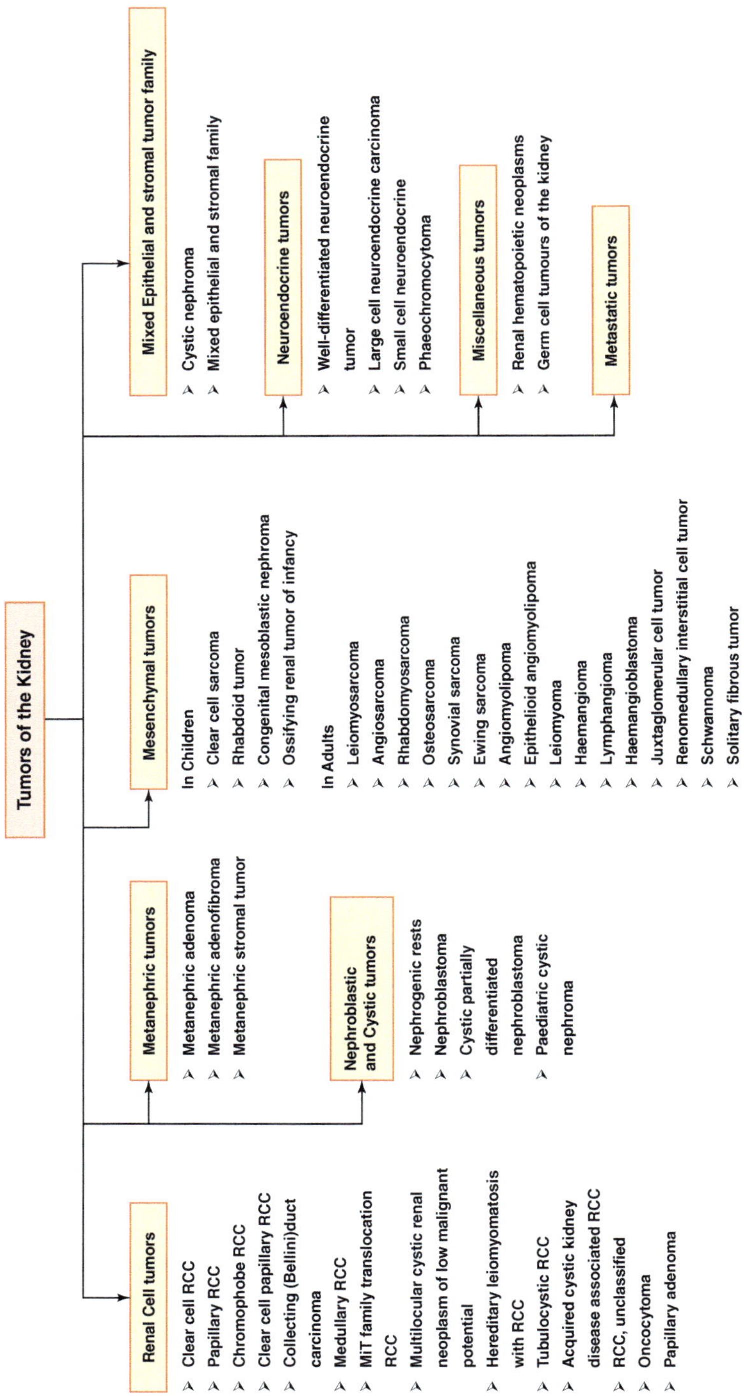

Fig. 9.1 WHO classification of tumors of the kidney

features, are categorized as "emerging/provisional tumors" in the 2016 WHO classification [22].

Tumor grading system: Histological tumor grading is a well-accepted prognostic factor in RCC. The Fuhrman grading system is one of the most popular grading systems for RCC, but it is difficult to apply in practice because each grade has three parameters that must be assessed simultaneously: nuclear size, shape, and nucleolar prominence [24, 25]. Deliberations at the 2012 ISUP Vancouver conference introduced a WHO/ISUP grading system that has been validated for clear cell RCC and papillary RCC [24–26].

Staging: According to the TNM system, staging of kidney cancer is as follows: primary tumor cannot be assessed (TX), no evidence of primary tumor (T0), tumors <7 cm (T1), with ≤4 cm (T1a) and > 4 cm but <7 cm (T1b), respectively. T2 tumors are ≥7 cm, with T2a measuring >4 cm and ≤ 7 cm, and pT2b > 10 cm, respectively. T1 and T2 stage tumors are confined to the kidney. T3 refers to the tumor that is spread to major veins or perinephric tissues. T3a refers to the tumor extending grossly into the renal vein or to the peri-renal or renal sinus fat, T3b refers to spreading to the infra-diaphragmatic IVC, and T3c refers to spreading to the supradiaphragmatic IVC or the IVC wall. T4 affects the ipsilateral adrenal gland or spreads beyond Gerota's fascia. The pNX refers to the tumor that cannot be evaluated, pN0 for no metastasis to regional lymph nodes, and pN1 for metastasis to regional lymph nodes. The pM1 refers to distant metastasis, which includes noncontiguous adrenal involvement. TNM staging groups include Stage I (Ia-T1 N0 M0, Ib-T2 N0 M0), Stage II (T2 N0 M0), Stage III (T1–3 N1 M0, T4 N1 M0), and Stage IV (T4 N1 M0, T any N any M1) [27, 28].

9.3 Pathophysiology

Kidneys are located retroperitoneally in the abdomen, on either side of the vertebral column. They are encased by the renal fascia/perirenal fascia/Gerota's fascia. The renal parenchyma is divided into cortex and medulla, both containing distinct structures of the nephron. The cortex is dark brown, granular, and contains renal corpuscles and the renal tubules. The cortex extends into the medulla and divides it into renal pyramids. Uriniferous tubules are the functional units of the kidney. Each tubule is made up of two unique morphological components: a nephron that creates filtrate and a collecting tubule that concentrates filtrate by further removing water. The nephron consists of a renal corpuscle, proximal tubules, thin limbs of Henle's loop, and a distal tubule (Fig. 9.2). Renal corpuscles are made up of a network of glomerular capillaries that filter blood before it enters the proximal convoluted tubule (PCT), composed of cuboidal epithelium with striated or brush border cells. PCT exits the cortex and enters the medulla as the thin descending limb (TDL), which is lined by cuboidal to squamous cells. The tubule then ascends towards the cortex, becoming the thick ascending limb (TAL) composed of cuboidal epithelium. The distal convoluted tubule (DCT) is formed after the TAL returns to the cortex (Fig. 9.2). The DCT connects the macula densa to the cortical collecting tubule

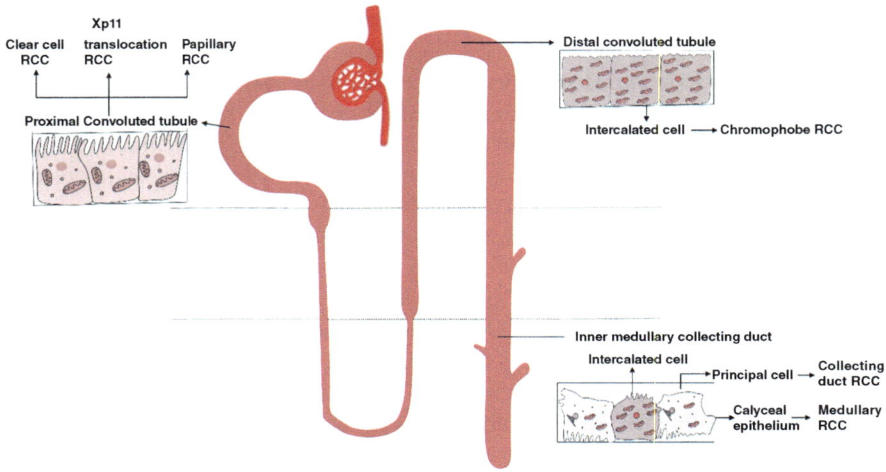

Fig. 9.2 Structure of nephron and the cell of origin of RCC subtypes

(CCT). Intercalated cells are present in the latter part of the DCT and persist throughout the collecting tubules. Collecting tubules connect to the distal convoluted tubules and then turn into collecting ducts. As they move from the outer to the inner medulla, the collecting duct cells go through a series of changes in their shapes, starting with squamous, then cuboidal, and finally columnar close to the renal papilla. Principal cells and intercalated cells are the two primary cell types found in collecting tubules and ducts. The principal cells contain several aquaporin channels, contributing to water permeability, while the intercalated cells secrete H^+ or HCO_3^-, helping to maintain acid-base balance [29, 30].

Cell of Origin: RCC develops from the epithelium of renal tubules. The cells of origin for clear cell RCC and papillary RCC have been proposed to be epithelial cells from the PCT (Fig. 9.2). Chromophobe RCC develops from intercalated cells in the DCT, whereas collecting duct RCC and medullary RCC develop from principal cells in the distal collecting duct and calyceal epithelium, respectively (Fig. 9.2). Rare RCC subtypes like Xp11 translocation RCC have also been linked to the proximal tubule epithelium (Fig. 9.2) [31].

Clear cell RCC (CCRCC): CCRCCs are typically yellow, with necrosis and hemorrhage. The cells have clear cytoplasm due to an abundance of glycogen and lipids, as well as thin-walled and staghorn-shaped vasculature [6, 32]. The loss of *VHL* function at 3p25–26 is very much common. According to the TCGA, 90% of sporadic cases have a mutated or silenced copy of *VHL*. In contrast, 3p deletions frequently result in the loss of another copy of *VHL* [33]. A pro-angiogenic gene expression pattern essential to the carcinogenesis of CCRCC is produced by the biallelic loss of *VHL*, which enables the improper stabilization of hypoxia-inducible factors (HIFs) and their incorrect stability [32, 34]. According to the TCGA, recurrent mutations in the PI3K/AKT/MTOR pathway, mutations in *SETD2* (linked to extensive DNA hypomethylation), and mutations affecting the SWI/SNF chromatin remodeling (*PBRM1*, *ARID1A*, and *SMARCA4*) are characteristics of CCRCCs [33].

Papillary RCC (PRCC): Macroscopically, PRCC appears friable with necrosis and hemorrhage [6]. They were traditionally classified into two subtypes based on their appearance [35]. In type 1 PRCC, the papillae are surrounded by cells containing scant cytoplasm, and a single layer of nuclei is positioned on the papillary core [35, 36]. Type 2 PRCCs commonly have papillary structures with true fibrovascular cores and cells with eosinophilic cytoplasm and large pseudostratified nuclei [35, 36]. Type 1 PRCCs are linked to hereditary PRCC syndrome and germline *MET* mutations [6]. PRCCs are characterized by the gain of chromosome 7 and/or 17 and loss of the Y chromosome [5]. According to the TCGA data, type 1 PRCCs have *MET* alterations, while type 2 PRCCs have *CDKN2A* silencing and *SETD2* mutations [36].

Chromophobe RCC (ChRCC): ChRCCs range from light tan to brown and have apparent cell membranes, irregularly shaped nuclei, and pale eosinophilic cytoplasm [5, 6]. They exhibit positive immunohistochemical staining for c-KIT and CK7 but negative staining for CAIX and CD10 [5, 6]. They show losses on chromosomes 1, 2, 6, 10, 13, 17, and 21; genetic losses may be fewer in eosinophilic variants [37, 38]. ChRCCs are more likely to develop in people with Birt-Hogg-Dube syndrome who have *FLCN* mutations. *TP53* and *PTEN* are two genes with high mutation rates [37, 38].

Clear cell papillary RCC (CCPRCC): The cells in CCPRCC have clear cytoplasm and a papillary structure with varying amounts of tubular, papillary, and solid patterns. CAIX and CK7 are typically positive in CCPRCC while CD10 is negative [39–41].

Collecting duct RCC: These tumors develop from collecting duct cells, and patients frequently present with hematuria [42, 43]. Chromosomes 1q, 8p, and 13q have been described as having cytogenetic changes and deletions (loss of heterozygosity) [44]. There is no specific mutation that defines this subtype, but approximately 30% of all patients have *NF2* mutations, while 24% have *SETD2* mutations [45]. Collecting duct RCC is immunohistochemically positive for PAX8, HMWCK, CK7, and SMARCB1/INI-1, and negative for OCT3/4, P63, and GATA3 [5].

Medullary duct RCC: Medullary carcinomas are uncommon tumors that develop in the renal medulla and are associated with sickle cell disease [5]. Adenoid cystic, reticular, and microcystic patterns are the most distinctive features of medullary RCC. Because of the small patient population, there are currently no known specific mutations; however, loss of *SMARCB1* [46] or *ALK* gene mutations have been reported in a few cases [47]. The expected immunoprofile for medullary duct RCC includes positive staining for PAX 8, CK7, and OCT 3/4, and negative staining for HMWCK and SMARCB1/INI-1 [5].

*MiT family translocation RCC (*MiT family TRCC): MiT family TRCC is an RCC subtype comprised of Xp11 TRCC and t (6;11) RCC [22]. TFE3 and TFEB (MiT transcription factors) rearrangement characterize both Xp11 translocation and t (6;11) RCC [6]. Xp11 TRCC accounts for less than 40% of pediatric RCC and about 4% of adult RCCs, with a mean onset age of 50 years [48, 49]. TFE3 and

TFEB nuclear immunostaining are particularly positive in Xp11 TRCC and t (6;11) RCC, respectively [50–52].

Multilocular cystic renal neoplasm of low malignant potential: This subtype has an excellent prognosis [53]. It is completely made up of cysts with isolated or clusters of clear cells, with no expansive growth [22]. The tumor is immunohistochemically positive for CAIX and CK7, as with CCPRCC [54]. The most common mutations are chromosome 3p deletions (74%), followed by *VHL* mutations (25%) [55, 56].

Hereditary leiomyomatosis with RCC (HLRCC): This subtype contains an abundance of eosinophilic cytoplasm, large nuclei with inclusion-like eosinophilic nucleoli [57]. It is characterized by negative immunohistochemical results for FH and positive results for 2SC (S-(2-succino)-cysteine) [58]. The germline mutation in *FH* distinguishes HLRCC from other RCCs. Because oxidative phosphorylation is impaired in HLRCC, tumor cells switch to aerobic glycolysis. Fumarate levels rise in the presence of *FH* deficiency, acting as an oncometabolite. Fumarate increases HIF1A levels by inhibiting HIF prolyl hydroxylase [6, 22].

Succinate dehydrogenase-deficient RCC (SDH-deficient RCC): People with inherited mutations in the *SDHA*, *SDHB*, *SDHC*, or *SDHD* genes are more likely to develop SDH-deficient RCC. Autosomal *SDH* genes encode proteins that form mitochondrial complex 2 at the inner mitochondrial membrane. SDH-deficient RCC can be distinguished from ChRCC because it typically tests negative for KIT and CK7 [59].

Mucinous tubular and spindle cell carcinoma (MTSCC): MTSCC is composed of a densely packed tubular component formed by cuboidal-shaped cells that transition to bland-appearing spindle-shaped cells. MTSCC and PRCC have overlapping morphologies as well as a similar immunoprofile. Both are CK7 and AMACR positive [5].

Tubulocystic RCC: Tubulocystic RCC is characterized by a single layer of abnormal cells arranged in a cubical pattern. Tumor cells have enlarged nuclei, visible nucleoli, and an abundance of eosinophilic cytoplasm [22, 60]. The immunohistochemical staining for CD10 and AMACR is positive [60]. Tubulocystic RCC with poorly differentiated foci is strongly linked to fumarate hydratase (FH) deficiency and aggressive behavior [6].

Acquired cystic disease (ACD)-associated RCC: RCC associated with ACD is more common in patients with advanced renal disease [22]. The structures of ACD-associated RCC vary and include papillary, macrocystic, tubulocystic, and cribriform patterns [60]. Tumor cells are larger, with granulated cytoplasm and a poorly-defined cell membrane. The tumor is positive for AMACR and CD10 [22].

Unclassified RCC: Tumors that exhibit features of more than one subtype may be grouped under unclassified RCC. Because unclassified RCCs are such a diverse group of tumors, there is no distinct immunohistochemical signature [25].

Oncocytomas: Oncocytomas contribute to 3–7% of all renal cell tumors [61]. They are uncommon in children and most prevalent in adults, particularly men over 50 years [62]. The tumor mass is composed of nests and tube-like structures formed by round to polygonal cells. Typically, oncocytomas have genetic defects such as chromosome 1 or Y loss or 11q13 rearrangement [63].

Papillary adenoma: Papillary adenoma has the same cytologic features as that of classic type 1 PRCC. The tumor is immunohistochemically positive for CK7 and AMARC [5]. They have cytogenetic abnormalities such as trisomy 7 and 17, and Y chromosome loss [64].

Oncocytic RCC occurring after Neuroblastoma: Oncocytic RCC that develops after neuroblastoma is reported in previous neuroblastoma patients who have undergone chemotherapy [22, 65]. However, it is believed that renal neoplasms in patients who had previously undergone neuroblastoma are a diverse group of RCCs rather than a single entity [65].

Thyroid-like follicular RCC: It is a sporadic RCC that resembles thyroid parenchyma and occurs predominantly in females and is indolent with only a few cases of metastases [66, 67]. The tumor usually appears tan-yellow macroscopically and is immunohistochemically positive for vimentin, cytokeratins CK20, and CK7 [68].

ALK rearrangement-associated RCC: It can affect both children and adults, regardless of sickle cell trait, and accounts for about 0.4% of all adult RCC [69]. The tumor stains positively for cytoplasmic ALK and nuclear TFE3 [69–71]. Genetic partners of *ALK* are *VCL*, *TPM3*, *EML4*, *STRN*, and *HOOK1* [72, 73].

RCC with (angio)leiomyomatous stroma: It was recently identified as an RCC subtype after previously being classified as either a CCRCC or a CCPRCC [74]. It is a rare subtype associated with tuberous sclerosis [75]. Immunohistochemically positive for CAIX, CD10, CK7, 34betaE12, and PAX8. The tumor lacks a 3p deletion and trisomies of 7 and 17 [76].

TCEB1 RCC: The gene *TCEB1* was found to be inactivated in a few cases of wt-VHL RCC. These tumors were frequently associated with a loss of chromosome 8 [77]. Similar to CCRCC, these new entities have thick fibromuscular bands that cross the tumor and clear cells with voluminous cytoplasm [78].

9.4 Treatment

Surgical ablation is the standard treatment option for localized RCC. Surgical interventions are the only long-term cure options for RCC [79]. In radical nephrectomy (RN), the kidney along with perinephric tissues is removed. Because of the widespread use of CT and MRI, the identification of incidental small tumors has increased significantly. This has transformed RCC surgical treatment, with overall survival increasing to around 65% in the case of localized RCC [79]. In partial nephrectomy (PN), only the tumor is surgically removed. In patients with known metastatic disease, cytoreductive nephrectomy (CN) is performed to remove the primary tumor, and metastasectomy is performed in some patients to remove metastatic cancers [80, 81]. Cryoablation is a process to destroy the kidney tumor by rapidly freezing it to −40 °C and then rapidly melting it. During this process, disruption of membranes and the inner machinery of the cells occurs. The process of cryoablation cycle can be repeated to destroy any remaining cellular processes. In radiofrequency ablation, a needle is inserted into the tumor during radiofrequency ablation (RFA) to destroy cancer with an electric current [82]. Direct contact with radiofrequency energy causes tissue destruction through thermal injury and tissue necrosis in 3–5 min [83].

Radiation and systemic therapy: This therapy is used as a follow-up treatment for cancer that has spread to the bone, brain, or spine. A focused beam of high-energy radiation is delivered to kidney cancer cells [82]. Radiation therapy is a "targeted" treatment that is as precise as possible at a specific area or tumor. Although RCC is radioresistant, radiation therapy can relieve bone or brain metastases [84]. TKIs that inhibit VEGFR have improved response rates and survival of mRCC [80]. Bevacizumab is used in treating advanced RCC in combination with interferon-alpha [80]. The approved combination therapy for mRCC includes (a) the combination of two ICIs (e.g., nivolumab + ipilimumab) and (b) the combination of antiangiogenic therapy and an ICI (e.g., pembrolizumab + axitinib and avelumab + axitinib) [85–87].

9.5 Conclusion

RCC is a diverse group of cancers with various subtypes, among which CCRCC is the most common, followed by PRCC and ChRCC. Following the new WHO classification of RCC, researchers have defined new and emerging renal entities, significantly deepening our understanding of renal tumors. RCC is becoming more common, with 30% of newly diagnosed cases being metastatic. Currently, antiangiogenic drugs that inhibit tyrosine kinases in combination with ICIs are used as first-line therapy for mRCC patients. Other TKIs, ICIs, and mTOR inhibitors are used as second-line therapies. Nonetheless, many patients treated with mTOR and TK inhibitors develop drug resistance, resulting in treatment relapse. As a result, finding novel targets for therapy is critical for improving the overall survival of mRCC patients. Another significant challenge is to discover new biomarkers for diagnosis to aid in treatment decisions.

References

1. Sung H, Ferlay J, Siegel RL, Laversanne M, Soerjomataram I, Jemal A, Bray F. Global cancer statistics 2020: GLOBOCAN estimates of incidence and mortality worldwide for 36 cancers in 185 countries. CA Cancer J Clin. 2021;71(3):209–49.
2. Scelo G, Larose TL. Epidemiology and risk factors for kidney cancer. J Clin Oncol. 2018;36(36):3574.
3. Padala SA, Barsouk A, Thandra KC, Saginala K, Mohammed A, Vakiti A, Rawla P, Barsouk A. Epidemiology of renal cell carcinoma. World J Oncol. 2020;11(3):79–87.
4. Ahrens M, Scheich S, Hartmann A, Bergmann L. IAG-N interdisciplinary working group kidney cancer of the German cancer society. Non-clear cell renal cell carcinoma-pathology and treatment options. Oncol Res Treat. 2019;42(3):128–35.
5. Athanazio DA, Amorim LS, da Cunha IW, Leite KR, da Paz AR, de Paula Xavier Gomes R, Tavora FR, Faraj SF, Cavalcanti MS, Bezerra SM. Classification of renal cell tumors–current

concepts and use of ancillary tests: recommendations of the Brazilian Society of Pathology. Surgical and experimental. Pathology. 2021;4(1):1–21.
6. Inamura K. Renal cell tumors: understanding their molecular pathological epidemiology and the 2016 WHO classification. Int J Mol Sci. 2017;18(10):2195.
7. Motzer RJ, Banchereau R, Hamidi H, Powles T, McDermott D, Atkins MB, Escudier B, Liu LF, Leng N, Abbas AR, Fan J. Molecular subsets in renal cancer determine outcome to checkpoint and angiogenesis blockade. Cancer Cell. 2020;38(6):803–17.
8. Koshkin VS, Barata PC, Zhang T, George DJ, Atkins MB, Kelly WJ, Vogelzang NJ, Pal SK, Hsu J, Appleman LJ, Ornstein MC. Clinical activity of nivolumab in patients with non-clear cell renal cell carcinoma. J Immunother Cancer. 2018;6(1):1–7.
9. Nakata K, Colombet M, Stiller CA, Pritchard-Jones K, Steliarova-Foucher E. IICC-3 contributors. Incidence of childhood renal tumours: an international population-based study. Int J Cancer. 2020;147(12):3313–27.
10. Du Z, Chen W, Xia Q, Shi O, Chen Q. Trends and projections of kidney cancer incidence at the global and national levels, 1990–2030: a Bayesian age-period-cohort modeling study. Biomark Res. 2020;8(1):1–10.
11. Batai K, Harb-De la Rosa A, Lwin A, Chaus F, Gachupin FC, Price E, Lee BR. Racial and ethnic disparities in renal cell carcinoma: an analysis of clinical characteristics. Clin Genitourin Cancer. 2019;17(1):e195–202.
12. Safiri S, Kolahi AA, Mansournia MA, Almasi-Hashiani A, Ashrafi-Asgarabad A, Sullman MJ, Bettampadi D, Qorbani M, Moradi-Lakeh M, Ardalan M, Mokdad A. The burden of kidney cancer and its attributable risk factors in 195 countries and territories, 1990–2017. Sci Rep. 2020;10(1):1–20.
13. Macleod LC, Hotaling JM, Wright JL, Davenport MT, Gore JL, Harper J, White E. Risk factors for renal cell carcinoma in the VITAL study. J Urol. 2013;190(5):1657–61.
14. Moore SC, Lee IM, Weiderpass E, Campbell PT, Sampson JN, Kitahara CM, Keadle SK, Arem H, De Gonzalez AB, Hartge P, Adami HO. Association of leisure-time physical activity with risk of 26 types of cancer in 1.44 million adults. JAMA Intern Med. 2016;176(6):816–25.
15. Hunt JD, Van der Hel OL, McMillan GP, Boffetta P, Brennan P. Renal cell carcinoma in relation to cigarette smoking: meta-analysis of 24 studies. Int J Cancer. 2005;114(1):101–8.
16. Cumberbatch MG, Rota M, Catto JW, La Vecchia C. The role of tobacco smoke in bladder and kidney carcinogenesis: a comparison of exposures and meta-analysis of incidence and mortality risks. Eur Urol. 2016;70(3):458–66.
17. Wirén S, Häggström C, Ulmer H, Manjer J, Bjørge T, Nagel G, Johansen D, Hallmans G, Engeland A, Concin H, Jonsson H. Pooled cohort study on height and risk of cancer and cancer death. Cancer Causes Control. 2014;25:151–9.
18. Gray RE, Harris GT. Renal cell carcinoma: diagnosis and management. Am Fam Physician. 2019;99(3):179–84.
19. Rossi SH, Klatte T, Usher-Smith J, Stewart GD. Epidemiology and screening for renal cancer. World J Urol. 2018;36:1341–53.
20. Maher ER. Hereditary renal cell carcinoma syndromes: diagnosis, surveillance and management. World J Urol. 2018;36:1891–8.
21. Stamatakis L, Metwalli AR, Middelton LA, Marston LW. Diagnosis and management of BHD-associated kidney cancer. Fam Cancer. 2013;12:397–402.
22. Moch H, Cubilla AL, Humphrey PA, Reuter VE, Ulbright TM. The 2016 WHO classification of tumours of the urinary system and male genital organs—part a: renal, penile, and testicular tumours. Eur Urol. 2016;70(1):93–105.
23. Lopez-Beltran A, Cheng L. Histologic variants of urothelial carcinoma: differential diagnosis and clinical implications. Hum Pathol. 2006;37(11):1371–88.
24. Samaratunga H, Gianduzzo T, Delahunt B. The ISUP system of staging, grading and classification of renal cell neoplasia. Journal of kidney cancer and VHL. 2014;1(3):26.
25. Warren AY, Harrison D. WHO/ISUP classification, grading and pathological staging of renal cell carcinoma: standards and controversies. World J Urol. 2018;36:1913–26.

26. Delahunt B, Eble JN, Egevad L, Samaratunga H. Grading of renal cell carcinoma. Histopathology. 2019;74(1):4–17.
27. Swami U, Nussenzveig RH, Haaland B, Agarwal N. Revisiting AJCC TNM staging for renal cell carcinoma: quest for improvement. Annals of translational medicine. 2019;7(Suppl 1):S18.
28. Delahunt B, Eble JN, Samaratunga H, Thunders M, Yaxley JW, Egevad L. Staging of renal cell carcinoma: current progress and potential advances. Pathology. 2021;53(1):120–8.
29. Madrazo-Ibarra A, Vaitla P. Histology, nephron. In: StatPearls. StatPearls Publishing; 2021.
30. McBride JM. Embryology, anatomy, and histology of the kidney. In: The Kidney: A Comprehensive Guide to Pathologic Diagnosis and Management; 2016. p. 1–8.
31. Dizman N, Philip EJ, Pal SK. Genomic profiling in renal cell carcinoma. Nature reviews nephrology. 2020;16(8):435–51.
32. Haake SM, Rathmell WK. Renal cancer subtypes: should we be lumping or splitting for therapeutic decision making? Cancer. 2017;123(2):200–9.
33. Cancer Genome Atlas Research Network. Comprehensive molecular characterization of clear cell renal cell carcinoma. Nature. 2013;499(7456):43–9.
34. Shen C, Kaelin Jr WG. The VHL/HIF axis in clear cell renal carcinoma. In Seminars in cancer biology 2013; (Vol. 23, 1, pp. 18-25). Academic Press.
35. Kim SS, Cho YM, Kim GH, Kee KH, Kim HS, Kim KM, Kim JH, Choi C. Recurrent KRAS mutations identified in papillary renal neoplasm with reverse polarity—a comparative study with papillary renal cell carcinoma. Mod Pathol. 2020;33(4):690–9.
36. Cancer Genome Atlas Research Network. Comprehensive molecular characterization of papillary renal-cell carcinoma. N Engl J Med. 2016;374(2):135–45.
37. Casuscelli J, Weinhold N, Gundem G, Wang L, Zabor EC, Drill E, Wang PI, Nanjangud GJ, Redzematovic A, Nargund AM, Manley BJ. Genomic landscape and evolution of metastatic chromophobe renal cell carcinoma. JCI Insight. 2017;2(12):e92688.
38. Davis C, Ricketts CJ, Wang M, Yang L, Cherniack A, Shen H, Buhay C, Kang H, Kim S, Fahey C, Hacker K. The somatic genomic landscape of chromophobe renal cell carcinoma. Cancer Cell. 2014;26(3):319–30.
39. Zhou H, Zheng S, Truong LD, Ro JY, Ayala AG, Shen SS. Clear cell papillary renal cell carcinoma is the fourth most common histologic type of renal cell carcinoma in 290 consecutive nephrectomies for renal cell carcinoma. Hum Pathol. 2014;45(1):59–64.
40. Yan WX, Cao WR, Zhao J, Zhang W, Wang XL, Yuan Q, Dang SQ. Clear cell papillary renal cell carcinoma: a clinicopathologic analysis of 6 cases. Int J Clin Exp Pathol. 2015;8(5):4595.
41. Aydin H, Chen L, Cheng L, Vaziri S, He H, Ganapathi R, Delahunt B, Magi-Galluzzi C, Zhou M. Clear cell tubulopapillary renal cell carcinoma: a study of 36 distinctive low-grade epithelial tumors of the kidney. Am J Surg Pathol. 2010;34(11):1608–21.
42. Tokuda N, Naito S, Matsuzaki O, Nagashima Y, Ozono S, Igarashi T, Japanese Society of Renal Cancer. Collecting duct (Bellini duct) renal cell carcinoma: a nationwide survey in Japan. J Urol. 2006;176(1):40–3.
43. Wright JL, Risk MC, Hotaling J, Lin DW. Effect of collecting duct histology on renal cell cancer outcome. J Urol. 2009;182(6):2595–600.
44. Schoenberg M, Brooks JD, Marshall FF, Epstein JI, Isaacs WB, Cairns P, Sidransky D. Frequent loss of chromosome arms 8p and 13q in collecting duct carcinoma (CDC) of the kidney. Genes Chromosom Cancer. 1995;12(1):76–80.
45. Pal SK, Choueiri TK, Wang K, Khaira D, Karam JA, Van Allen E, Palma NA, Stein MN, Johnson A, Squillace R, Elvin JA. Characterization of clinical cases of collecting duct carcinoma of the kidney assessed by comprehensive genomic profiling. Eur Urol. 2016;70(3):516–21.
46. Carlo MI, Chaim J, Patil S, Kemel Y, Schram AM, Woo K, Coskey D, Nanjangud GJ, Voss MH, Feldman DR, Hsieh JJ. Genomic characterization of renal medullary carcinoma and treatment outcomes. Clin Genitourin Cancer. 2017;15(6):e987–94.
47. Seo AN, Yoon G, Ro JY. Clinicopathologic and molecular pathology of collecting duct carcinoma and related renal cell carcinomas. Adv Anat Pathol. 2017;24(2):65–77.
48. Kmetec A, Jeruc J. Xp 11.2 translocation renal carcinoma in young adults; recently classified distinct subtype. Radiol Oncol. 2014;48(2):197–202.

49. Sukov WR, Hodge JC, Lohse CM, Akre MK, Leibovich BC, Thompson RH, Cheville JC. ALK alterations in adult renal cell carcinoma: frequency, clinicopathologic features and outcome in a large series of consecutively treated patients. Mod Pathol. 2012;25(11):1516–25.
50. Zou H, Kang X, Pang LJ, Hu W, Zhao J, Qi Y, Hu J, Liu C, Li H, Liang W, Yuan X. Xp11 translocation renal cell carcinoma in adults: a clinicopathological and comparative genomic hybridization study. Int J Clin Exp Pathol. 2014;7(1):236.
51. Inamura K, Fujiwara M, Togashi Y, Nomura K, Mukai H, Fujii Y, Yamamoto S, Yonese J, Fukui I, Ishikawa Y. Diverse fusion patterns and heterogeneous clinicopathologic features of renal cell carcinoma with t (6; 11) translocation. Am J Surg Pathol. 2012;36(1):35–42.
52. Argani P, Lal P, Hutchinson B, Lui MY, Reuter VE, Ladanyi M. Aberrant nuclear immunoreactivity for TFE3 in neoplasms with TFE3 gene fusions: a sensitive and specific immunohistochemical assay. Am J Surg Pathol. 2003;27(6):750–61.
53. Eble JN, Sauter G, Epstein JI, Sesterhenn IA, editors. World Health Organization classification of Tumours. Pathology and genetics of Tumours of the urinary systems and male genital. Organs.-Lyon: IARC Press; 2004. p. 359.
54. Williamson SR, Halat S, Eble JN, Grignon DJ, Lopez-Beltran A, Montironi R, Tan PH, Wang M, Zhang S, MacLennan GT, Baldridge LA. Multilocular cystic renal cell carcinoma: similarities and differences in immunoprofile compared with clear cell renal cell carcinoma. Am J Surg Pathol. 2012;36(10):1425–33.
55. Halat S, Eble JN, Grignon DJ, Lopez-Beltran A, Montironi R, Tan PH, Wang M, Zhang S, MacLennan GT, Cheng L. Multilocular cystic renal cell carcinoma is a subtype of clear cell renal cell carcinoma. Mod Pathol. 2010;23(7):931–6.
56. Teichman AV, Compérat E, Behnke S, Storz M, Moch H, Schraml P. VHL mutations and dysregulation of pVHL-and PTEN-controlled pathways in multilocular cystic renal cell carcinoma. Mod Pathol. 2011;24(4):571–8.
57. Merino MJ, Torres-Cabala C, Pinto P, Linehan WM. The morphologic spectrum of kidney tumors in hereditary leiomyomatosis and renal cell carcinoma (HLRCC) syndrome. Am J Surg Pathol. 2007;31(10):1578–85.
58. Trpkov K, Hes O, Agaimy A, Bonert M, Martinek P, Magi-Galluzzi C, Kristiansen G, Lüders C, Nesi G, Compérat E, Sibony M. Fumarate hydratase–deficient renal cell carcinoma is strongly correlated with fumarate hydratase mutation and hereditary leiomyomatosis and renal cell carcinoma syndrome. Am J Surg Pathol. 2016;40(7):865–75.
59. Gill AJ. Succinate dehydrogenase (SDH) and mitochondrial driven neoplasia. Pathology. 2012;44(4):285–92.
60. Srigley JR, Delahunt B, Eble JN, Egevad L, Epstein JI, Grignon D, Hes O, Moch H, Montironi R, Tickoo SK, Zhou M. The International Society of Urological Pathology (ISUP) Vancouver classification of renal neoplasia. Am J Surg Pathol. 2013;37(10):1469–89.
61. Abualjadayel MH, Safdar OY, Banjari MA, El Desoky S, Mokhtar GA, Azhar RA. A rare benign tumor in a 14-year-old girl. Case Rep Nephrol. 2018;2018:1548283.
62. Gudbjartsson T, Hardarson S, Petursdottir V, Thoroddsen A, Magnusson J, Einarsson GV. Renal oncocytoma: a clinicopathological analysis of 45 consecutive cases. BJU Int. 2005;96(9):1275–9.
63. Wobker SE, Williamson SR. Modern pathologic diagnosis of renal oncocytoma. J Kidney Cancer VHL. 2017;4(4):1.
64. Grande JP, Fidler ME. Renal cell cancer. In: Reference module in biomedical sciences; 2015.
65. Falzarano SM, McKenney JK, Montironi R, Eble JN, Osunkoya AO, Guo J, Zhou S, Xiao H, Dhanasekaran SM, Shukla S, Mehra R. Renal cell carcinoma occurring in patients with prior neuroblastoma. Am J Surg Pathol. 2016;40(7):989–97.
66. Amin MB, Gupta R, Ondrej H, McKenney JK, Michal M, Young AN, Paner GP, Junker K, Epstein JI. Primary thyroid-like follicular carcinoma of the kidney: report of 6 cases of a histologically distinctive adult renal epithelial neoplasm. Am J Surg Pathol. 2009;33(3):393–400.
67. Eble JN, Delahunt B. Emerging entities in renal cell neoplasia: thyroid-like follicular renal cell carcinoma and multifocal oncocytoma-like tumours associated with oncocytosis. Pathology. 2018;50(1):24–36.

68. Wang H, Yu J, Xu Z, Li G. Clinicopathological study on thyroid follicular carcinoma-like renal tumor related to serious hypertension: case report and review of the literature. Medicine. 2017;96(12):e6419.
69. Sugawara E, Togashi Y, Kuroda N, Sakata S, Hatano S, Asaka R, Yuasa T, Yonese J, Kitagawa M, Mano H, Ishikawa Y. Identification of anaplastic lymphoma kinase fusions in renal cancer: large-scale immunohistochemical screening by the intercalated antibody-enhanced polymer method. Cancer. 2012;118(18):4427–36.
70. Cajaiba MM, Jennings LJ, Rohan SM, Perez-Atayde AR, Marino-Enriquez A, Fletcher JA, Geller JI, Leuer KM, Bridge JA, Perlman EJ. ALK-rearranged renal cell carcinomas in children. Genes Chromosom Cancer. 2016;55(5):442–51.
71. Kusano H, Togashi Y, Akiba J, Moriya F, Baba K, Matsuzaki N, Yuba Y, Shiraishi Y, Kanamaru H, Kuroda N, Sakata S. Two cases of renal cell carcinoma harboring a novel STRN-ALK fusion gene. Am J Surg Pathol. 2016;40(6):761–9.
72. Mariño-Enríquez A, Ou WB, Weldon CB, Fletcher JA, Pérez-Atayde AR. ALK rearrangement in sickle cell trait-associated renal medullary carcinoma. Genes Chromosom Cancer. 2011;50(3):146–53.
73. Debelenko LV, Raimondi SC, Daw N, Shivakumar BR, Huang D, Nelson M, Bridge JA. Renal cell carcinoma with novel VCL–ALK fusion: new representative of ALK-associated tumor spectrum. Mod Pathol. 2011;24(3):430–42.
74. Kuhn E, De Anda J, Manoni S, Netto G, Rosai J. Renal cell carcinoma associated with prominent angioleiomyoma-like proliferation: report of 5 cases and review of the literature. Am J Surg Pathol. 2006;30(11):1372–81.
75. Guo J, Tretiakova MS, Troxell ML, Osunkoya AO, Fadare O, Sangoi AR, Shen SS, Lopez-Beltran A, Mehra R, Heider A, Higgins JP. Tuberous sclerosis–associated renal cell carcinoma: a clinicopathologic study of 57 separate carcinomas in 18 patients. Am J Surg Pathol. 2014;38(11):1457–67.
76. Williamson SR, Eble JN, Amin MB, Gupta NS, Smith SC, Sholl LM, Montironi R, Hirsch MS, Hornick JL. Succinate dehydrogenase-deficient renal cell carcinoma: detailed characterization of 11 tumors defining a unique subtype of renal cell carcinoma. Mod Pathol. 2015;28(1):80–94.
77. Shah RB, Stohr BA, Tu ZJ, Gao Y, Przybycin CG, Nguyen J, Cox RM, Rashid-Kolvear F, Weindel MD, Farkas DH, Trpkov K. "Renal cell carcinoma with leiomyomatous stroma" harbor somatic mutations of TSC1, TSC2, MTOR, and/or ELOC (TCEB1): clinicopathologic and molecular characterization of 18 sporadic tumors supports a distinct entity. Am J Surg Pathol. 2020;44(5):571–81.
78. Batavia AA, Schraml P, Moch H. Clear cell renal cell carcinoma with wild-type von Hippel-Lindau gene: a non-existent or new tumour entity? Histopathology. 2019;74(1):60–7.
79. Krabbe LM, Bagrodia A, Margulis V, Wood CG. Surgical management of renal cell carcinoma. In Seminars in interventional radiology 2014 31, 01, pp. 027–032. Thieme Medical Publishers.
80. Choueiri TK, Motzer RJ. Systemic therapy for metastatic renal-cell carcinoma. N Engl J Med. 2017;376(4):354–66.
81. Alt AL, Boorjian SA, Lohse CM, Costello BA, Leibovich BC, Blute ML. Survival after complete surgical resection of multiple metastases from renal cell carcinoma. Cancer. 2011;117(13):2873–82.
82. Thakur A, Jain SK. Kidney cancer: current progress in treatment. World J Oncol. 2011;2(4):158.
83. Nakada SY, Jerde TJ, Warner TF, Wright AS, Haemmerich D, Mahvi DM, Lee FT Jr. Bipolar radiofrequency ablation of the kidney: comparison with monopolar radiofrequency ablation. J Endourol. 2003;17(10):927–33.
84. Shaikh T, Handorf EA, Murphy CT, Kutikov A, Uzzo RG, Hallman M, Horwitz EM, Smaldone MC. Contemporary trends in the utilization of radiotherapy in patients with renal cell carcinoma. Urology. 2015;86(6):1165–73.
85. Albiges L, Powles T, Staehler M, Bensalah K, Giles RH, Hora M, Kuczyk MA, Lam TB, Ljungberg B, Marconi L, Merseburger AS. Updated European Association of Urology guidelines on renal cell carcinoma: immune checkpoint inhibition is the new backbone in first-line treatment of metastatic clear-cell renal cell carcinoma. Eur Urol. 2019;76(2):151–6.

86. Rassy EE, Khoury Abboud RM, Ibrahim N, Assi T, Aoun F, Kattan J. The current state of immune checkpoint inhibitors in the first-line treatment of renal cancer. Immunotherapy. 2018;10(12):1047–52.
87. Motzer RJ, Tannir NM, McDermott DF, Arén Frontera O, Melichar B, Choueiri TK, Plimack ER, Barthélémy P, Porta C, George S, Powles T. Nivolumab plus ipilimumab versus sunitinib in advanced renal-cell carcinoma. N Engl J Med. 2018;378(14):1277–90.

Bladder Cancer

10

Nusrath Banu, Anil Kumar Pasupulati,
Anvesh Karthik Yalavarthy, Satya Dattatreya Palanki,
and Rama Krishna Kancha

10.1 Introduction

Epidemiology: Bladder cancer (BC) is the tenth most prevalent malignancy and ranks thirteenth for cancer-related deaths [1]. Urothelial carcinoma (UC) accounts for approximately 90% of BC cases. Approximately 75% of the newly diagnosed BC cases were nonmuscle invasive, while 25% were muscle invasive [2]. The incidence and mortality rates of BC were highest in Eastern Asia (132,316 cases and 54,206 deaths), followed by Northern America (89,997 cases and 21,045 deaths), and Western Europe (68,143 cases and 20,866 deaths) [3]. Further, the global incidence and mortality rates were significantly higher in males (440,864 cases, cumulative risk 1.05; 158,785 deaths, cumulative risk 0.30) than in females (132,414 cases, cumulative risk 0.26; 53,751 deaths, cumulative risk 0.08). The age-standardized incidence rate of BC was highest in Southern Europe with 15.3 cases per 100,000, followed by Western Europe and Northern America (13.0 and 10.9 per 100,000 respectively) [3]. The least incidence rate was observed in Middle Africa followed by South-Central Asia and Western Africa [3]. The 5-year survival rate depends on the stage of malignancy, with the highest rate of survival in the in-situ stage (95.8%), compared to the localized (69.5%), regional (36.3%), and metastatic cases (4.6%) [1].

N. Banu · R. K. Kancha (✉)
Molecular Medicine and Therapeutics Laboratory, CPMB, Osmania University, Hyderabad, India
e-mail: ramakancha@osmania.ac.in

A. K. Pasupulati
Deptartment of Biochemistry, School of Life Sciences, University of Hyderabad, Hyderabad, India

A. K. Yalavarthy · S. D. Palanki
Renovo Soumya Cancer Centre, Hyderabad, India

R. K. Kancha (ed.), *Biomedical Aspects of Solid Cancers*,
https://doi.org/10.1007/978-981-97-1802-3_10

Risk factors: Smoking, exposure to carcinogenic chemicals, age (above 55 years), gender (four times more common in men), genetic factors, pathogens, red meat, obesity, and alcohol consumption were associated with the incidence of BC [1]. Smoking is the primary cause, accounting for 50–65% of cases each year [4]. A synergistic impact of smoking and arsenic at high concentrations increases the incidence of BC [5]. *GSTM1* and *NAT2* genes, which are involved in the metabolism of cancer-causing agents, enhance the risk of BC [2]. BC cases of the squamous cell subtype are more common in the Middle-East and Africa because of the widespread parasitic disease (schistosomiasis) [6]. According to a meta-analysis, high consumption of red meat raises the incidence of BC by 17% [7]. A linear correlation was observed between Body mass index (BMI) and BC incidence [8].

Screening and Diagnosis: The early symptoms include painless hematuria, while macrohematuria is associated with the advanced stage [9]. BC (in-situ carcinoma) frequently exhibits symptoms of the lower urinary tract such as urinary urgency, incomplete emptying of the bladder, dripping, delayed micturition, urinary hesitancy, and nocturia [9]. If the results of the cystoscopy are negative, additional testing options include urine cytology, computed tomography (CT) or urography/intravenous urography (if CT is not an option) [9]. Urine-based biomarkers are an alternative for detecting BC because they are noninvasive with high specificity and sensitivity [10]. FDA-approved tests for BC patients include NMP22 as a protein biomarker [10, 11], bladder tumor antigen (BTA) test [11], ImmunoCytTM/uCyt+TM test to identify CEA (carcinoembryonic antigen) and mucins on the cancerous urothelial cells [12], and (d) UroVysionTM uses FISH probes to analyze urothelial cancer cells for genetic alterations, which include aneuploidy of chromosome 3, 7, 17, and del (9p21) [13, 14]. Non-FDA approved urine biomarkers are categorized as: (a) urine protein biomarkers that include BLCA-1, BLCA-4 [15, 16], Hyaluronidase [17], Cytokeratins-8, 18, 19 [18], Survivin [19], ProEGF, SAA4, APOA1–2, APOB & E, APOC2–3 [20], CCL18, PAI-1, and CD44 [21], (b) urine metabolite markers that include lactate, beta-hydroxypyruvate, arachidonate, BCAAs, adenosine, and succinate [22], (c) urine genetic biomarkers that include *FGFR3*, *p53* [23], *CDK1*, *HOXA13*, *MDK*, *IGFBP5* [24], *PON2* [25], miR-26a, miR-191, miR-940 [26], and methylated *TWIST1*, *MEIS1*, *OSR1*, *OTX1*, *SIM2*, and *ONECUT2* [10, 27].

10.2 Classification

There are several classifications for BC. (A) BC is classified into (a) nonmuscle invasive (NMIBC) and (b) muscle invasive (MIBC) [28]. Further, NMIBC and MIBC are categorized into (i) early BC subtyping, (ii) NMIBC subtyping, and (iii) MIBC subtyping (Fig. 10.1) [28]. (B) The BOLD 2018 subtyping system of BC consists of the following subtypes: neural-like, luminal-like, papillary-like, HER2-like, SSC-like, and mesenchymal-like [28]. (C) According to the 2016 WHO classification, urothelial tract tumors are classified into ten groups. UC (urothelial

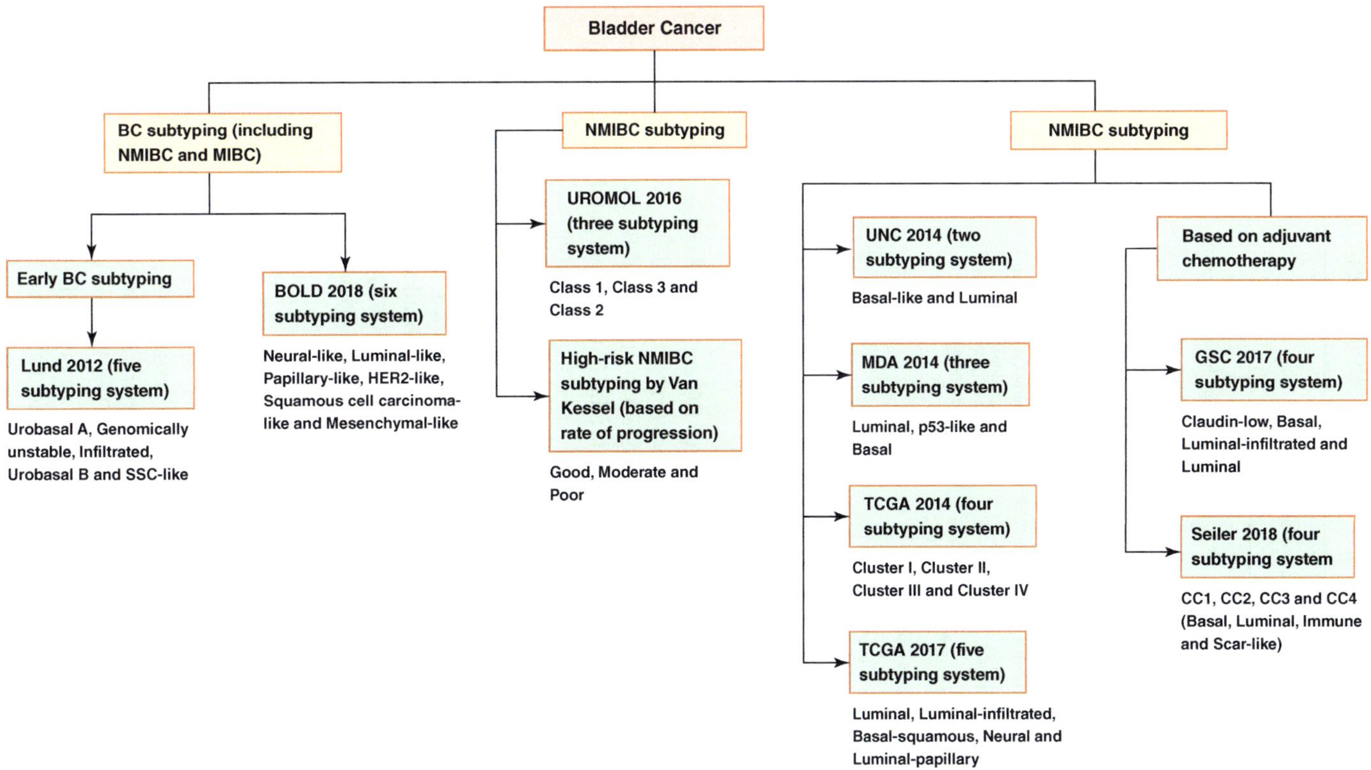

Fig. 10.1 Molecular subtyping of bladder cancer

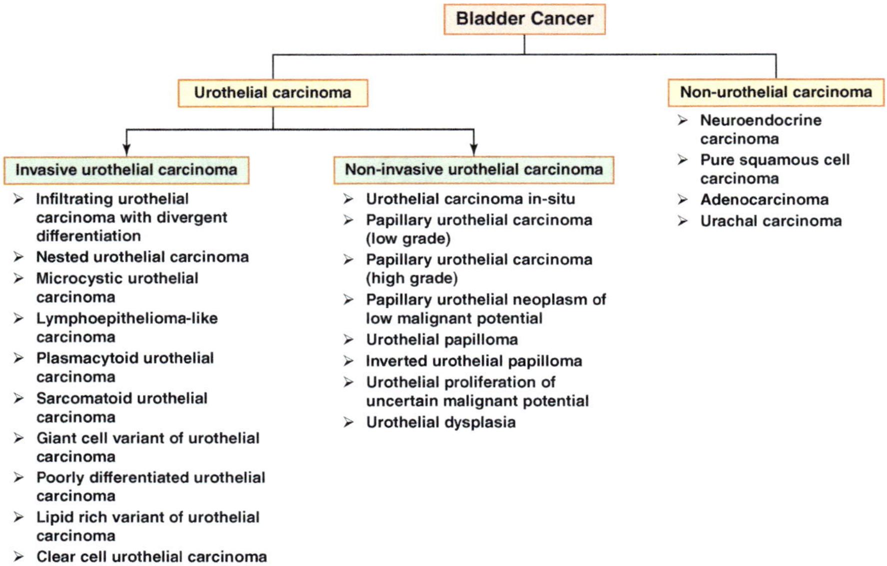

Fig. 10.2 Histological classification of bladder cancer

carcinoma) is the most prevalent type of BC and is further divided into invasive and noninvasive, each with several subtypes (Fig. 10.2) [29].

Staging: According to the TNM system of staging of BC, TX: Tumor cannot be assessed; T0: No sign of primary tumor; Ta: Noninvasive papillary carcinoma; Tis: Carcinoma in situ; T1: Tumor invades into the lamina propria; T2: Invasion into the muscularis propria; T2a: Infiltration into superficial muscle; T2b: Invasion into deep muscle; T3: Invades perivesical soft tissue; T3a and T3b: Tumor invasion is microscopic and macroscopic, respectively; T4: Tumor invades any organ; NX: Regional lymph nodes cannot be graded; N0: Absence of local metastasis; N1: Infiltration of a single lymph node in the pelvic cavity; N2: Infiltration of multiple lymph nodes in the pelvic cavity; N3: Invasion into common iliac lymph nodes; M0: No distant metastasis; M1a: Nonregional lymph nodes metastasis; M1b: Distant metastasis [2, 30].

10.3 Pathophysiology

Anatomy: The bladder is divided into two parts: (i) The upper part consists of apex and dome, which are present above the ureteric orifices, and (ii) the lower part comprises of fundus, trigone, and neck [31]. The bladder wall consists of urothelium, lamina propria, musculus propria, and serosa layers (Fig. 10.3) [32]. (a) The urothelium is a stratified epithelium that has three distinct cell layers: basal, intermediate, and superficial (Fig. 10.3). The basal layer comprises of small cuboidal cells, while

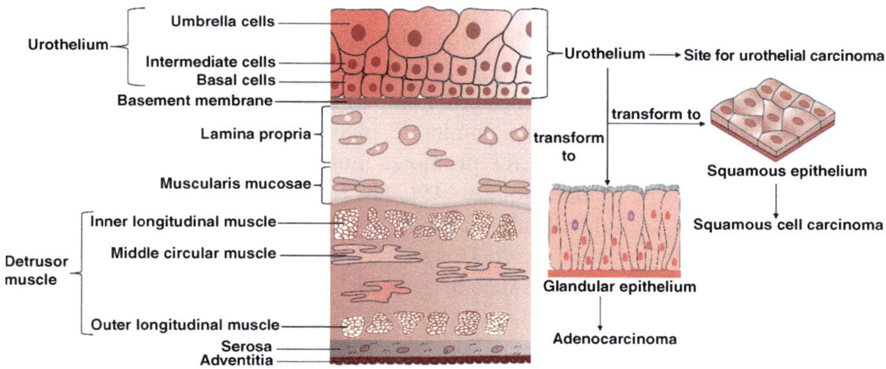

Fig. 10.3 Anatomy of bladder and the pathogenesis of various bladder cancer subtypes

the intermediate layers are polygonal in shape and can stretch and flatten [33]. The superficial layer is made up of large, occasionally multinucleated cells, which serve as a protective impermeable sheath, preventing urine reabsorption across the urothelium into the bloodstream. (b) The extracellular matrix of the lamina propria is made up of several important components along with the muscularis mucosae. The lamina propria and urothelium are sensory centers that regulate the afferent limb of the micturition reflex [34]. Because of the presence of specialized cells, it serves as a functional center and capacitance layer of the bladder [35]. (c) The muscularis propria (detrusor muscle) is made up of three layers: the inner (longitudinal muscle), middle (circular muscle), and outer (longitudinal muscle) (Fig. 10.3) [36]. (d) The bladder is partly enclosed by the serosa, which has a mesothelium lining on the outside and varying amounts of vascularized adipose tissue underneath, frequently penetrating the muscularis propria.

Cell of Origin: The majority of BC subtypes originate in the urothelium. UC is defined as the invasion of tumor cells with urothelial origin into the basement membrane and lamina propria [37]. The conversion of transitional cells to squamous cells occurs during the histogenesis of bladder SCC (Fig. 10.3). Adenocarcinoma develops from glandular neoplasia of the urothelium (Fig. 10.3) [38]. The urachal remnant, which originates from the allantoic fibrous connection between the bladder and the umbilical cord, gives rise to urachal adenocarcinoma (Fig. 10.3) [38].

Invasive Urothelial Carcinoma: It is the most prevalent UC subtype that has spread beyond the basement membrane [39]. Mutations are more common in *TP53*, *FGFR3*, *PIK3CA*, *RB1*, and *HRAS* genes along with *TERT* promoter mutations [29]. Uroplakin III, GATA3, CK7, CK20, high-molecular-weight cytokeratin, thrombomodulin, p40, and p63 are the common immunohistochemical markers for UC [40, 41]. The most crucial prognostic factor is invasion depth, especially the penetration of the muscularis propria [39].

Infiltrating urothelial carcinoma with divergent differentiation: It is a common subtype with varying amounts of UC, which include squamous differentiation, glandular differentiation, and trophoblastic differentiation [29]. Squamous differentiation makes up to 40% of invasive UC cases, followed by glandular differentiation with 18% of cases, while trophoblastic differentiation is a rare subtype [42–44].

Nested urothelial carcinoma: It is a rare variant consisting of small nested architecture, minimal cytologic atypia, moderate pleomorphism, and a conspicuous nucleolus. The presence of a *TERT* promoter mutation distinguishes benign UC from nested UC in low-grade cytology [45]. The transcriptional phenotype of this variant is similar to the luminal subtype [46].

Microcystic urothelial carcinoma: This subtype accounts for 1% of the BC cases, which is characterized by the presence of cysts and tubules [47]. Similar to conventional UC, this variant also exhibits GATA3, CK7, CK20, and p63 expression. As the tubules and cysts resemble glandular structures, microcystic UC can be confused with bladder adenocarcinoma [48].

Micropapillary urothelial carcinoma (MUC): A rare variant of UC characterized by numerous small nests of cancer cells without true fibrovascular cores. This subtype makes up to 0.7–8% of all instances, is more frequent in men, and often coexists with conventional UC [49]. MUC is linked to miRNA-296 downregulation, which plays a role in regulating the inflammatory response [50]. Furthermore, activation of RUVBL1 seems to contribute to the development of MUC [50]. *HER2/ERBB2* overexpression and amplification are more common in MUC than in conventional UC [51, 52]. Most MUC cancers are of the luminal subtype because of the expression of the FOXA1 biomarker [46, 52].

Lymphoepithelioma-like carcinoma (LELC): This is a rare subtype of BC that is characterized by syncytial undifferentiated carcinoma cells mixed with a polymorphic inflammatory infiltrate [53]. The expression of cytokeratin AE1/AE3, CK7, p53, and GATA3 is more common in LELC [54, 55]. PD-L1 expression acts as a potential biomarker for immunotherapy [56].

Plasmacytoid urothelial carcinoma: It is a rare subtype of UC, which is characterized by eccentric nuclei [57]. The molecular characteristic of this variant is a nonsense mutation in the *CDH1* gene [58]. It has been demonstrated that *CDH1* mutations increase cellular migration, which may enhance tumor spread into the peritoneum [58].

Sarcomatoid urothelial carcinoma: This variant accounts for 0.3% of all urothelial neoplasms [59]. The presence of high-grade spindle tumor cells as well as epithelial and mesenchymal differentiation is a distinguishing feature of this variant [60, 61]. The expression of immunohistochemical biomarkers such as p63, GATA3, pan-keratin, and cytokeratins (903, 7, 5/6) is more common [62]. Mutations in genes such as *TP53*, *RB1*, and *PIK3CA* were relatively high when compared to the conventional UC [63].

Giant cell variant of urothelial carcinoma: This is a rare variant with unusual pleomorphic cells that look similar to giant cell carcinoma of the lungs and pancreas [47]. The expression of immunohistochemical biomarkers such as CK7, CAM 5.2, AE1/AE3, and epithelial membrane antigen is more common [64].

Lipid-rich variant of urothelial carcinoma: This is a rare variant distinguished by clear cytoplasmic vacuoles with irregularly positioned nuclei resembling large lipoblasts or signet-ring cells. Cytokeratin AE1/AE3 staining is a characteristic feature of this variant [65, 66].

Clear cell urothelial carcinoma: This variant is distinguished by large clear cells that are rich in glycogen [47, 67]. Due to the immunoprofile overlap caused by the expression of CK7 and CK20, it is challenging to distinguish clear cell UC from conventional UC [68, 69].

Urothelial carcinoma in situ *(CIS)*: This is a noninvasive flat urothelial lesion which accounts for less than 3% of all BC cases [29, 70]. CIS is commonly associated with high-grade papillary or invasive UC [71]. Immunohistochemistry involves nuclear staining of p53 and positive CK20 throughout the thickness of CIS [70].

Noninvasive papillary urothelial carcinoma-low grade: These lesions have fine papillae with extensive branching, which exhibit an ordered appearance with prominent modifications in architectural and cytological aspects at low-power magnification [72]. At medium power, altered polarity, irregular nucleus, and pleomorphism are clearly visible [39]. Mitoses are typically observed away from the basement membrane [39].

Noninvasive papillary urothelial carcinoma-high grade: The papillae are frequently fused in high-grade lesions, forming apparent solid masses [72]. Abnormal or frequent mitoses can be found at any level of the epithelium [39]. Similar to invasive cancers, this tumor frequently exhibits loss of p21 or p27 and overexpression of the genes *p53*, *HER2*, or *EGFR* [73]. About 60% of high-grade carcinomas usually relapse, with a 25% rate of progression to the lamina propria compared to a 5% rate of progression to the muscularis propria [39].

Papillary urothelial neoplasm of low malignant potential (PUNLMP): These tumors feature delicate papillae enveloped by thick urothelium [72]. The nuclei of tumor cells are uniformly shaped, slightly enlarged, and highly packed [39]. PUNLMPs have a considerably low risk of relapse and stage advancement when compared to low-grade papillary UC [74].

Urothelial papilloma: This tumor comprises of a fine fibrovascular core that is lined by thick urothelium [74]. Papillomas are diploid with low proliferation, frequent *FGFR3* mutation (75%), whereas cytokeratin 20 is only expressed in the superficial (umbrella) cells [73]. The most effective course of treatment is complete transurethral resection [74].

Inverted urothelial papilloma: It accounts for less than 1% of all bladder neoplasms [72]. It arises from the surface epithelium and invades the lamina propria [73]. With minimal cytological atypia, it appears as a complex trabecular and inverted growth pattern [72]. Transurethral resection is used to treat inverted papilloma, which has a very low relapse rate [39].

Urothelial proliferation with uncertain malignant potential: It is a flat lesion with a thick urothelium but no cytologic atypia and fine papillary structures [29]. Patients with prior papillary urothelial lesions frequently develop this malignancy [39].

Urothelial dysplasia: It is described as a flat lesion with significant cytological abnormalities but does not meet the specifications of urothelial CIS [29]. It exhibits slightly altered polarity, focal nuclear crowding, and enlarged nuclei with irregularities [72]. Loss of alleles and alterations in chromosome 9 and *p53* have been observed [73]. Expression of cytokeratin 20 may be helpful in diagnosis [72], and the progression rate has been reported to be 15 to 19% [39].

Nonurothelial carcinomas: They constitute less than 5% of all BC cases. The majority of these carcinomas originate from the epithelium, including neuroendocrine carcinoma, pure squamous cell carcinoma, adenocarcinoma, and urachal carcinoma [75].

Neuroendocrine carcinoma: The different types of neuroendocrine carcinoma include small-cell carcinoma, large-cell neuroendocrine carcinoma, paraganglioma, and well-differentiated neuroendocrine tumors [29]. CD56, chromogranin, and synaptophysin are neuroendocrine biomarkers expressed by both small and large cell carcinomas [47]. Gene expression profiling and immunohistochemistry revealed that *DLL3*, *PD-L1*, *CD56*, and *ASCL1* have distinct expressions in small-cell bladder cancers [76].

Pure squamous cell carcinoma: This subtype is more prevalent in areas (Egypt and Sudan) where Schistosomiasis is endemic [77]. It can be distinguished by the abundance of keratin production as pearl formations and intracytoplasmic granules [78]. The majority of cases are diagnosed at an advanced stage with an increased risk of local recurrence [79].

Adenocarcinoma: This tumor is made up of malignant glandular epithelium [80]. Primary adenocarcinoma is a very rare subtype, accounting for 0.5–2% of cases, whereas secondary adenocarcinoma is the most prevalent form that develops as a result of direct infiltration or metastasized from distant organs [78]. Many genes in the *MAPK*, *mTOR*, *Wnt*, and *Tp53/Rb1* pathways have been altered in primary bladder adenocarcinomas, with *TP53*, *PIK3CA*, and *KRAS* mutations being more common [81].

Urachal carcinoma: These tumors may have cells with mucin, enteric, unspecified, or signet ring-like morphological characteristics [82]. The urachal remnant gives rise to urachal carcinomas, which affect the bladder dome. Mutations in *TP53*, *KRAS*, *BRAF*, and *PIK3CA* were more common [83].

10.4 Treatment

Surgery: NMIBC treatment typically involves transurethral resection of bladder tumor (TURBT). TURBT has received severe criticism because it may result in the implantation of tumor cells in the healthy bladder mucosa [84]. To lower the relapse rate in cases of NMIBC, a single dose of chemotherapy is administered shortly following TURBT [85]. Transurethral en-bloc resection of nonmuscle invasive bladder tumor (EBRT) was developed in order to prevent the spillage of cancerous cells, thereby reducing the risk of bladder perforation [86]. In contrast to standard resection, the results of EBRT did not significantly lower the risk. Therefore, the use of EBRT may not be recommended for tumors larger than 3 cm in size that are flat, multifocal, particularly those that occur on the bladder dome [87].

Radical cystectomy (RC) and lymph node dissection (LND): In RC, the entire bladder is removed along with surrounding tissues and organs [88]. For MIBC patients, RC and LND have been the standard treatment options [89]. To lower the risk of local recurrence and improve survival rates in MIBC patients, RC is performed with wider resection of perivesical soft tissue and extended lymph node dissection [89]. A robot-assisted laparoscopic technique is used for cystectomy and lymphadenectomy with extra-corporeal reconstruction of the urinary diversion [90]. After cystectomy, a variety of urinary diversions have been used, ranging from the stomach to the colon [91].

Chemotherapy: NMIBC patients with moderate risk are administered with a dose of intravesical chemotherapy within 24 h following TURBT in order to eliminate free-floating cancer cells and thus reduce urothelium seeding [92]. Mitomycin C, gemcitabine, valrubicin, and epirubicin are among the primary and secondary treatment options for NMIBC patients [93, 94]. The combination of drugs used in neoadjuvant chemotherapy, such as gemcitabine + cisplatin or dose-dense MVAC (methotrexate + vinblastine + doxorubicin + cisplatin), resulted in improved survival in patients with metastatic disease [95, 96].

Immunotherapy: BCG is the widely used treatment for high-risk and moderate-risk NMIBC patients. BCG is thought to adhere to the urothelium, become internalized, and then cause immune responses via antigen-presenting cells [97, 98]. During the initial stage, BCG will be injected into the bladder once a week for the first 6 weeks, lasting 1–2 h. If a patient tolerates and responds well to the therapy as determined by postinduction cystoscopy, a maintenance regimen of 1–3 years should be continued [92]. When compared to various intravesical chemotherapy treatments, BCG is more effective in terms of response rate and reduced risk of recurrence [99]. In particular, immune checkpoint inhibitors (ICIs) and monoclonal antibodies against PD-1 and PD-L1 are effective immunotherapies for BC because of its increased mutational load. The intrinsic checkpoint pathways that control autoimmunity are often utilized by cancer cells to escape the immunological response [100]. Patients with advanced metastatic disease who progressed on first-line therapy and were given pembrolizumab as second-line therapy had better survival than patients who received second-line chemotherapy [101]. Anti-PD-L1 drugs such as avelumab and durvalumab, and anti-PD-1 drug nivolumab have been approved as second-line agents for the treatment of metastatic cancer [102–104].

Targeted Therapies and Antibody-Drug Conjugates: Patients with metastatic BC responded well to treatment with erdafitinib [105, 106]. Enfortumab-vedotin is used to treat metastatic UC that combines an anti-nectin-4 antibody with auristatin E [107]. The FDA also authorized a combination therapy of enfortumab-vedotin and pembrolizumab to treat metastatic BC in patients who are ineligible for cisplatin-containing chemotherapy [108]. Another drug called sacituzumab-govitecan, which combines a topoisomerase inhibitor with an antibody against trophoblast cell surface marker 2, demonstrated an overall response rate of 29% in patients who received chemotherapy and immunotherapy [109].

10.5 Conclusion

BC is a heterogeneous disease that includes both pure UC and its histological variants, as well as nonurothelial carcinoma, which includes squamous and glandular carcinomas. Most BC cases with UC histology make up to about 75% of all cases, while the remaining cases exhibit other histological subtypes. The determination of UC variants is crucial for deciding appropriate treatment as they are related to a poor prognosis and may possess therapeutic complications. With the goal of developing effective therapies, considerable attempts are being made to incorporate histological subtypes of UC into clinical research. The approval of ICIs and erdafitinib has led to a significant improvement in the treatment of BC. Despite the benefits of these therapies, there are still significant challenges due to the poor response rate and drug resistance. As a result, new combination therapies are being studied to overcome these limitations. The combination of both immunotherapy and targeted therapy can be a promising treatment strategy for improving response rates and decreasing resistance in bladder cancer management.

References

1. Saginala K, Barsouk A, Aluru JS, Rawla P, Padala SA, Barsouk A. Epidemiology of bladder cancer. Med Sci. 2020;8(1):15.
2. Sanli O, Dobruch J, Knowles MA, Burger M, Alemozaffar M, Nielsen ME, Lotan Y. Bladder cancer. Nat Rev Dis Primers. 2017;3(1):1–9.
3. Sung H, Ferlay J, Siegel RL, Laversanne M, Soerjomataram I, Jemal A, Bray F. Global cancer statistics 2020: GLOBOCAN estimates of incidence and mortality worldwide for 36 cancers in 185 countries. CA Cancer J Clin. 2021;71(3):209–49.
4. Freedman ND, Silverman DT, Hollenbeck AR, Schatzkin A, Abnet CC. Association between smoking and risk of bladder cancer among men and women. JAMA. 2011;306(7):737–45.
5. Kurttio P, Pukkala E, Kahelin H, Auvinen A, Pekkanen J. Arsenic concentrations in well water and risk of bladder and kidney cancer in Finland. Environ Health Perspect. 1999;107(9):705–10.
6. Mostafa MH, Sheweita SA, O'Connor P. Relationship between schistosomiasis and bladder cancer. Clin Microbiol Rev. 1999;12(1):97–111.
7. Li F, An S, Hou L, Chen P, Lei C, Tan W. Red and processed meat intake and risk of bladder cancer: a meta-analysis. Int J Clin Exp Med. 2014;7(8):2100.
8. Sun JW, Zhao LG, Yang Y, Ma X, Wang YY, Xiang YB. Obesity and risk of bladder cancer: a dose-response meta-analysis of 15 cohort studies. PLoS One. 2015;10(3):e0119313.
9. Ulamec M, Murgić J, Novosel L, Tomić M, Terlević R, Tomašković I, Jazvić M, Froebe A, Krušlin B. New insights into the diagnosis, molecular taxonomy, and treatment of bladder cancer. Acta Medica Academica. 2021;50(1):143.
10. Oeyen E, Hoekx L, De Wachter S, Baldewijns M, Ameye F, Mertens I. Bladder cancer diagnosis and follow-up: the current status and possible role of extracellular vesicles. Int J Mol Sci. 2019;20(4):821.
11. Chou R, Gore JL, Buckley D, Fu R, Gustafson K, Griffin JC, Grusing S, Selph S. Urinary biomarkers for diagnosis of bladder cancer: a systematic review and meta-analysis. Ann Intern Med. 2015;163(12):922–31.
12. Greene KL, Berry A, Konety BR. Diagnostic utility of the ImmunoCyt/uCyt+ test in bladder cancer. Reviews in urology. 2006;8(4):190–7.

13. Halling KC, Kipp BR. Bladder cancer detection using FISH (UroVysion assay). Adv Anat Pathol. 2008;15(5):279–86.
14. Darwiche F, Parekh DJ, Gonzalgo ML. Biomarkers for non-muscle invasive bladder cancer: current tests and future promise. Indian J Urol. 2015;31(4):273.
15. Cai Q, Wu Y, Guo Z, Gong R, Tang Y, Yang K, Li X, Guo X, Niu Y, Zhao Y. Urine BLCA-4 exerts potential role in detecting patients with bladder cancers: a pooled analysis of individual studies. Oncotarget. 2015;6(35):37500.
16. Myers-Irvin JM, Landsittel D, Getzenberg RH. Use of the novel marker BLCA-1 for the detection of bladder cancer. J Urol. 2005;174(1):64–8.
17. Lokeshwar VB, Block NL. HA-HAase urine test: a sensitive and specific method for detecting bladder cancer and evaluating its grade. Urol Clin N Am. 2000;27(1):53–61.
18. Sánchez-Carbayo M, Herrero E, Megías J, Mira A, Soria F. Initial evaluation of the new urinary bladder cancer rapid test in the detection of transitional cell carcinoma of the bladder. Urology. 1999;54(4):656–61.
19. Margulis V, Lotan Y, Shariat SF. Survivin: a promising biomarker for detection and prognosis of bladder cancer. World J Urol. 2008;26:59–65.
20. Chen CL, Lin TS, Tsai CH, Wu CC, Chung T, Chien KY, Wu M, Chang YS, Yu JS, Chen YT. Identification of potential bladder cancer markers in urine by abundant-protein depletion coupled with quantitative proteomics. J Proteome. 2013;85:28–43.
21. Urquidi V, Kim J, Chang M, Dai Y, Rosser CJ, Goodison S. CCL18 in a multiplex urine-based assay for the detection of bladder cancer. PLoS One. 2012;7(5):e37797.
22. Wittmann BM, Stirdivant SM, Mitchell MW, Wulff JE, McDunn JE, Li Z, Dennis-Barrie A, Neri BP, Milburn MV, Lotan Y, Wolfert RL. Bladder cancer biomarker discovery using global metabolomic profiling of urine. PLoS One. 2014;9(12):e115870.
23. Van Rhijn BW, Van Der Kwast TH, Liu L, Fleshner NE, Bostrom PJ, Vis AN, Alkhateeb SS, Bangma CH, Jewett MA, Zwarthoff EC, Zlotta AR. The FGFR3 mutation is related to favorable pT1 bladder cancer. J Urol. 2012;187(1):310–4.
24. Breen V, Kasabov N, Kamat AM, Jacobson E, Suttie JM, O'Sullivan PJ, Kavalieris L, Darling DG. A holistic comparative analysis of diagnostic tests for urothelial carcinoma: a study of Cxbladder detect, UroVysion® FISH, NMP22® and cytology based on imputation of multiple datasets. BMC Med Res Methodol. 2015;15(1):1–2.
25. Bacchetti T, Sartini D, Pozzi V, Cacciamani T, Ferretti G, Emanuelli M. Exploring the role of Paraoxonase-2 in bladder cancer: analyses performed on tissue samples, urines and cell cultures. Oncotarget. 2017;8(17):28785.
26. De Long J, Sullivan TB, Humphrey J, Logvinenko T, Summerhayes KA, Kozinn S, Harty N, Summerhayes IC, Libertino JA, Holway AH, Rieger-Christ KM. A non-invasive miRNA based assay to detect bladder cancer in cell-free urine. Am J Transl Res. 2015;7(11):2500.
27. van Kessel KE, Van Neste L, Lurkin I, Zwarthoff EC, Van Criekinge W. Evaluation of an epigenetic profile for the detection of bladder cancer in patients with hematuria. J Urol. 2016;195(3):601–7.
28. Zhu S, Yu W, Yang X, Wu C, Cheng F. Traditional classification and novel subtyping systems for bladder cancer. Front Oncol. 2020;10:102.
29. Humphrey PA, Moch H, Cubilla AL, Ulbright TM, Reuter VE. The 2016 WHO classification of tumours of the urinary system and male genital organs—part B: prostate and bladder tumours. Eur Urol. 2016;70(1):106–19.
30. Raj KK, Taneja Y, Ramdev P, Dhaked SK, Singh CK, Shekar AP. A prospective observational study to evaluate the role of restaging transurethral resection of bladder tumour in patients with non-muscle invasive bladder cancer. International Journal of Research in Medical Sciences. 2019;7(11):4134.
31. Sánchez Freire V, Burkhard FC, Schmitz A, Kessler TM, Monastyrskaya K. Structural differences between the bladder dome and trigone revealed by mRNA expression analysis of cold-cut biopsies. BJU Int. 2011;108(2b):E126–35.
32. Chai TC, Russo A, Yu S, Lu M. Mucosal signaling in the bladder. Auton Neurosci. 2016;200:49–56.

33. Abelson B, Sun D, Que L, Nebel RA, Baker D, Popiel P, Amundsen CL, Chai T, Close C, DiSanto M, Fraser MO. Sex differences in lower urinary tract biology and physiology. Biol Sex Differ. 2018;9(1):1–3.
34. Vannucchi MG, Traini C, Guasti D, Giulio DP, Faussone-Pellegrini MS. Telocytes subtypes in human urinary bladder. J Cell Mol Med. 2014;18(10):2000–8.
35. Andersson KE, McCloskey KD. Lamina propria: the functional center of the bladder? Neurourol Urodyn. 2014;33(1):9–16.
36. Sam P, Nassereddin A, LaGrange CA. Anatomy, abdomen and pelvis, bladder detrusor muscle. In: StatPearls. StatPearls Publishing; 2021.
37. Kaseb H, Aeddula NR. Bladder cancer. In: StatPearls. Treasure Island (FL); 2024.
38. Yu EM, Belay S, Li W, Aragon-Ching JB. Non-urothelial and urothelial variants of bladder cancer. Cancer Treatment and Research Communications. 2022;33:100661.
39. Kim YA, Moon KC. Histological classification of bladder tumors. In: Bladder cancer. Academic Press; 2018. p. 147–80.
40. Chang A, Amin A, Gabrielson E, Illei P, Roden RB, Sharma R, Epstein JI. Utility of GATA3 immunohistochemistry in differentiating urothelial carcinoma from prostate adenocarcinoma and squamous cell carcinomas of the uterine cervix, anus, and lung. Am J Surg Pathol. 2012;36(10):1472–6.
41. Leivo MZ, Elson PJ, Tacha DE, Delahunt B, Hansel DE. A combination of p40, GATA-3 and uroplakin II shows utility in the diagnosis and prognosis of muscle-invasive urothelial carcinoma. Pathology. 2016;48(6):543–9.
42. Mitra AP, Bartsch CC, Bartsch G Jr, Miranda G, Skinner EC, Daneshmand S. Does presence of squamous and glandular differentiation in urothelial carcinoma of the bladder at cystectomy portend poor prognosis? An intensive case-control analysis. Urol Oncol. 2014;32(2):117–27.
43. Lopez-Beltran A, Henriques V, Montironi R, Cimadamore A, Raspollini MR, Cheng L. Variants and new entities of bladder cancer. Histopathology. 2019;74(1):77–96.
44. Dick B, Olubowale O, Kim J, Krane S. Urothelial carcinoma: highlights and reviews on various pathologies. EMJ Urol. 2020;8(1):46–53.
45. Zhong M, Tian W, Zhuge J, Zheng X, Huang T, Cai D, Zhang D, Yang XJ, Argani P, Fallon JT, Epstein JI. Distinguishing nested variants of urothelial carcinoma from benign mimickers by TERT promoter mutation. Am J Surg Pathol. 2015;39(1):127–31.
46. Warrick JI, Sjödahl G, Kaag M, Raman JD, Merrill S, Shuman L, Chen G, Walter V, DeGraff DJ. Intratumoral heterogeneity of bladder cancer by molecular subtypes and histologic variants. Eur Urol. 2019;75(1):18–22.
47. Alderson M, Grivas P, Milowsky MI, Wobker SE. Histologic variants of urothelial carcinoma: morphology, molecular features and clinical implications. Bladder Cancer. 2020;6(2):107–22.
48. Lopez Beltran A, Montironi R, Cheng L. Microcystic urothelial carcinoma: morphology, immunohistochemistry and clinical behaviour. Histopathology. 2014;64(6):872–9.
49. Wang JK, Boorjian SA, Cheville JC, Kim SP, Tarrell RF, Thapa P, Frank I. Outcomes following radical cystectomy for micropapillary bladder cancer versus pure urothelial carcinoma: a matched cohort analysis. World J Urol. 2012;30:801–6.
50. Guo CC, Dadhania V, Zhang LI, Majewski T, Bondaruk J, Sykulski M, Wronowska W, Gambin A, Wang Y, Zhang S, Fuentes-Mattei E. Gene expression profile of the clinically aggressive micropapillary variant of bladder cancer. Eur Urol. 2016;70(4):611–20.
51. Zinnall U, Weyerer V, Compérat E, Camparo P, Gaisa NT, Knuechel-Clarke R, Perren A, Lugli A, Toma M, Baretton G, Kristiansen G. Micropapillary urothelial carcinoma: evaluation of HER2 status and immunohistochemical characterization of the molecular subtype. Hum Pathol. 2018;80:55–64.
52. Ching CB, Amin MB, Tubbs RR, Elson P, Platt E, Dreicer R, Fergany A, Hansel DE. HER2 gene amplification occurs frequently in the micropapillary variant of urothelial carcinoma: analysis by dual-color in situ hybridization. Mod Pathol. 2011;24(8):1111–9.
53. Raphael V, Jitani AK, Sailo SL, Vakha M. Lymphoepithelioma-like carcinoma of the urinary bladder: a rare case report. Urology Annals. 2015;7(4):516.

54. Lopez-Beltran A, Paner G, Blanca A, Montironi R, Tsuzuki T, Nagashima Y, Chuang SS, Win KT, Madruga L, Raspollini MR, Cheng L. Lymphoepithelioma-like carcinoma of the upper urinary tract. Virchows Arch. 2017;470:703–9.
55. Williamson SR, Zhang S, Lopez-Beltran A, Shah RB, Montironi R, Tan PH, Wang M, Baldridge LA, MacLennan GT, Cheng L. Lymphoepithelioma-like carcinoma of the urinary bladder: clinicopathologic, immunohistochemical, and molecular features. Am J Surg Pathol. 2011;35(4):474–83.
56. Manocha U, Kardos J, Selitsky S, Zhou M, Johnson SM, Breslauer C, Epstein JI, Kim WY, Wobker SE. RNA expression profiling of lymphoepithelioma-like carcinoma of the bladder reveals a basal-like molecular subtype. Am J Pathol. 2020;190(1):134–44.
57. Sood S, Paner GP. Plasmacytoid urothelial carcinoma: an unusual variant that warrants aggressive management and critical distinction on transurethral resections. Arch Pathol Lab Med. 2019;143(12):1562–7.
58. Al-Ahmadie HA, Iyer G, Lee BH, Scott SN, Mehra R, Bagrodia A, Jordan EJ, Gao SP, Ramirez R, Cha EK, Desai NB. Frequent somatic CDH1 loss-of-function mutations in plasmacytoid variant bladder cancer. Nat Genet. 2016;48(4):356–8.
59. Cheng L, Zhang S, Alexander R, MacLennan GT, Hodges KB, Harrison BT, Lopez-Beltran A, Montironi R. Sarcomatoid carcinoma of the urinary bladder: the final common pathway of urothelial carcinoma dedifferentiation. Am J Surg Pathol. 2011;35(5):e34–46.
60. Ikegami H, Iwasaki H, Ohjimi Y, Takeuchi T, Ariyoshi A, Kikuchi M. Sarcomatoid carcinoma of the urinary bladder: a clinicopathologic and immunohistochemical analysis of 14 patients. Hum Pathol. 2000;31(3):332–40.
61. Sanfrancesco J, McKenney JK, Leivo MZ, Gupta S, Elson P, Hansel DE. Sarcomatoid urothelial carcinoma of the bladder: analysis of 28 cases with emphasis on clinicopathologic features and markers of epithelial-to-mesenchymal transition. Arch Pathol Lab Med. 2016;140(6):543–51.
62. Guo CC, Majewski T, Zhang L, Yao H, Bondaruk J, Wang Y, Zhang S, Wang Z, Lee JG, Lee S, Cogdell D. Dysregulation of EMT drives the progression to clinically aggressive sarcomatoid bladder cancer. Cell Rep. 2019;27(6):1781–93.
63. Wang X, Lopez-Beltran A, Osunkoya AO, Wang M, Zhang S, Davidson DD, Emerson RE, Williamson SR, Tan PH, Kaimakliotis HZ, Baldridge LA. TERT promoter mutation status in sarcomatoid urothelial carcinomas of the upper urinary tract. Future Oncol. 2017;13(8):705–14.
64. Lopez-Beltran A, Blanca A, Montironi R, Cheng L, Regueiro JC. Pleomorphic giant cell carcinoma of the urinary bladder. Hum Pathol. 2009;40(10):1461–6.
65. Kojima Y, Takasawa A, Murata M, Akagashi K, Inoue T, Hara M, Tokunaga Y, Minase T, Hasegawa T, Sawada N. A case of urothelial carcinoma, lipid cell variant. Pathol Int. 2013;63(3):183–7.
66. Lopez-Beltran A, Amin MB, Oliveira PS, Montironi R, Algaba F, McKenney JK, de Torres I, Mazerolles C, Wang M, Cheng L. Urothelial carcinoma of the bladder, lipid cell variant: clinicopathologic findings and LOH analysis. Am J Surg Pathol. 2010;34(3):371–6.
67. Yamashita RY, Yamaguchi R, Yuen K, Niwakawa M, Tobisu K. Urothelial carcinoma (clear cell variant) diagnosed with useful immunohistochemistry stain. Int J Urol. 2006;13(11):1448–50.
68. Sung MT, Zhang S, MacLennan GT, Lopez-Beltran A, Montironi R, Wang M, Tan PH, Cheng L. Histogenesis of clear cell adenocarcinoma in the urinary tract: evidence of urothelial origin. Clin Cancer Res. 2008;14(7):1947–55.
69. Oliva E, Amin MB, Jimenez R, Young RH. Clear cell carcinoma of the urinary bladder: a report and comparison of four tumors of mullerian origin and nine of probable urothelial origin with discussion of histogenesis and diagnostic problems. Am J Surg Pathol. 2002;26(2):190–7.
70. Nese N, Gupta R, Bui MH, Amin MB. Carcinoma in situ of the urinary bladder: review of clinicopathologic characteristics with an emphasis on aspects related to molecular diagnostic techniques and prognosis. J Natl Compr Cancer Netw. 2009;7(1):48–57.

71. Gofrit ON, Pode D, Pizov G, Zorn KC, Katz R, Duvdevani M, Shapiro A. The natural history of bladder carcinoma in situ after initial response to bacillus Calmette-Gúerin immunotherapy. Urol Oncol. 2009;27(3):258–62.
72. Eble JN, Sauter G, Epstein JI, Sesterhenn IA, (eds.). World Health Organization classification of Tumours. Pathology and genetics of Tumours of the urinary systems and male genital. Organs.-Lyon: IARC Press; 2004. p. 359.
73. Lopez-Beltran A, Montironi R. Non-invasive urothelial neoplasms: according to the most recent WHO classification. Eur Urol. 2004;46(2):170–6.
74. Amin MB, McKenney JK, Paner GP, Hansel DE, Grignon DJ, Montironi R, Lin O, Jorda M, Jenkins LC, Soloway M, Epstein JI. ICUD-EAU international consultation on bladder cancer 2012: pathology. Eur Urol. 2013;63(1):16–35.
75. Ravi K, Kumar T, Bakshi H, Desai J, Sen S, Yadav V. Non urothelial bladder cancers: a case series. Indian J Surg Oncol. 2013;4:2–8.
76. Koshkin VS, Garcia JA, Reynolds J, Elson P, Magi-Galluzzi C, McKenney JK, Isse K, Bishop E, Saunders LR, Balyimez A, Rashid S. Transcriptomic and protein analysis of small-cell bladder cancer (SCBC) identifies prognostic biomarkers and DLL3 as a relevant therapeutic TargetMolecular profiling of small-cell bladder cancer. Clin Cancer Res. 2019;25(1):210–21.
77. Felix AS, Soliman AS, Khaled H, Zaghloul MS, Banerjee M, El-Baradie M, El-Kalawy M, Abd-Elsayed AA, Ismail K, Hablas A, Seifeldin IA. The changing patterns of bladder cancer in Egypt over the past 26 years. Cancer Causes Control. 2008;19:421–9.
78. Processali T, Diminutto A, Cerruto MA, Antonelli A. The impact of histological variants on bladder cancer outcomes. AME Med J. 2020;5(4)
79. Matulay JT, Woldu SL, Lim A, Narayan VM, Li G, Kamat AM, Anderson CB. The impact of squamous histology on survival in patients with muscle-invasive bladder cancer. Urol Oncol. 2019;37(6):e17–353.e24.
80. Zhong M, Gersbach E, Rohan SM, Yang XJ. Primary adenocarcinoma of the urinary bladder: differential diagnosis and clinical relevance. Arch Pathol Lab Med. 2013;137(3):371–81.
81. Roy S, Pradhan D, Ernst WL, Mercurio S, Najjar Y, Parikh R, Parwani AV, Pai RK, Dhir R, Nikiforova MN. Next-generation sequencing-based molecular characterization of primary urinary bladder adenocarcinoma. Mod Pathol. 2017;30(8):1133–43.
82. Dhillon J, Liang Y, Kamat AM, Siefker-Radtke A, Dinney CP, Czerniak B, Guo CC. Urachal carcinoma: a pathologic and clinical study of 46 cases. Hum Pathol. 2015;46(12):1808–14.
83. Reis H, van der Vos KE, Niedworok C, Herold T, Módos O, Szendrői A, Hager T, Ingenwerth M, Vis DJ, Behrendt MA, de Jong J. P athogenic and targetable genetic alterations in 70 urachal adenocarcinomas. Int J Cancer. 2018;143(7):1764–73.
84. Dobruch J, Oszczudłowski M. Bladder cancer: current challenges and future directions. Medicina. 2021;57(8):749.
85. Dobruch J, Herr H. Should all patients receive single chemotherapeutic agent instillation after bladder tumour resection? BJU Int. 2009;104(2):170–4.
86. Mori K, D'Andrea D, Enikeev DV, Egawa S, Shariat SF. En bloc resection for nonmuscle invasive bladder cancer: review of the recent literature. Curr Opin Urol. 2020;30(1):41–7.
87. Grimberg DC, Shah A, Inman BA. En bloc resection of bladder tumors: style or substance? Eur Urol. 2020;78:570.
88. Joensen UN, Maibom SL, Poulsen AM. Surgical management of muscle invasive bladder cancer: a review of current recommendations. Semin Oncol Nurs. 2021;37(1):151104.
89. Yafi FA, Kassouf W. Radical cystectomy is the treatment of choice for invasive bladder cancer. Can Urol Assoc J. 2009;3(5):409.
90. Catto JW, Khetrapal P, Ambler G, Sarpong R, Khan MS, Tan M, Feber A, Dixon S, Goodwin L, Williams NR, McGrath J. Robot-assisted radical cystectomy with intracorporeal urinary diversion versus open radical cystectomy (iROC): protocol for a randomised controlled trial with internal feasibility study. BMJ Open. 2018;8(8):e020500.
91. Lee RK, Abol-Enein H, Artibani W, Bochner B, Dalbagni G, Daneshmand S, Fradet Y, Hautmann RE, Lee CT, Lerner SP, Pycha A. Urinary diversion after radical cystectomy for bladder cancer: options, patient selection, and outcomes. BJU Int. 2014;113(1):11–23.

92. Chang SS, Boorjian SA, Chou R, Clark PE, Daneshmand S, Konety BR, Pruthi R, Quale DZ, Ritch CR, Seigne JD, Skinner EC. Diagnosis and treatment of non-muscle invasive bladder cancer: AUA/SUO guideline. J Urol. 2016;196(4):1021–9.
93. Messing EM, Tangen CM, Lerner SP, Sahasrabudhe DM, Koppie TM, Wood DP, Mack PC, Svatek RS, Evans CP, Hafez KS, Culkin DJ. Effect of intravesical instillation of gemcitabine vs saline immediately following resection of suspected low-grade non–muscle-invasive bladder cancer on tumor recurrence: SWOG S0337 randomized clinical trial. JAMA. 2018;319(18):1880–8.
94. Tomaszewski JJ, Smaldone MC. Emerging intravesical therapies for management of non-muscle invasive bladder cancer. Open Access Journal of Urology. 2010;2:67.
95. Teply BA, Kim JJ. Systemic therapy for bladder cancer–a medical oncologist's perspective. Journal of solid tumors. 2014;4(2):25.
96. Merseburger AS, Apolo AB, Chowdhury S, Hahn NM, Galsky MD, Milowsky MI, Petrylak D, Powles T, Quinn DI, Rosenberg JE, Siefker-Radtke A. SIU-ICUD recommendations on bladder cancer: systemic therapy for metastatic bladder cancer. World J Urol. 2019;37:95–105.
97. Babjuk M, Böhle A, Burger M, Capoun O, Cohen D, Compérat EM, Hernández V, Kaasinen E, Palou J, Rouprêt M, van Rhijn BW. EAU guidelines on non–muscle-invasive urothelial carcinoma of the bladder: update 2016. Eur Urol. 2017;71(3):447–61.
98. Pettenati C, Ingersoll MA. Mechanisms of BCG immunotherapy and its outlook for bladder cancer. Nat Rev Urol. 2018;15(10):615–25.
99. Sylvester RJ, van der MEIJDEN AP, Witjes JA, Kurth K. Bacillus calmette-guerin versus chemotherapy for the intravesical treatment of patients with carcinoma in situ of the bladder: a meta-analysis of the published results of randomized clinical trials. J Urol. 2005;174(1):86–91.
100. Donin NM, Lenis AT, Holden S, Drakaki A, Pantuck A, Belldegrun A, Chamie K. Immunotherapy for the treatment of urothelial carcinoma. J Urol. 2017;197(1):14–22.
101. Bellmunt J, De Wit R, Vaughn DJ, Fradet Y, Lee JL, Fong L, Vogelzang NJ, Climent MA, Petrylak DP, Choueiri TK, Necchi A. Pembrolizumab as second-line therapy for advanced urothelial carcinoma. N Engl J Med. 2017;376(11):1015–26.
102. Apolo AB, Infante JR, Balmanoukian A, Patel MR, Wang D, Kelly K, Mega AE, Britten CD, Ravaud A, Mita AC, Safran H. Avelumab, an anti–programmed death-ligand 1 antibody, in patients with refractory metastatic urothelial carcinoma: results from a multicenter, phase ib study. J Clin Oncol. 2017;35(19):2117.
103. Powles T, O'Donnell PH, Massard C, Arkenau HT, Friedlander TW, Hoimes CJ, Lee JL, Ong M, Sridhar SS, Vogelzang NJ, Fishman MN. Efficacy and safety of durvalumab in locally advanced or metastatic urothelial carcinoma: updated results from a phase 1/2 open-label study. JAMA Oncol. 2017;3(9):e172411.
104. Sharma P, Retz M, Siefker-Radtke A, Baron A, Necchi A, Bedke J, Plimack ER, Vaena D, Grimm MO, Bracarda S, Arranz JÁ. Nivolumab in metastatic urothelial carcinoma after platinum therapy (CheckMate 275): a multicentre, single-arm, phase 2 trial. Lancet Oncol. 2017;18(3):312–22.
105. Loriot Y, Necchi A, Park SH, Garcia-Donas J, Huddart R, Burgess E, Fleming M, Rezazadeh A, Mellado B, Varlamov S, Joshi M. Erdafitinib in locally advanced or metastatic urothelial carcinoma. N Engl J Med. 2019;381(4):338–48.
106. Robinson BD, Vlachostergios PJ, Bhinder B, Liu W, Li K, Moss TJ, Bareja R, Park K, Tavassoli P, Cyrta J, Tagawa ST. Upper tract urothelial carcinoma has a luminal-papillary T-cell depleted contexture and activated FGFR3 signaling. Nat Commun. 2019;10(1):2977.
107. Rosenberg JE, O'Donnell PH, Balar AV, McGregor BA, Heath EI, Evan YY, Galsky MD, Hahn NM, Gartner EM, Pinelli JM, Liang SY. Pivotal trial of enfortumab vedotin in urothelial carcinoma after platinum and anti-programmed death 1/programmed death ligand 1 therapy. J Clin Oncol. 2019;37(29):2592.
108. Rosenberg JE, Flaig TW, Friedlander TW, Milowsky MI, Srinivas S, Petrylak DP, Merchan JR, Bilen MA, Carret AS, Yuan N, Sasse C. Study EV-103: Preliminary durability results of

enfortumab vedotin plus pembrolizumab for locally advanced or metastatic urothelial carcinoma. J Clin Oncol. 2020;38(6):441.

109. Tagawa ST, Balar A, Petrylak DP, Grivas P, Agarwal N, Sternberg CN, Hong Q, Gladden A, Kanwal C, Siemon-Hryczyk P, Goswami T. Initial results from TROPHY-U-01: a phase II open-label study of sacituzumab govitecan in patients (pts) with metastatic urothelial cancer (mUC) after failure of platinum-based regimens (PLT) or immunotherapy. Ann Oncol. 2019;30:v890–1.

Ovarian Cancer

11

Sai Charitha Mullaguri, Bindu Madhava Reddy Aramati, Krishna Chaitanya Puligundla, and Rama Krishna Kancha

11.1 Introduction

Epidemiology: Globally, ovarian cancer ranks eighteenth in incidence (313,959 new cases in the year 2020) and fourteenth in terms of mortality (207,252 deaths in the year 2020) [1]. Among all cancers in women, it ranks eighth (3.4%) and second (4.7%) in incidence and mortality, respectively [1, 2]. The incidence rate was reduced from 3.6% in 2018 to 1.6% in 2020 and the mortality rate was reduced from 4.3% to 2.1% [1, 2]. According to the GLOBOCAN, the incidence and mortality rates were high in Asia (170,759 new cases and 112,936 deaths) that contribute to 54.4% and 54.5% of world-wide diagnoses and deaths, respectively. Ovarian cancer in Europe (66,693 new cases and 44,053 deaths) accounts to 21.2% and 21.3% of all global ovarian cancer cases and deaths, respectively. According to the SEER database for the year 2020, the estimated number of new diagnoses and mortality due to ovarian cancer were 21,750 and 13,940, respectively [3]. The 5-year survival rate is mainly based on the cancer stage at which the patient is diagnosed; the highest (92%) was in patients with stage I localized cancer and the lowest (29%) was in stage IV patients [3, 4]. The 5-year survival rates for localized and distant stages of cancer, respectively were 93% and 30% in white women, and 86% and 22% in black

S. C. Mullaguri · R. K. Kancha (✉)
Molecular Medicine and Therapeutics Laboratory, CPMB, Osmania University, Hyderabad, India
e-mail: ramakancha@osmania.ac.in

B. M. R. Aramati
Department of Animal Biotechnology, School of Life Sciences, University of Hyderabad, Hyderabad, India

K. C. Puligundla (✉)
Department of Medical Oncology, MNJ Institute of Oncology and Regional Cancer Centre, Hyderabad, India

R. K. Kancha (ed.), *Biomedical Aspects of Solid Cancers*,
https://doi.org/10.1007/978-981-97-1802-3_11

women [3]. In Europe, the incidence rates were 4.0%, 3.9%, and 3.1% and mortality rates were 5.7%, 6.9%, and 4.5% for the age groups 0–44, 45–64, and 65 or above, respectively [5]. Among children and adolescents in the age group of 0–18 years, the incidence was high (87.5%) when compared to the other gynecological malignancies [6].

Risk Factors: Major risk factors include family history of any gynecological cancers, sporadic alterations in genes, various syndromes, endometriosis, usage of hormone replacement therapy (HRT) after menopause, nulliparity, older age, obesity, poor diet and nutrition, smoking and perineal talc application [2, 7, 8]. Individuals with *BRCA1* mutations have about 44% risk while with *BRCA2* mutations have about 17% risk of developing ovarian cancer [9]. First-degree female relatives of a woman diagnosed with ovarian cancer are at a greater risk of developing ovarian cancer though they do not possess *BRCA1* and *BRCA2* mutations [10]. Vaginal infections caused due to *Neisseria gonorrhea* or *Chlamydia trachomatis* increase the risk of OC [11]. Additionally, a meta-analysis of epidemiological data revealed that the risk of ovarian cancer increases with multiple miscarriages and decreasing menarcheal age [12, 13].

Diagnosis and Screening: Ovarian cancers are hard to diagnose at the early stages as the symptoms are vague and not specific to ovarian cancers [14]. The diagnosis is usually in the later stages of tumor due to lack of proper initial screening. Rectovaginal examination and transvaginal ultrasonography can be used to detect solid abnormal mass of cells in ovary [15]. The sensitivity of transvaginal ultrasonography in detecting benign and malignant ovarian lesions is 86–94% and the specificity is 94–96% [16]. The most common screening method is detecting the levels of CA125 in the blood [7, 17, 18]. About 80% of patients with Epithelial ovarian carcinoma (EOC) have elevated levels of CA125 [15]. Screening for autoantibodies, ctDNA (circulating tumor DNA), DNA methylation in blood, microRNA, and thickness of cervical mucus improves detection of the initial phase of the disease while magnetic relaxometry and autofluorescence improve visualizing the tumor better in the later phase [17]. Circulating tumor cells (CTCs) act as an important prognostic and/or diagnostic marker for both primary and metastatic cancers [19, 20]. Analysis of serum samples revealed that there is a CTCs positive rate of 82%, 85%, 91%, and 100% in patients with stage I, II, III, and IV ovarian cancers, respectively [21]. FASN, a lipogenic enzyme is significantly elevated in ovarian cancers and is considered as a metabolic marker [22].

11.2 Classification

Different classifications were made based on (i) histology, (ii) staging, and (iii) proliferative status of the tumor. (i) Based on histology, ovarian cancer is classified into (a) epithelial ovarian carcinoma, (b) germ cell tumors, (c) sex-cord stromal tumors, (d) small cell carcinoma, (e) ovarian sarcoma, (f) carcinosarcoma, and (g) undifferentiated carcinomas (Fig. 11.1) [2, 23, 24]. (a) EOC is the predominant subtype in the population [2]. Globally, it accounts for over 95% of all ovarian

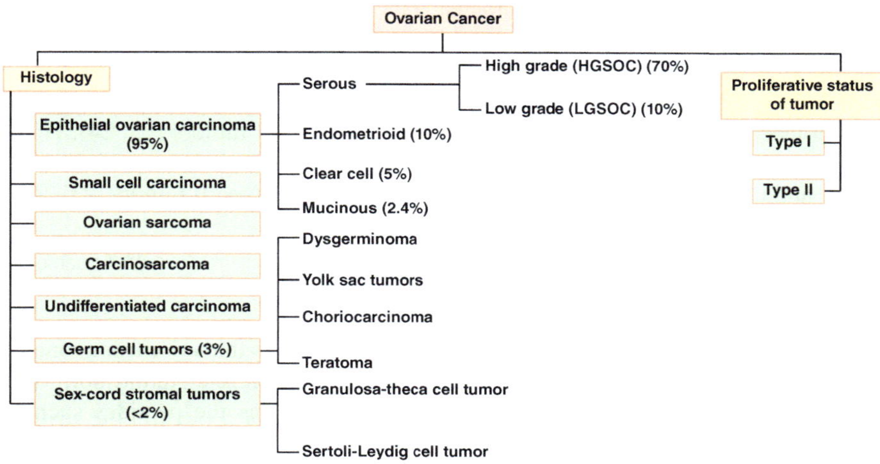

Fig. 11.1 Classification of ovarian cancer based on histology and proliferative status of tumors

cancer cases [25]. EOC is further classified into high-grade serous ovarian carcinoma (HGSOC), low-grade serous ovarian carcinoma (LGSOC), clear cell carcinoma (CCC), endometrioid, and mucinous ovarian carcinomas (MOC) (Fig. 11.1) [2]. HGSOC accounts for 70% of all EOCs followed by LGSOC, endometrioid, CCC, and MOC with frequencies of 10%, 10%, 5%, and 2.4%, respectively [2, 26, 27]. (b) Germ cell tumors are rare ovarian tumors accounting to 3% of all ovarian cancer cases and are frequently diagnosed at an early age with an average age of diagnosis of 10–30 years [4]. Germ cell tumors are further classified into dysgerminoma, yolk sac tumors (endodermal sinus tumors), choriocarcinoma, and teratoma (Fig. 11.1) [28]. (c) Sex-cord stromal tumors are rarely malignant tumors and the average age of diagnosis is 50 years [4]. These tumors are further classified into granulosa-theca and Sertoli-Leydig cell tumors (Fig. 11.1) [29].

(ii) According to the 2014 FIGO staging, ovarian cancer is classified into different stages [30]. Stage IA refers to tumor confinement to one ovary while IB indicates tumor confinement to both the ovaries [30]. Stage IC is further divided into three stages: IC1 refers to tumor within one or two ovaries with a spill of tumor cells upon surgery, IC2 indicates the presence of tumor on the ovarian surface and IC3 indicates malignant cells in accumulated fluid in the peritoneal cavity [30]. Stage IIA specifies the extension of tumors from ovaries to the uterus and stage IIB indicates extension of tumors into other pelvic intraperitoneal tissues [30]. Stage IIIA is further divided into IIIA1, which shows tumor metastasis from ovaries to retroperitoneal lymph nodes at a distance of $\geq$10 mm and IIIA2 indicates microscopic extrapelvic metastasis [30]. Stage IIIB indicates macroscopic metastasis to peritoneum with a dimension of $\leq$2 cm beyond pelvis with or without spread to retroperitoneal lymph nodes [30]. Stage IIIC specifies metastasis to peritoneum with a dimension of greater than 2 cm beyond pelvis with or without spread to retroperitoneal lymph nodes and includes metastasis of tumor to liver and spleen [30]. Stage IVA indicates distant metastasis with pleural effusion and stage IVB specifies metastasis to extra-abdominal organs [30].

(iii) The WHO classified ovarian cancers into (a) type I and (b) type II (Fig. 11.1) [23]. Low-grade, less aggressive tumors of serous, endometrioid, clear cell, and mucinous epithelial carcinomas are classified under type I tumors [23, 24]. High-grade, highly proliferative and metastatic tumors of serous carcinoma, carcinosarcoma, and undifferentiated carcinoma are classified under type II tumors [23, 24].

11.3 Pathophysiology

Anatomy and Cell of Origin: Ovaries are a pair of structures that arise from gonadal primordia. These are the primary endocrine glands that secrete steroid hormones such as estrogen, progesterone, and androgens, as well as the peptides such as inhibin, activin, and relaxin. The ovaries are located in the lower pelvic region along the sacroiliac joint. A superior pole and an inferior pole exist in each ovary. The fallopian tubes' infundibulum is located along the superior pole (also known as the tubal pole). The inferior pole (also known as uterine pole) is directed toward the uterus and is attached by the ovarian ligaments. Each ovary has an anterior border (also known as the mesovarian margin) and a posterior border. The ovaries are positioned in the pelvic region with the help of three ligaments: (a) proper ligament connects uterus to the ovary and is also called as utero-ovarian ligament, (b) suspensory ligament is a thin fold of parietal peritoneum that attaches the ovary to the pelvic wall and is also called as the infundibulopelvic ligament, and (c) mesovarium is a thin peritoneal fold that connects the anterior border of the ovary to the posterior of the uterine broad ligament. The surface of ovary is covered by tunica albuginea and germinal epithelium. Each ovary is divided into three regions namely surface, cortex, and medulla (Fig. 11.2). The surface is mainly made up of simple cuboidal epithelial cells and is called as the germinal epithelium (Fig. 11.2). The cortex contains numerous ovarian follicles and connective tissue called as stroma while medulla consists of loose connective tissue and neurovascular network (Fig. 11.2). Serous Tubal Intraepithelial Carcinoma (STIC) lesions are the precursor cells that arise in fallopian tube [2]. These lesions are found in about 80% of early stage HGSC and 18–60% of advanced stage HGSC [2]. LGSOC and MOC develop from atypical proliferative (borderline) tumor while CCC and endometrioid tumors arise from precursor cells of transformed endometrioid origin [2]. Majority of EOCs have extrauterine mullerian (embryonic duct that develops into female reproductive tract) epithelium as the site of origin [31].

Genetics: Mutant p53 is considered as a crucial and early characteristic feature of developing HGSOC and occurs in more than 90% of EOC patients [32–34]. About 20% of HGSOC patients have *BRCA1* and *BRCA2* gene mutations [2]. A 13% frequency of *BRCA1* and *BRCA2* mutations was observed in invasive ovarian cancer [35]. Additional genes with alterations in HGSOC include *FXM1* (84%), *Rb1* (67%), and *Notch1* (22%) [2]. In MOC, mutations in *KRAS* occur in 25–50% of patients [36–38] while *HER2* amplifications occur in about 19% of cases [38]. In

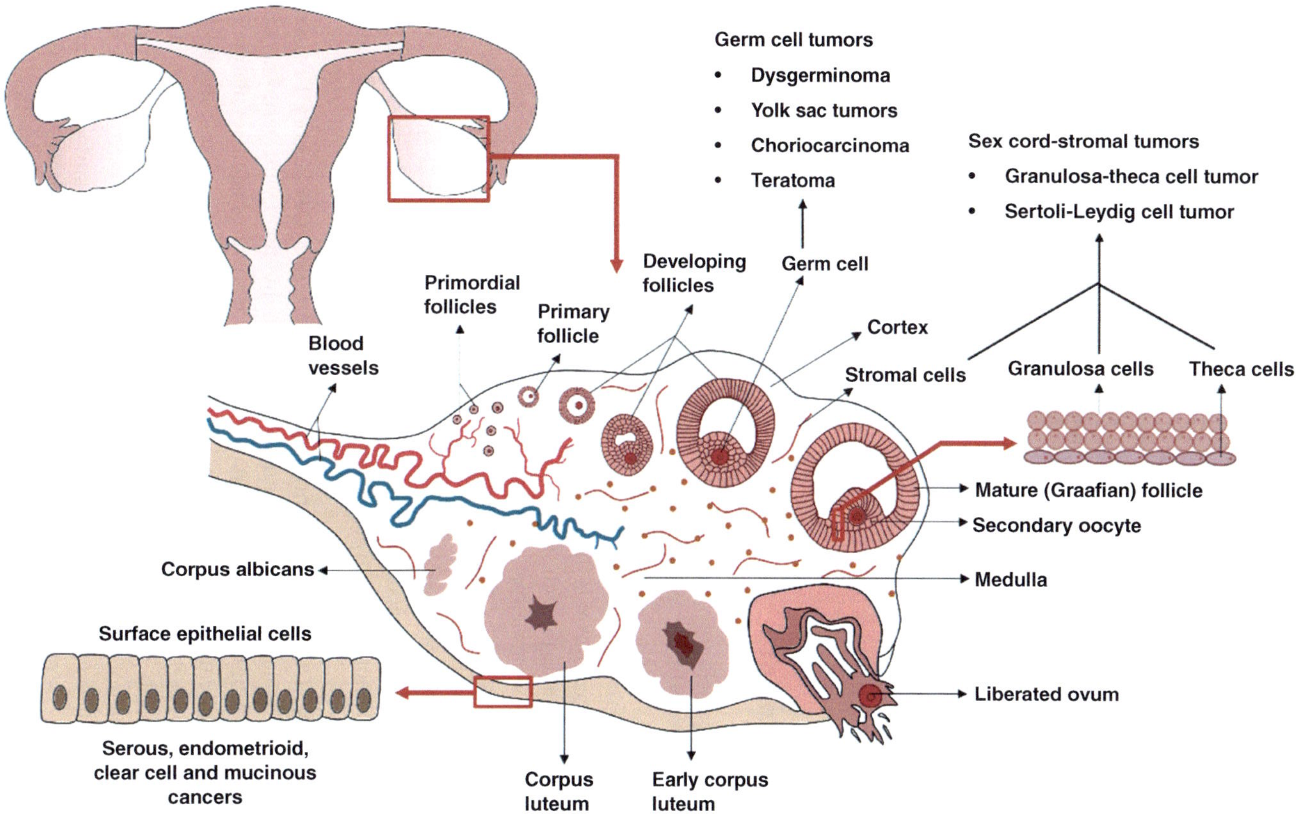

Fig. 11.2 Cell of origin of different types of ovarian cancers. The anatomy of female reproductive system and the process of ovulation were depicted in the figure. The cells that develop into different histological subtypes of ovarian cancer were shown

LGSOC, mutations in *BRAF* (38%) and *KRAS* (19%) are the most common genetic alterations [2, 39]. Ovarian serous borderline tumors (OSBTs) that are associated with adenofibroma are most common borderline tumors in ovary and about 6.8% of OSBTs give rise to LGSOC [40]. Mutations in *KRAS* range from 23% to 48% in OSBTs and 0%–33% in LGSOC whereas mutations in *BRAF* range from 17% to 36% in OSBTs and 19%–54.5% in LGSOCs [40]. Mutations in *ARID1A* were observed in about 50% of CCC patients [41–43]. Mutations in *CTNNB1* and *PTEN* are most common in endometroid tumors [44] while mutations in *PIK3CA* (33%) are frequently observed in CCC [43, 45]. Integrated molecular profiling of endometrioid ovarian cancer samples revealed that the tumors have a distinct heterogenous mutational profiles [46]. In a study of ovarian carcinoma, 15% of patients had inherited *BRCA1* or *BRCA2* mutations [47]. The relative risk (RR) for women with mutations in *PALB2* was 2.91 for ovarian cancer [48] while the RR for women with mutations in *BRIP1* was 11.22 for invasive EOC and 14.09 for HGSOC [49]. A number of lncRNAs (long noncoding RNAs) are found to play important roles in tumor growth [50].

11.4 Treatment

Debulking surgery followed chemotherapy is the primary treatment for ovarian, fallopian tube or primary peritoneal cancer and neoadjuvant chemotherapy for advanced-stage ovarian cancer [51–53]. Recent studies report that the PARP inhibitors were increasingly used for the treatment of ovarian cancer [54]. The use of carboplatin plus paclitaxel is the preferred first-line therapy and cisplatin therapy is considered in suitable patients and full adjuvant therapy for early-stage HGSOC are among the key recommendations [55]. A recent study observed that the median survival rate increased by 5.5% for every 10% increase in maximal cytoreduction [56]. Maintenance therapy following first-line primary/adjuvant chemotherapy is a significant development in the treatment of advance stage cancer [57]. In patients with recurrent ovarian cancer, the overall survival (OS) was higher in cytoreductive surgery and chemotherapy group when compared to the chemotherapy alone group [58].

According to NCCN compendium, olaparib maintenance is a category 1 recommendation and a category 2A recommendation for individuals with germline and somatic *BRCA* mutations, respectively for patients who responded to platinum-based first-line chemotherapy with or without bevacizumab [57]. According to the clinical trials undertook by FDA, bevacizumab (Avastin), and PARP inhibitors (rucaparib, olaparib, and niraparib) appeared to slow down the more advanced ovarian cancers. The combination of olaparib and bevacizumab was used for maintenance treatment of ovarian cancers; niraparib was used to keep epithelial ovarian cancers at bay. Bevacizumab treatment is a therapeutic option for stage II–IV patients, having either complete or partial response to surgery and with wild-type or unknown *BRCA1/2* mutation status but not for patients with *BRCA1/2* mutations [58]. In a phase 3 trial of olaparib plus bevacizumab, the progression-free survival

(PFS) was higher for olaparib plus bevacizumab treated patients than in placebo plus bevacizumab group (16.6 months) [59]. In another randomized phase 3 trial in 733 patients, the median PFS and OS rate were higher in patients treated with niraparib (PFS: 21.9 months; OS: 84%) than in placebo group (PFS: 10.4 months; OS: 77%) [60]. In a randomized phase 3 trial of 295 *BRCA1/2* mutation-positive patients, the PFS was 51.7 months in olaparib group as compared to 38.8 months in the placebo group [61]. Higher PFS (56.0 months) was observed in patients when treated with olaparib than in placebo group (13.8 months) [62]. In addition, treatment with decitabine has shown antitumor responses in 18–30% of cases in EOC patients with prior chemotherapy and either resistant or refractory illness [63]. In KEYNOTE-028 PHASE Ib multicohort study, pembrolizumab was given to patients who were resistant to platinum-based treatment and the patients' objective response rate (ORR) was observed to be 11.5% and about 23% of them had a stable disease [34]. In a phase 2 trial, an ORR of 47.5% and a median PFS of 10.0 months were observed with a combination of pembrolizumab, bevacizumab, and oral metronomic cyclophosphamide [64]. In a phase I/II trial of veliparib in platinum-resistant or partially sensitive EOC patients with germline *BRCA1/2* mutations, an OS of 13.7 months and PFS of 5.6 months were observed [65].

11.5 Conclusion

Ovarian cancers are one of the most common gynecological malignancies that are often not diagnosed at early stages. Certain biomarkers such as elevated levels of CA125 can be used for the diagnosis of ovarian cancers at early stages. Nevertheless, it still remains a challenge to detect the ovarian cancer onset at early stages. Among the histological subtypes, EOC accounts to more than 95% of ovarian cancer cases and about 90% of EOC patients were found to have mutations in the *TP53* gene. Importantly, the cancerous cells are reported to invade other parts of the body by breaking off from the initial tumor leading to metastasis. Hence, screening the type II tumors before the metastasis is necessary. Treatment strategies including cytoreductive debulking surgery followed by chemotherapy, use of PARP inhibitors, and bevacizumab were found to be successful in reducing the frequency of relapse of ovarian cancer.

References

1. Sung H, Ferlay J, Siegel RL, Laversanne M, Soerjomataram I, Jemal A, Bray F. Global cancer statistics 2020: GLOBOCAN estimates of incidence and mortality worldwide for 36 cancers in 185 countries. CA Cancer J Clin. 2021;71(3):209–49.
2. Lheureux S, Braunstein M, Oza AM. Epithelial ovarian cancer: evolution of management in the era of precision medicine. CA Cancer J Clin. 2019;69(4):280–304.
3. Siegel RL, Miller KD, Jemal A. Cancer statistics, 2020. CA Cancer J Clin. 2020;70(1):7–30.
4. Stewart C, Ralyea C, Lockwood S. Ovarian cancer: an integrated review. Sem Oncol Nurs. 2019;35(2):151–6.

5. Dyba T, Randi G, Bray F, Martos C, Giusti F, Nicholson N, Gavin A, Flego M, Neamtiu L, Dimitrova N, Carvalho RN. The European cancer burden in 2020: Incidence and mortality estimates for 40 countries and 25 major cancers. Eur J Cancer. 2021;157:308–47.
6. Wohlmuth C, Wohlmuth-Wieser I. Gynecologic malignancies in children and adolescents: how common is the uncommon? J Clin Med. 2021;10(4):722.
7. Lheureux S, Gourley C, Vergote I, Oza AM. Epithelial ovarian cancer. Lancet. 2019;393(10177):1240–53.
8. El-Sherif A, El-Sherif S, Taylor AH, Ayakannu T. Ovarian cancer: lifestyle, diet and nutrition. Nutr Cancer. 2021;73(7):1092–107.
9. Kuchenbaecker KB, Hopper JL, Barnes DR, Phillips KA, Mooij TM, Roos-Blom MJ, Jervis S, Van Leeuwen FE, Milne RL, Andrieu N, Goldgar DE. Risks of breast, ovarian, and contralateral breast cancer for BRCA1 and BRCA2 mutation carriers. JAMA. 2017;317(23):2402–16.
10. Jervis S, Song H, Lee A, Dicks E, Tyrer J, Harrington P, Easton DF, Jacobs IJ, Pharoah PP, Antoniou AC. Ovarian cancer familial relative risks by tumour subtypes and by known ovarian cancer genetic susceptibility variants. J Med Genet. 2014;51(2):108–13.
11. Sipos A, Ujlaki G, Mikó E, Maka E, Szabó J, Uray K, Krasznai Z, Bai P. The role of the microbiome in ovarian cancer: Mechanistic insights into oncobiosis and to bacterial metabolite signaling. Mol Med. 2021;27(1):1–20.
12. Gong TT, Wu QJ, Vogtmann E, Lin B, Wang YL. Age at menarche and risk of ovarian cancer: a meta-analysis of epidemiological studies. Int J Cancer. 2013;132(12):2894–900.
13. Braem MG, Onland-Moret NC, Schouten LJ, Kruitwagen RF, Lukanova A, Allen NE, Wark PA, Tjønneland A, Hansen L, Braüner CM, Overvad K. Multiple miscarriages are associated with the risk of ovarian cancer: results from the European Prospective Investigation into Cancer and Nutrition. PLoS One. 2012;7(5):e37141.
14. Jacobs IJ, Menon U. Progress and challenges in screening for early detection of ovarian cancer. Mol Cell Proteomics. 2004;3(4):355–66.
15. Doubeni CA, Doubeni AR, Myers AE. Diagnosis and management of ovarian cancer. Am Fam Physician. 2016;93(11):937–44.
16. Timmerman D, Ameye L, Fischerova D, Epstein E, Melis GB, Guerriero S, Van Holsbeke C, Savelli L, Fruscio R, Lissoni AA, Testa AC. Simple ultrasound rules to distinguish between benign and malignant adnexal masses before surgery: prospective validation by IOTA group. BMJ. 2010:341.
17. Nebgen DR, Lu KH, Bast RC. Novel approaches to ovarian cancer screening. Curr Oncol Rep. 2019;21:1–1.
18. Gaona-Luviano P, Medina-Gaona LA, Magaña-Pérez K. Epidemiology of ovarian cancer. Chin Clin Oncol. 2020;9(4):47.
19. Asante DB, Calapre L, Ziman M, Meniawy TM, Gray ES. Liquid biopsy in ovarian cancer using circulating tumor DNA and cells: ready for prime time? Cancer Lett. 2020;468:59–71.
20. Yang F, Tang J, Zhao Z, Zhao C, Xiang Y. Circulating tumor DNA: A noninvasive biomarker for tracking ovarian cancer. Reprod Biol Endocrinol. 2021;19:1–2.
21. Zhang X, Li H, Yu X, Li S, Lei Z, Li C, Zhang Q, Han Q, Li Y, Zhang K, Wang Y. Analysis of circulating tumor cells in ovarian cancer and their clinical value as a biomarker. Cell Physiol Biochem. 2018;48(5):1983–94.
22. Yoon H, Lee S. Fatty acid metabolism in ovarian cancer: therapeutic implications. Int J Mol Sci. 2022;23(4):2170.
23. Kurman RJ, Shih IM. The dualistic model of ovarian carcinogenesis: revisited, revised, and expanded. Am J Pathol. 2016;186(4):733–47.
24. Torre LA, Trabert B, DeSantis CE, Miller KD, Samimi G, Runowicz CD, Gaudet MM, Jemal A, Siegel RL. Ovarian cancer statistics, 2018. CA Cancer J Clin. 2018;68(4):284–96.
25. Prat J. Ovarian carcinomas: five distinct diseases with different origins, genetic alterations, and clinicopathological features. Virchows Arch. 2012;460(3):237–49.
26. Kurman RJ. Origin and molecular pathogenesis of ovarian high-grade serous carcinoma. Ann Oncol. 2013;24:x16–21.

27. Kaldawy A, Segev Y, Lavie O, Auslender R, Sopik V, Narod SA. Low-grade serous ovarian cancer: a review. Gynecol Oncol. 2016;143(2):433–8.
28. Nogales FF, Dulcey I, Preda O. Germ cell tumors of the ovary: an update. Arch Pathol Lab Med. 2014;138(3):351–62.
29. Al Harbi R, McNeish IA, El-Bahrawy M. Ovarian sex cord-stromal tumors: an update on clinical features, molecular changes, and management. Int J Gynecol Cancer. 2021;31(2).
30. Berek JS, Kehoe ST, Kumar L, Friedlander M. Cancer of the ovary, fallopian tube, and peritoneum. Int J Gynecol Obstet. 2018;143:59–78.
31. Dubeau L, Drapkin R. Coming into focus: the nonovarian origins of ovarian cancer. Ann Oncol. 2013;24:viii28–35.
32. Cancer Genome Atlas Research Network. Integrated genomic analyses of ovarian carcinoma. Nature. 2011;474(7353):609.
33. Ottevanger PB. Ovarian cancer stem cells more questions than answers. Sem Cancer Biol. 2017;44:67–71.
34. Moufarrij S, Dandapani M, Arthofer E, Gomez S, Srivastava A, Lopez-Acevedo M, Villagra A, Chiappinelli KB. Epigenetic therapy for ovarian cancer: promise and progress. Clin Epigenetics. 2019;11(1):1–1.
35. Zhang S, Royer R, Li S, McLaughlin JR, Rosen B, Risch HA, Fan I, Bradley L, Shaw PA, Narod SA. Frequencies of BRCA1 and BRCA2 mutations among 1,342 unselected patients with invasive ovarian cancer. Gynecol Oncol. 2011;121(2):353–7.
36. Enomoto T, Weghorst CM, Inoue M, Tanizawa O, Rice JM. K-ras activation occurs frequently in mucinous adenocarcinomas and rarely in other common epithelial tumors of the human ovary. Am J Pathol. 1991;139(4):777.
37. Gemignani ML, Schlaerth AC, Bogomolniy F, Barakat RR, Lin O, Soslow R, Venkatraman E, Boyd J. Role of KRAS and BRAF gene mutations in mucinous ovarian carcinoma. Gynecol Oncol. 2003;90(2):378–81.
38. Perren TJ. Mucinous epithelial ovarian carcinoma. Ann Oncol. 2016;27:i53–7.
39. Singer G, Oldt R III, Cohen Y, Wang BG, Sidransky D, Kurman RJ, Shih IM. Mutations in BRAF and KRAS characterize the development of low-grade ovarian serous carcinoma. J Natl Cancer Inst. 2003;95(6):484–6.
40. Malpica A, Wong KK. The molecular pathology of ovarian serous borderline tumors. Ann Oncol. 2016;27:i16–9.
41. Jones S, Wang TL, Shih IM, Mao TL, Nakayama K, Roden R, Glas R, Slamon D, Diaz LA Jr, Vogelstein B, Kinzler KW. Frequent mutations of chromatin remodeling gene ARID1A in ovarian clear cell carcinoma. Science. 2010;330(6001):228–31.
42. Wiegand KC, Shah SP, Al-Agha OM, Zhao Y, Tse K, Zeng T, Senz J, McConechy MK, Anglesio MS, Kalloger SE, Yang W. ARID1A mutations in endometriosis-associated ovarian carcinomas. N Engl J Med. 2010;363(16):1532–43.
43. Wei W, Dizon D, Vathipadiekal V, Birrer MJ. Ovarian cancer: genomic analysis. Ann Oncol. 2013;24:x7–15.
44. Wright K, Wilson P, Morland S, Campbell I, Walsh M, Hurst T, Ward B, Cummings M, Chenevix-Trench G. β-Catenin mutation and expression analysis in ovarian cancer: Exon 3 mutations and nuclear translocation in 16% of endometrioid tumours. Int J Cancer. 1999;82(5):625–9.
45. Kuo KT, Mao TL, Jones S, Veras E, Ayhan A, Wang TL, Glas R, Slamon D, Velculescu VE, Kuman RJ, Shih IM. Frequent activating mutations of PIK3CA in ovarian clear cell carcinoma. Am J Pathol. 2009;174(5):1597–601.
46. Pierson WE, Peters PN, Chang MT, Chen LM, Quigley DA, Ashworth A, Chapman JS. An integrated molecular profile of endometrioid ovarian cancer. Gynecol Oncol. 2020;157(1):55–61.
47. Norquist BM, Harrell MI, Brady MF, Walsh T, Lee MK, Gulsuner S, Bernards SS, Casadei S, Yi Q, Burger RA, Chan JK. Inherited mutations in women with ovarian carcinoma. JAMA Oncol. 2016;2(4):482–90.

48. Yang X, Leslie G, Doroszuk A, Schneider S, Allen J, Decker B, Dunning AM, Redman J, Scarth J, Plaskocinska I, Luccarini C. Cancer risks associated with germline PALB2 pathogenic variants: an international study of 524 families. J Clin Oncol. 2020;38(7):674.
49. Ramus SJ, Song H, Dicks E, Tyrer JP, Rosenthal AN, Intermaggio MP, Fraser L, Gentry-Maharaj A, Hayward J, Philpott S, Anderson C. Germline mutations in the BRIP1, BARD1, PALB2, and NBN genes in women with ovarian cancer. J Natl Cancer Inst. 2015;107(11):djv214.
50. Wang JY, Lu AQ, Chen LJ. LncRNAs in ovarian cancer. Clin Chim Acta. 2019;490:17–27.
51. Ledermann JA, Raja FA, Fotopoulou C, Gonzalez-Martin A, Colombo N, Sessa C. Newly diagnosed and relapsed epithelial ovarian carcinoma: ESMO Clinical Practice Guidelines for diagnosis, treatment and follow-up. Ann Oncol. 2013;24:vi24–32.
52. Fleming GF, Seidman J, Lengyel E, et al. Epithelial ovarian cancer. In: Chi DS, Berchuck A, Dizon DS, editors. Principles and practice of gynecologic oncology. 7th ed. Philadelphia, PA: Lippincott Williams & Wilkins; 2017. p. 611–705.
53. Van Meurs HS, Tajik P, Hof MH, Vergote I, Kenter GG, Mol BW, Buist MR, Bossuyt PM. Which patients benefit most from primary surgery or neoadjuvant chemotherapy in stage IIIC or IV ovarian cancer? An exploratory analysis of the European Organisation for Research and Treatment of Cancer 55971 randomised trial. Eur J Cancer. 2013;49(15):3191–201.
54. Tew WP, Lacchetti C, Ellis A, Maxian K, Banerjee S, Bookman M, Jones MB, Lee JM, Lheureux S, Liu JF, Moore KN. PARP inhibitors in the management of ovarian cancer: ASCO guideline. J Clin Oncol Off J Am Soc Clin Oncol. 2020;38(30):3468.
55. Bookman MA. Optimal primary therapy of ovarian cancer. Ann Oncol. 2016;27:i58–62.
56. Kuroki L, Guntupalli SR. Treatment of epithelial ovarian cancer. BMJ. 2020:371.
57. O'Malley DM. New therapies for ovarian cancer. J Natl Compr Canc Netw. 2019;17(5.5):619–21.
58. Garcia A, Singh H. Bevacizumab and ovarian cancer. Therap Adv Med Oncol. 2013;5(2):133–41.
59. Ray-Coquard I, Pautier P, Pignata S, Pérol D, González-Martín A, Berger R, Fujiwara K, Vergote I, Colombo N, Mäenpää J, Selle F. Olaparib plus bevacizumab as first-line maintenance in ovarian cancer. N Engl J Med. 2019;381(25):2416–28.
60. González-Martín A, Pothuri B, Vergote I, DePont Christensen R, Graybill W, Mirza MR, McCormick C, Lorusso D, Hoskins P, Freyer G, Baumann K. Niraparib in patients with newly diagnosed advanced ovarian cancer. N Engl J Med. 2019;381(25):2391–402.
61. Poveda A, Floquet A, Ledermann JA, Asher R, Penson RT, Oza AM, Korach J, Huzarski T, Pignata S, Friedlander M, Baldoni A. Olaparib tablets as maintenance therapy in patients with platinum-sensitive relapsed ovarian cancer and a BRCA1/2 mutation (SOLO2/ENGOT-Ov21): a final analysis of a double-blind, randomised, placebo-controlled, phase 3 trial. Lancet Oncol. 2021;22(5):620–31.
62. Banerjee S, Moore KN, Colombo N, Scambia G, Kim BG, Oaknin A, Friedlander M, Lisyanskaya A, Floquet A, Leary A, Sonke GS. Maintenance olaparib for patients with newly diagnosed advanced ovarian cancer and a BRCA mutation (SOLO1/GOG 3004): 5-year follow-up of a randomised, double-blind, placebo-controlled, phase 3 trial. Lancet Oncol. 2021;22(12):1721–31.
63. Natanzon Y, Goode EL, Cunningham JM. Epigenetics in ovarian cancer. Semin Cancer Biol. 2018;51:160–9.
64. Zsiros E, Lynam S, Attwood KM, Wang C, Chilakapati S, Gomez EC, Liu S, Akers S, Lele S, Frederick PJ, Odunsi K. Efficacy and safety of pembrolizumab in combination with bevacizumab and oral metronomic cyclophosphamide in the treatment of recurrent ovarian cancer: a phase 2 nonrandomized clinical trial. JAMA Oncol. 2021;7(1):78–85.
65. Steffensen KD, Adimi P, Jakobsen A. Veliparib monotherapy to patients with BRCA germ line mutation and platinum-resistant or partially platinum-sensitive relapse of epithelial ovarian cancer: a phase I/II study. In J Gynecol Cancer. 2017;27(9):1842–9.

Endometrial Cancer

12

Sai Charitha Mullaguri, Prapthi Bathini,
Sri Charitha Gorantla, Bindu Madhava Reddy Aramati,
and Rama Krishna Kancha

12.1 Introduction

Epidemiology: Endometrial cancer (EC), also called as cancer of the corpus uteri ranks sixth in terms of cancer incidence in women (4.5% of all cancer cases). It ranks fifteenth in global cancer incidence with 417,367 new cases accounting to 2.2% of all cancer cases, but ranks nineteenth in mortality with 97,370 deaths accounting to 1% of all cancer-related deaths in the year 2020 [1]. The age-standardized rate of incidence is significantly higher (8.7/100,000) than the age-standardized mortality rate (1.8/100,000). Based on the statistics from GLOBOCAN factsheet for the year 2020, the 5-year prevalence was high in Asia (35.9%) and Europe (34.1%). According to the US-SEER database in the year 2020 for endometrial cancer, the estimated new cases and deaths were 65,620 and 12,590, respectively [2]. In Europe for the year 2020, the incidence was 6.8% (1,30,100 new cases; cumulative risk 2.05) and mortality was 3.5% (30,000 new cases; cumulative risk 0.35) [3]. Unimproved survival rates for EC patients are mainly due to the absence of effective treatment strategies for metastatic cancers [4]. The 5-year survival rates for localized, regional, and distant stages of cancer were 96%, 71%, and 17% in white women, and 85%, 49%, and 9% in black women, respectively [2]. Among children and adolescents in United States, the relative frequency of endometrial cancer was 2.5% when compared to other gynecological malignancies [5].

S. C. Mullaguri · R. K. Kancha (✉)
Molecular Medicine and Therapeutics Laboratory, CPMB, Osmania University, Hyderabad, India
e-mail: ramakancha@osmania.ac.in

P. Bathini
Apollo Institute of Medical Sciences and Research, Hyderabad, India

S. C. Gorantla · B. M. R. Aramati (✉)
Department of Animal Biotechnology, School of Life Sciences, University of Hyderabad, Hyderabad, India

R. K. Kancha (ed.), *Biomedical Aspects of Solid Cancers*,
https://doi.org/10.1007/978-981-97-1802-3_12

Risk Factors: Major risk factors include obesity, genetic alterations, family history of ECs, polycystic ovarian syndrome (PCOS), diabetes and excess use of tamoxifen after breast cancer [6, 7]. Other risk factors include old age, early menarche (menstruating at an early age), late menopause, exposure to radiation, and increased exogenous estrogen usage [8]. According to the ACS, about 2 out of 3 cases of endometrial cancer are found in women aged 55 or older. Young women with obesity are at a greater risk due to the increased aromatase levels resulting in the increased production of estrogen [7, 9]. The relative risk (RR) of endometrial cancer increases with an increase in the body mass index (BMI) [10, 11]. A case-control study concluded that the BMI is directly proportional and the physical activity is inversely proportional to the risk of uterine cancer [12]. Women who have been exposed to high levels of estrogen are at a greater risk for endometrial cancer. This includes nulliparous women (never had children), early menarche, and late menopause [13]. Women with PCOS are at a higher risk of developing endometrial cancer when compared to that of ovarian and breast cancers [14]. Additionally, diabetic women have a greater risk of endometrial cancer [15, 16]. Larger duration of tamoxifen usage (≥10 years) following breast cancer diagnosis led to an increased risk of endometrial cancer [17]. Women with a family history of EC, colon cancer or hereditary nonpolyposis colorectal cancer (HNPCC) are at an increased risk of developing endometrial cancer [18]. The intentional weight loss by postmenopausal women and the use of oral bisphosphonates to treat osteoporosis are associated with a reduced risk of endometrial cancer [19, 20]. The use of oral contraceptives reduced the risk of endometrial cancer by as much as 33% compared to nonusers of combined oral contraceptives (COC), and the risk reduction continued beyond 30 years of COC termination [21].

Diagnosis and Screening: Endometrial biopsy is the most common method of obtaining tissue for diagnosis [22, 23]. Pelvic ultrasonography and sentinel node biopsy are also used to detect endometrial cancer [24]. Contrast-enhanced MRI and CT are widely used to detect the extent of tumor and invasion of endometrial tumors into surrounding tissues [25]. A meta-analysis revealed that ultrasonography has a sensitivity and specificity of 90% and 54%, respectively when endometrium thickness of ≥5 mm is considered [26]. Blood-based infrared spectroscopy, an alternative approach to detect endometrial cancer has a sensitivity of 87% and a specificity of 78% [27]. A multicentered cohort study revealed that the sentinel lymph node (SLN) mapping and biopsy were observed to have higher diagnostic value and can safely replace lymphadenectomy in staging [28]. Single-cell RNA sequencing (scRNA-seq) analysis of endometrial cancer as well as normal endometrium samples revealed that a high level of intertumoral heterogeneity exists in the immune microenvironment and the presence of vascular cancer-associated fibroblasts (vCAFs) may be responsible for the poor prognosis of endometrial cancer [29]. The number of mesenchymal stem cells in tumor microenvironment directly correlate with the stage of disease and might help to envisage the prognosis of endometrial cancer [30].

12.2 Classification

Endometrial cancer is classified based on (i) clinical, metabolic, and endocrine characteristics, (ii) histology, (iii) staging, and (iv) molecular markers (Fig. 12.1). (i) Based on the characteristics of tumors, endometrial cancer is broadly classified into type I and type II (Fig. 12.1) [24, 31–34]. Type I tumors are low grade, moderately or highly differentiated with a favorable prognosis. They are associated with obesity, hormone-receptor (estrogen and progesterone) positivity, high levels of estrogen, and endometrial hyperplasia [31]. Type II tumors are poorly differentiated with poor prognosis and are associated with an atrophic endometrium [31]. These tumors may arise in the absence of endocrine (estrogen) and metabolic changes and are mostly observed in nonobese women [31].

(ii) Based on the histology, EC is classified into following subtypes: (a) endometrioid and its variants, accounts to about 85% of all endometrial cancer cases and is the most common subtype (Fig. 12.1) [35]. The variants of endometrioid carcinoma are squamous, mucinous, and villoglandular differentiation (Fig. 12.1) [35]. (b) Serous carcinoma is an aggressive form and accounts to 3–10% of endometrial cancers, (c) clear cell carcinoma is an uncommon form of EC that accounts to less than 5% of all endometrial cancer cases, and (d) undifferentiated and dedifferentiated carcinoma (Fig. 12.1) [35]. Undifferentiated carcinoma has no differentiation of cells and is further classified into dedifferentiated carcinoma where tumor cells of endometrioid carcinoma are observed along with undifferentiated cells [35, 36].

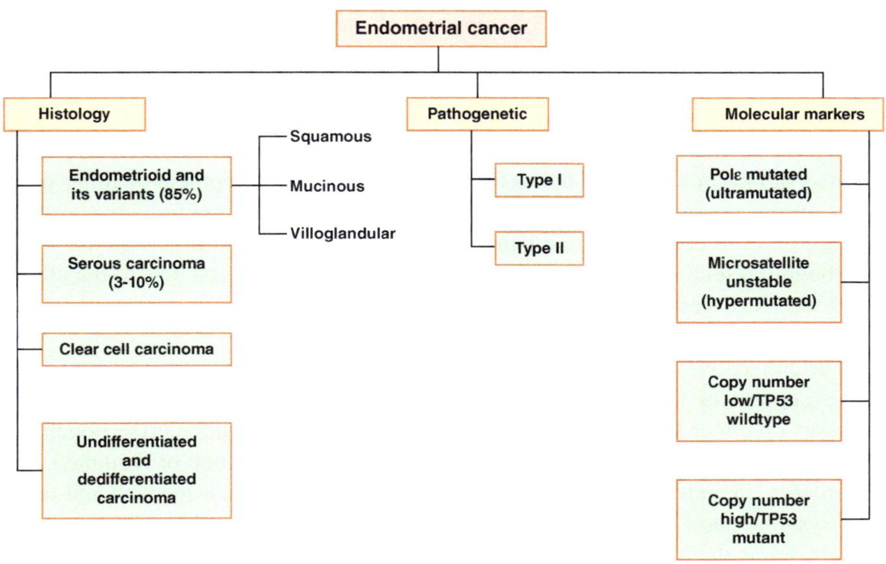

Fig. 12.1 Classification of endometrial cancer based on histology, pathogenetic nature, and molecular markers

(iii) FIGO has classified endometrial cancer into different stages in the year 2009 [37, 38]. Stage I, an initial stage in tumor development is subdivided into two stages: stage IA refers to tumor confinement to uterus with less than 50% invasion into myometrium and stage IB indicates tumor confinement to uterus with ≥50% myometrial invasion [37]. Stage II indicates invasion of cancer into cervical stroma and stage III is further subdivided into IIIA, IIIB, IIIC1, and IIIC2 [37]. In stage IIIA, tumor invasion occurs into the fallopian tubes and ovaries, and in stage IIIB, invaded tumor appears in the vaginal area [37]. Stage IIIC1 results in tumor invasion into pelvic nodes whereas in stage IIIC2, paraaortic nodes are involved [37]. Stage IV is further subdivided into IVA and IVB where tumor invades into bladder or bowel mucosa in IVA while distant metastasis occurs in stage IVB [37].

(iv) Based on the somatic mutation rate, microsatellite instability (MSI) status, and somatic copy number status, EC is classified into four different subtypes by The Cancer Genome Atlas (TCGA) (Fig. 12.1) [35, 39, 40]. The subtypes include (i) POLε mutated (ultra-mutated) with any of the five hotspot mutations that include P286R, S297F, V411L, A456P, and S459F [41], (ii) microsatellite unstable (hyper mutated), (iii) copy number low (CNL)/TP53 wild-type (also called as endometrioid-like), and (iv) copy number high (CNH)/TP53 mutant (also called as serous-like) [39].

12.3 Pathophysiology

Anatomy and Cell of Origin: The uterus (womb) is a fibromuscular structure in the female pelvic region, measures about 8 cm in length, and is present superioanterior to the bladder. The anatomical components of uterus include the fundus, corpus, isthmus, and cervix. Fundus is the widest portion of the uterus that connects to fallopian tube. Corpus is also called as the body of uterus (uterine cavity), lies intraperitoneally and starts directly below the level of fallopian tubes. Isthmus is a 1 cm long passage that connects uterus and cervix, and Cervix is the tubular portion located sub-peritoneally and opens into the vagina. The development of embryo and fetus during pregnancy is carried out in uterus of the female reproductive system. During embryo development, a pair of paramesonephric (Müllerian) ducts, which are the initial fetal structures of the female reproductive tract give rise to the uterus. At 9 weeks of gestation period, the uterine body can be clearly observed for the first time.

The connective tissue that encircles the uterus is called as the parametrium. With the exception of the ventral portion of the cervix, the parametrium forms two recesses on either side of the uterus: the ventrally located vesicouterine pouch and the dorsally located rectouterine pouch (also called as the pouch of Douglas). The vasculature includes uterine arteries that branches within the uterine wall and forms two systems named as anterior and posterior arcuate arteries. The uterine venous plexus drains the blood into internal iliac vein. The lymph from the body of uterus is drained into the iliac and external iliac (also called as obturator) lymph nodes while the lymph from fundus is drained into the para-aortic lymph nodes.

Sympathetic nerve fibers, which generate uterine muscle contraction and blood vessel constriction and parasympathetic (sacral) nerve fibers, which reduce muscle activity and widen blood vessels, are the two types of nerves that supply the uterus.

The uterus has three distinct layers of tissue namely perimetrium (serosa or adventitia), myometrium (uterine muscularis), and endometrium (uterine mucosa) (Fig. 12.2). Perimetrium is the outer most layer made up of epithelial cells and is surrounded by a thin connective tissue layer. Myometrium is the middle layer made up of smooth muscle tissue and is further subdivided into three sub-layers namely sub-vascular layer (thin layer present immediate to the endometrium), vascular layer (strong layer that plays a major role in the labor), and a supra vascular layer (thin sheet that stabilizes uterine wall). Endometrium is the innermost mucous membrane that lines the uterine cavity and continues with the lining of the cervical canal. Endometrium mainly consists of simple columnar epithelial cells and numerous tubular glands namely endometrial glands present in the functional portion of endometrium (Fig. 12.2). Endometrial atypical hyperplasia/endometrioid intraepithelial neoplasia (EAH/EIN) are the precursor lesions for almost all endometrioid endometrial cancers and some serous carcinomas [42]. These lesions have highly proliferated endometrial glands, which are lined by a number of atypical cells [43]. Serous intraepithelial carcinoma (SIEC), the precursor lesions for serous carcinoma have pleomorphic cells, show nucleomegaly, and are highly proliferative, but are not invasive [44–46]. Among molecular subtypes, the copy number high (CNH)/TP53 mutant has SIEC as precursors [47] while EAH/EIN are precursors for POLε-mutated subtype [48].

Genetics: In a cohort study that included 466 samples from endometrioid endometrial cancer patients, the genes with higher mutational frequency were *PIK3CA*

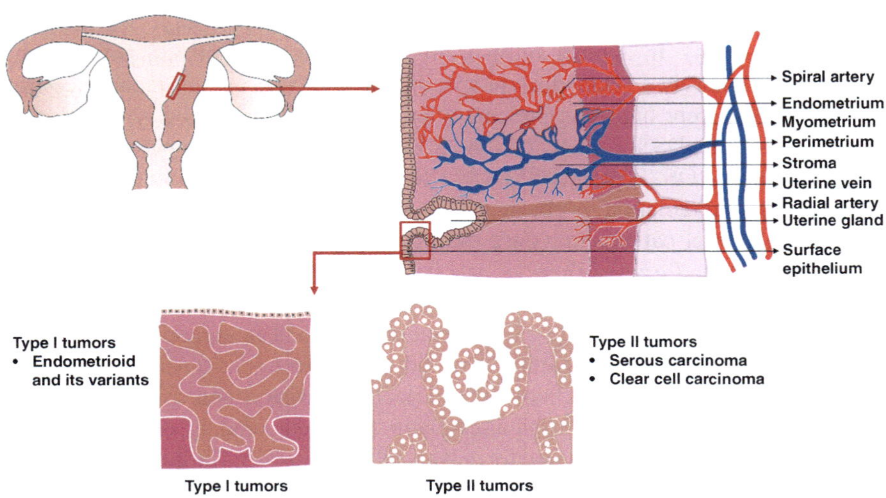

Fig. 12.2 Pathophysiology of endometrial cancer. The three layers of uterine wall and the origin of different histological subtypes from the endometrium

(22%), *CTNNB1* (19%), *KRAS* (19%), *FGFR2* (10%) and the MSI was observed in 34% of the patients [49]. When the MSI positive tumors were compared with microsatellite stable (MSS) tumors, frequency of mutations was higher in *KRAS* (MSI: 28%; MSS: 14%) and *FGFR2* (MSI: 15%; MSS: 8%) while the frequency of mutations was lower in *CTNNB1* (MSI: 11%; MSS: 24%) [49]. Exon-sequencing of *PIK3R1* from 42 endometrioid endometrial carcinomas (EECs) and nonendometrioid endometrial cancers (NEECs) revealed that the somatic mutations were observed in 43% of EECs and 12% of NEECs [50]. In EECs, the mutations in *PIK3R1* co-occur with mutations in *PTEN* and *KRAS* while mutually exclusive with mutations in the *PIK3CA* [50]. In proteogenomic characterization of 95 endometrial carcinoma samples, higher rates of microsatellite indels were observed in *PTEN* (92%), *ARID1A* (76%), *RPL22* (64%), *INPPL1* (56%), *KMT2B* (56%), and *JAK1* (44%) in MSI subtype of endometrioid tumors (25 samples) [51]. About 25–30% of endometrial serous carcinomas have overexpressed HER2 protein and/or *HER2* gene amplifications, which makes HER2 an important therapeutic target in endometrial serous carcinomas [52]. In a study to assess the incidence of homologous recombination deficiency (HRD) in endometrial cancers, about 46% of nonendometrioid endometrial cancer samples exhibited HRD while none of the endometrioid endometrial cancer samples showed HRD [53].

12.4 Treatment

Surgery and Radiation Therapy: The standard first-line therapeutic strategy is the total hysterectomy along with bilateral salpingo-oophorectomy (removing the ovaries and fallopian tubes) and lymphadenectomy [34]. A study in 12,333 patients revealed that the extent or increased number of lymph nodes removal improves the disease-specific survival of the patients having intermediate or high risk of recurrence of ECs [54]. In another retrospective cohort analysis of 328 patients, the 5-year overall survival (OS), disease-specific survival (DSS), and recurrence-free survival (RFS) were higher in patients with pelvic and para-aortic lymphadenectomy (OS: 83.2%; DSS: 84.9%; RFS: 80.7%) than in patients with pelvic lymphadenectomy alone (OS: 72.6%; DSS: 73%; RFS: 64.8%) [55]. Brachytherapy (also called as internal radiation) is considered as a standard therapy in surgically treated endometrial cancer patients to reduce the risk of vaginal recurrence [56].

Chemotherapy, Targeted Therapy, and Immunotherapy: The most common combinations include carboplatin/paclitaxel and cisplatin/doxorubicin that are also commonly used for high-grade cancer patients who had undergone surgery. In a phase III open-label trial of carboplatin and paclitaxel for advanced endometrial cancer, the treatment with carboplatin and paclitaxel was found to be noninferior alternative to paclitaxel-doxorubicin-cisplatin treatment, and is considered as a global first-line standard therapy for advanced cancer [57]. Targeted therapeutic drugs are currently used to treat high-risk endometrial cancers or those that have metastasized or recurred after treatment. In a phase IB/II trial of lenvatinib (targeted therapy) plus pembrolizumab (immune checkpoint inhibitor), the objective response rate (ORR) at 24 weeks was observed to be 52% [58]. Further, the OS and PFS (progression-free survival) were higher in lenvatinib plus pembrolizumab group (OS: 17.4 months; PFS: 6.6 months) than in patients undergoing chemotherapy (OS: 12 months; PFS: 3.8 months) [59]. Another clinical trial of pembrolizumab in patients with MSI and mismatch repair deficient (MRD) endometrial cancer showed 48% of ORR and PFS of 13.1 months [60]. In a multicentered phase 1 trial of dostarlimab in recurrent or advanced MRD ECs, the ORR was observed to be 42%, of which 13% of patients showed complete response and 30% showed partial response [61].

12.5 Conclusion

In conclusion, endometrial cancer is a common gynecologic cancer that arises from the lining of the uterus. The diagnosis of endometrial cancer involves a combination of clinical history and examination, imaging studies, and biopsy, with histological examination of the endometrial tissue. Screening for EC is done in women with risk factors such as obesity, diabetes or a family history of endometrial or colorectal cancer. Early identification and adoption of healthy lifestyle by reducing the weight and eating a healthy diet should be advised. Understanding the molecular mechanisms behind the signaling mechanisms involved in ECs especially estrogen and progesterone receptor signaling and their downstream targets help us to find out better ways to prevent or therapeutically target them. Treatment strategies such as targeted therapy combined with immunotherapy are under various clinical trials to treat patients with high-grade endometrial cancers.

References

1. Sung H, Ferlay J, Siegel RL, Laversanne M, Soerjomataram I, Jemal A, Bray F. Global cancer statistics 2020: GLOBOCAN estimates of incidence and mortality worldwide for 36 cancers in 185 countries. CA Cancer J Clin. 2021;71(3):209–49.
2. Siegel RL, Miller KD, Jemal A. Cancer statistics, 2020. CA Cancer J Clin. 2020;70(1):7–30.
3. Dyba T, Randi G, Bray F, Martos C, Giusti F, Nicholson N, Gavin A, Flego M, Neamtiu L, Dimitrova N, Carvalho RN. The European cancer burden in 2020: incidence and mortality estimates for 40 countries and 25 major cancers. Eur J Cancer. 2021;157:308–47.
4. McAlpine JN, Temkin SM, Mackay HJ. Endometrial cancer: not your grandmother's cancer. Cancer. 2016;122(18):2787–98.
5. Wohlmuth C, Wohlmuth-Wieser I. Gynecologic malignancies in children and adolescents: how common is the uncommon? J Clin Med. 2021;10(4):722.
6. Raglan O, Kalliala I, Markozannes G, Cividini S, Gunter MJ, Nautiyal J, Gabra H, Paraskevaidis E, Martin-Hirsch P, Tsilidis KK, Kyrgiou M. Risk factors for endometrial cancer: an umbrella review of the literature. Int J Cancer. 2019;145(7):1719–30.
7. Lu KH, Broaddus RR. Endometrial cancer. N Engl J Med. 2020;383(21):2053–64.
8. MacMahon B. Risk factors for endometrial cancer. Gynecol Oncol. 1974;2(2–3):122–9.
9. Kerr J, Anderson C, Lippman SM. Physical activity, sedentary behaviour, diet, and cancer: an update and emerging new evidence. Lancet Oncol. 2017;18(8):e457–71.

10. Renehan AG, Zwahlen M, Egger M. Adiposity and cancer risk: new mechanistic insights from epidemiology. Nat Rev Cancer. 2015;15(8):484–98.
11. Lauby-Secretan B, Scoccianti C, Loomis D, Grosse Y, Bianchini F, Straif K. Body fatness and cancer—viewpoint of the IARC working group. N Engl J Med. 2016;375(8):794–8.
12. Nunez C, Bauman A, Egger S, Sitas F, Nair-Shalliker V. Obesity, physical activity and cancer risks: results from the cancer, lifestyle and evaluation of risk study (CLEAR). Cancer Epidemiol. 2017;47:56–63.
13. Kitson SJ, Evans DG, Crosbie EJ. Identifying high-risk women for endometrial cancer prevention strategies: proposal of an endometrial cancer risk prediction model. Cancer Prev Res. 2017;10(1):1–3.
14. Barry JA, Azizia MM, Hardiman PJ. Risk of endometrial, ovarian and breast cancer in women with polycystic ovary syndrome: a systematic review and meta-analysis. Hum Reprod Update. 2014;20(5):748–58.
15. Liao C, Zhang D, Mungo C, Tompkins DA, Zeidan AM. Is diabetes mellitus associated with increased incidence and disease-specific mortality in endometrial cancer? A systematic review and meta-analysis of cohort studies. Gynecol Oncol. 2014;135(1):163–71.
16. Saed L, Varse F, Baradaran HR, Moradi Y, Khateri S, Friberg E, Khazaei Z, Gharahjeh S, Tehrani S, Sioofy-Khojine AB, Najmi Z. The effect of diabetes on the risk of endometrial cancer: an updated a systematic review and meta-analysis. BMC Cancer. 2019;19(1):527.
17. Swerdlow AJ, Jones ME. Tamoxifen treatment for breast cancer and risk of endometrial cancer: a case–control study. J Natl Cancer Inst. 2005;97(5):375–84.
18. Lynch HT, Snyder CL, Shaw TG, Heinen CD, Hitchins MP. Milestones of Lynch syndrome: 1895–2015. Nat Rev Cancer. 2015;15(3):181–94.
19. Luo J, Chlebowski RT, Hendryx M, Rohan T, Wactawski-Wende J, Thomson CA, Felix AS, Chen C, Barrington W, Coday M, Stefanick M. Intentional weight loss and endometrial cancer risk. J Clin Oncol. 2017;35(11):1189.
20. Newcomb PA, Passarelli MN, Phipps AI, Anderson GL, Wactawski-Wende J, Ho GY, O'Sullivan MJ, Chlebowski RT. Oral bisphosphonate use and risk of postmenopausal endometrial cancer. J Clin Oncol. 2015;33(10):1186.
21. Iversen L, Sivasubramaniam S, Lee AJ, Fielding S, Hannaford PC. Lifetime cancer risk and combined oral contraceptives: the Royal College of General Practitioners' Oral Contraception Study. Am J Obstet Gynecol. 2017;216(6):580–e1.
22. Faria SC, Devine CE, Rao B, Sagebiel T, Bhosale P. Imaging and staging of endometrial cancer. Sem Ultrasound CT MRI. 2019;40(4):287–94.
23. Huvila J, Pors J, Thompson EF, Gilks CB. Endometrial carcinoma: molecular subtypes, precursors and the role of pathology in early diagnosis. J Pathol. 2021;253(4):355–65.
24. Morice P, Leary A, Creutzberg C, Abu-Rustum N, Darai E. Endometrial cancer. Lancet. 2016;387(10023):1094–108.
25. Andreano A, Rechichi G, Rebora P, Sironi S, Valsecchi MG, Galimberti S. MR diffusion imaging for preoperative staging of myometrial invasion in patients with endometrial cancer: a systematic review and meta-analysis. Eur Radiol. 2014;24:1327–38.
26. Timmermans A, Opmeer BC, Khan KS, Bachmann LM, Epstein E, Clark TJ, Gupta JK, Bakour SH, Van Den Bosch T, Van Doorn HC, Cameron ST. Endometrial thickness measurement for detecting endometrial cancer in women with postmenopausal bleeding: a systematic review and meta-analysis. Obstet Gynecol. 2010;116(1):160–7.
27. Paraskevaidi M, Morais CL, Ashton KM, Stringfellow HF, McVey RJ, Ryan NA, O'Flynn H, Sivalingam VN, Kitson SJ, MacKintosh ML, Derbyshire AE. Detecting endometrial cancer by blood spectroscopy: a diagnostic cross-sectional study. Cancers. 2020;12(5):1256.
28. Rossi EC, Kowalski LD, Scalici J, Cantrell L, Schuler K, Hanna RK, Ade M, Ivanova A, Boggess JF. A comparison of sentinel lymph node biopsy to lymphadenectomy for endometrial cancer staging (FIRES trial): a multicentre, prospective, cohort study. Lancet Oncol. 2017;18(3):384–92.

29. Yu Z, Zhang J, Zhang Q, Wei S, Shi R, Zhao R, An L, Grose R, Feng D, Wang H. Single-cell sequencing reveals the heterogeneity and intratumoral crosstalk in human endometrial cancer. Cell Prolif. 2022;55(6):e13249.
30. Wang KH, Chang YH, Harnod T, Ding DC. Endometrial cancer-infiltrating mesenchymal stem cells exhibit immunosuppressive effects. Cell Transplant. 2022;31:09636897221104452.
31. Bokhman JV. Two pathogenetic types of endometrial carcinoma. Gynecol Oncol. 1983;15(1):10–7.
32. Murali R, Soslow RA, Weigelt B. Classification of endometrial carcinoma: more than two types. Lancet Oncol. 2014;15(7):e268–78.
33. Passarello K, Kurian S, Villanueva V. Endometrial cancer: an overview of pathophysiology, management, and care. Sem Oncol Nurs. 2019;35(2):157–65.
34. Brooks RA, Fleming GF, Lastra RR, Lee NK, Moroney JW, Son CH, Tatebe K, Veneris JL. Current recommendations and recent progress in endometrial cancer. CA Cancer J Clin. 2019;69(4):258–79.
35. Bell DW, Ellenson LH. Molecular genetics of endometrial carcinoma. Annu Rev Pathol. 2019;14:339–67.
36. Silva EG, Deavers MT, Malpica A. Undifferentiated carcinoma of the endometrium: a review. Pathology. 2007;39(1):134–8.
37. Pecorelli S. Revised FIGO staging for carcinoma of the vulva, cervix, and endometrium. Int J Gynaecol Obstet. 2009;105(2):103–4.
38. Koskas M, Amant F, Mirza MR, Creutzberg CL. Cancer of the corpus uteri: 2021 update. Int J Gynecol Obstet. 2021;155:45–60.
39. Levine DA, Cancer Genome Atlas Research Network Genome sequencing centres: Broad Institute Getz Gad 1 Gabriel Stacey B. 1 Cibulskis Kristian 1 Lander Eric 1 Sivachenko Andrey 1 Sougnez Carrie 1 Lawrence Mike 1, Washington University in St Louis Kandoth Cyriac 2 Dooling David 2 Fulton Robert 2 Fulton Lucinda 2 Kalicki-Veizer Joelle 2 McLellan Michael D. 2 O'Laughlin Michelle 2 Schmidt Heather 2 Wilson Richard K. 2 Ye Kai 2 Ding Li 2 Mardis Elaine R. 2, University of Southern California & Johns Hopkins Baylin Stephen B. 21 Bootwalla Moiz S. 22 Lai Phillip H. 22 Triche Jr Timothy J. 22 Van Den Berg David J. 22 Weisenberger Daniel J. 22 Laird Peter W. 22 Shen Hui 22, Institute for Systems Biology Reynolds Sheila M. 23 Shmulevich Ilya 23. Integrated genomic characterization of endometrial carcinoma. Nature. 2013;497(7447):67–73.
40. Akhtar M, Al Hyassat S, Elaiwy O, Rashid S, Al-Nabet AD. Classification of endometrial carcinoma: new perspectives beyond morphology. Adv Anat Pathol. 2019;26(6):421–7.
41. Vermij L, Smit V, Nout R, Bosse T. Incorporation of molecular characteristics into endometrial cancer management. Histopathology. 2020;76(1):52–63.
42. Conlon N, Paula AD, Ashley CW, Segura S, De Brot L, da Silva EM, Soslow RA, Weigelt B, DeLair DF. Endometrial carcinomas with a "serous" component in young women are enriched for DNA mismatch repair deficiency, lynch syndrome, and POLE exonuclease domain mutations. Am J Surg Pathol. 2020;44(5):641.
43. World Health Organization. Female genital tumours. International Agency for Research on Cancer; 2020.
44. Wheeler DT, Bell KA, Kurman RJ, Sherman ME. Minimal uterine serous carcinoma: diagnosis and clinicopathologic correlation. Am J Surg Pathol. 2000;24(6):797–806.
45. Baergen RN, Warren CD, Isacson C, Ellenson LH. Early uterine serous carcinoma: clonal origin of extrauterine disease. Int J Gynecol Pathol. 2001;20(3):214–9.
46. Pathiraja P, Dhar S, Haldar K. Serous endometrial intraepithelial carcinoma: a case series and literature review. Cancer Manag Res. 2013;5:117–22.
47. Sherman ME, Bur ME, Kurman RJ. p53 in endometrial cancer and its putative precursors: evidence for diverse pathways of tumorigenesis. Hum Pathol. 1995;26(11):1268–74.
48. Temko D, Van Gool IC, Rayner E, Glaire M, Makino S, Brown M, Chegwidden L, Palles C, Depreeuw J, Beggs A, Stathopoulou C. Somatic POLE exonuclease domain mutations are early events in sporadic endometrial and colorectal carcinogenesis, determining driver mutational landscape, clonal neoantigen burden and immune response. J Pathol. 2018;245(3):283–96.

49. Byron SA, Gartside M, Powell MA, Wellens CL, Gao F, Mutch DG, Goodfellow PJ, Pollock PM. FGFR2 point mutations in 466 endometrioid endometrial tumors: relationship with MSI, KRAS, PIK3CA, CTNNB1 mutations and clinicopathological features. PLoS One. 2012;7(2):e30801.
50. Urick ME, Rudd ML, Godwin AK, Sgroi D, Merino M, Bell DW. PIK3R1 (p85α) is somatically mutated at high frequency in primary endometrial cancer. Cancer Res. 2011;71(12):4061–7.
51. Dou Y, Kawaler EA, Zhou DC, Gritsenko MA, Huang C, Blumenberg L, Karpova A, Petyuk VA, Savage SR, Satpathy S, Liu W. Proteogenomic characterization of endometrial carcinoma. Cell. 2020;180(4):729–48.
52. Buza N. HER2 testing in endometrial serous carcinoma: time for standardized pathology practice to meet the clinical demand. Arch Pathol Lab Med. 2021;145(6):687–91.
53. de Jonge MM, Auguste A, van Wijk LM, Schouten PC, Meijers M, Ter Haar NT, Smit VT, Nout RA, Glaire MA, Church DN, Vrieling H. Frequent homologous recombination deficiency in high-grade endometrial Carcinomas homologous recombination deficiency in endometrial cancer. Clin Cancer Res. 2019;25(3):1087–97.
54. Chan JK, Cheung MK, Huh WK, Osann K, Husain A, Teng NN, Kapp DS. Therapeutic role of lymph node resection in endometrioid corpus cancer: a study of 12,333 patients. Cancer. 2006;107(8):1823–30.
55. Todo Y, Kato H, Kaneuchi M, Watari H, Takeda M, Sakuragi N. Survival effect of Para-aortic lymphadenectomy in endometrial cancer (SEPAL study): a retrospective cohort analysis. Lancet. 2010;375(9721):1165–72.
56. Chargari C, Deutsch E, Blanchard P, Gouy S, Martelli H, Guérin F, Dumas I, Bossi A, Morice P, Viswanathan AN, Haie-Meder C. Brachytherapy: an overview for clinicians. CA Cancer J Clin. 2019;69(5):386–401.
57. Miller DS, Filiaci VL, Mannel RS, Cohn DE, Matsumoto T, Tewari KS, DiSilvestro P, Pearl ML, Argenta PA, Powell MA, Zweizig SL. Carboplatin and paclitaxel for advanced endometrial cancer: final overall survival and adverse event analysis of a phase III trial (NRG Oncology/GOG0209). J Clin Oncol. 2020;38(33):3841.
58. Taylor MH, Lee CH, Makker V, Rasco D, Dutcus CE, Wu J, Stepan DE, Shumaker RC, Motzer RJ. Phase IB/II trial of lenvatinib plus pembrolizumab in patients with advanced renal cell carcinoma, endometrial cancer, and other selected advanced solid tumors. J Clin Oncol. 2020;38(11):1154.
59. Makker V, Colombo N, Casado Herráez A, Santin AD, Colomba E, Miller DS, Fujiwara K, Pignata S, Baron-Hay S, Ray-Coquard I, Shapira-Frommer R. Lenvatinib plus pembrolizumab for advanced endometrial cancer. N Engl J Med. 2022;386(5):437–48.
60. O'Malley DM, Bariani GM, Cassier PA, Marabelle A, Hansen AR, De Jesus AA, Miller WH, Safra T, Italiano A, Mileshkin L, Xu L. Pembrolizumab in patients with microsatellite instability–high advanced endometrial cancer: results from the KEYNOTE-158 study. J Clin Oncol. 2022;40(7):752–61.
61. Oaknin A, Tinker AV, Gilbert L, Samouëlian V, Mathews C, Brown J, Barretina-Ginesta MP, Moreno V, Gravina A, Abdeddaim C, Banerjee S. Clinical activity and safety of the anti–programmed death 1 monoclonal antibody dostarlimab for patients with recurrent or advanced mismatch repair–deficient endometrial cancer: a nonrandomized phase 1 clinical trial. JAMA Oncol. 2020;6(11):1766–72.

Cervical Cancer

13

Sai Charitha Mullaguri, Sandhya Annamaneni,
Anvesh Karthik Yalavarthy, Satya Dattatreya Palanki,
and Rama Krishna Kancha

13.1 Introduction

Epidemiology: In the year 2020, cervical cancer or the cancer of cervix uteri ranks seventh in global incidence of all cancers with 6,04,127 new cases accounting to 3.1% and ninth in mortality with 3,41,831 deaths accounting to 3.4% [1]. In females, it is the fourth among cancers in incidence (6.5%) and mortality (7.7%) [1]. The incidence and mortality rates were very high in south central Asia (1,48,128 new cases and 91,985 deaths) and eastern Asia (1,29,567 new cases and 66,436 deaths) followed by south eastern Asia (68,623 new cases and 38,530 deaths) and eastern Africa (54,560 new cases and 36,497 deaths). In European countries, 58,200 new diagnoses and 26,000 deaths with incidence and mortality rates of 3% each were observed [2]. The 5-year survival rate is generally based on the cancer stage at which the patient is diagnosed; the highest rate (92%) was in patients diagnosed with stage I localized cancer and the lowest (17%) was in patients with stage IV cancer [3]. The 5-year survival rates for localized, regional metastatic, and distant metastatic stages of cancer were 92%, 57%, and 19%, respectively in white women, and 87%, 49%, and 11%, respectively in black women [3]. In United States, the median age of cervical cancer diagnosis is 47 years [4]. The delayed age of diagnosis is largely due to lack of screening, poor awareness, and poor diagnostic measures in many countries. Further, lack of possible effective treatments for recurrent and/or

S. C. Mullaguri · R. K. Kancha (✉)
Molecular Medicine and Therapeutics Laboratory, CPMB, Osmania University,
Hyderabad, India
e-mail: ramakancha@osmania.ac.in

S. Annamaneni
Department of Genetics, Osmania University, Hyderabad, India

A. K. Yalavarthy · S. D. Palanki (✉)
Renovo Soumya Cancer Centre, Hyderabad, India

R. K. Kancha (ed.), *Biomedical Aspects of Solid Cancers*,
https://doi.org/10.1007/978-981-97-1802-3_13

metastatic cervical cancers resulted in still or reduced survival rates [5]. Among children and adolescents in the age group of 0–18 years in United States, the incidence of cervical cancer was observed to be 3.9% [6].

Risk Factors: Major risk factors include human papilloma virus (HPV) infection, cervix dysplasia, smoking, early age of sexual intercourse, multiple partners, and continuous use of oral contraceptives [7]. An analysis of 78 studies that included 1,57,879 women concluded that about 10.4% women with normal cervical cytology are infected with the HPV [8]. About 10% of patients with HPV develop precancerous lesions, which later develop into cervical cancer [9]. An analysis of eleven studies that included 1918 cervical cancer patients revealed that about 90.7% of cervical cancers were developed due to HPV infection [10]. Among various HPV types, 16, 18, and 45 are observed to be most prevalent and high-risk variants across the world [11, 12]. Further, a meta-analysis of 23 epidemiological studies revealed that the smokers are at a greater risk of developing squamous cell carcinoma than adenocarcinoma [13].

Diagnosis and Screening: The most common screening method is papanicolaou cytology (pap) smear test [7]. Colposcopy is usually done in patients with abnormal pap test results [14]. Pelvic examination must be carried out in women with visible lesions upon colposcopy [14]. mRNA testing of *E6* and *E7* oncogenes of HPV can act as a predictive marker for detecting cervical carcinoma [15]. Further, mRNA testing of high-risk HPV types in women with normal cervical cytology resulted in early detection of risk of cervical lesions that can lead to cancer [16].

13.2 Classification

Two different classifications of cervical cancer were made based on (i) histology and (ii) staging. (i) Based on histological evaluation of cervical biopsy, cervical cancer is classified into (a) squamous cell carcinoma (SCC), which accounts to 70% of cervical carcinomas (Fig. 13.1) [17, 18]. (b) Adenocarcinoma (AC), which accounts to 25% of all cervical cancer cases (Fig. 13.1) [17, 18]. (c) Adenosquamous, a mixed cancer type with tumor cells of both adenocarcinoma and squamous cell carcinoma accounts to 3% of total cervical cancer patients (Fig. 13.1) [7]. Additional subtypes of cervical cancer include neuroendocrine carcinoma [19], clear cell carcinoma, and gastric-type adenocarcinoma, which together constitute less than 2% of all cervical carcinomas (Fig. 13.1) [7]. (ii) Based on the FIGO staging, cervical cancer is mainly divided into four stages [9, 20]. Stages IA and IB refers to invasive carcinomas with maximum depth of invasion of less than 5 mm and greater than or equal to 5 mm, respectively [20]. Further, stages IA1 and IA2 refer to measured

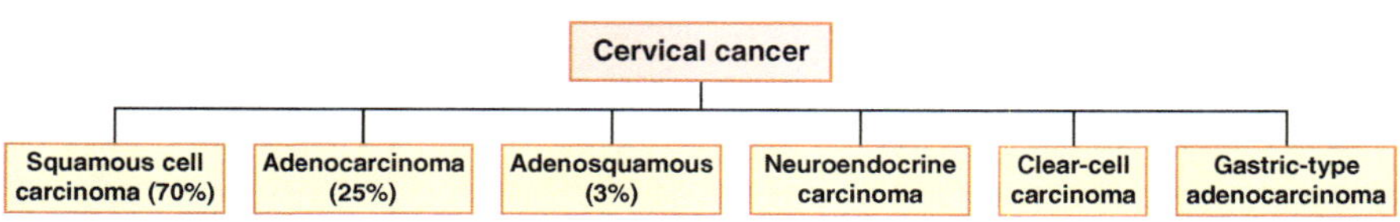

Fig. 13.1 Histological classification of cervical cancer

depth of stromal invasion of less than 3 mm, and in between 3 mm and 5 mm, respectively [20]. Stages IB1, IB2, and IB3 refers to a measured depth of invasion of ≥5 mm and <2 cm in stage IB1, ≥2 cm and <4 cm in stage IB2, and ≥4 cm in stage IB3 [20]. In stage II, tumor invasion occurs into upper two-thirds of vagina with an invasion depth of <4 cm (stage IIA1) and ≥4 cm (stage IIA2) [20]. Stage III describes carcinoma extension into lower one-third of vagina, pelvic wall, pelvic lymph nodes, and para-aortic lymph nodes, which are described as stage IIIA, IIIB, IIIC1, and IIIC2, respectively [20]. In stage IV, the carcinoma has metastasized to adjacent pelvic organs (stage IVA) and to distant organs (stage IVB) [20].

13.3 Pathophysiology

Anatomy: The cervix is a sphincter-shaped region of the uterus that connects uterus to the vagina. It consists of folds and crypts, and acts as a barrier separating the uterus resulting in the protection of embryo when implanted. The cervical rings are the most prominent structures that are supported by a thick layer of smooth muscle fibers, which allow cervix to contract or relax during the childbirth. The lining of the cervix is a thick layer of mucosa containing secretory cells that secrete cervical mucus. The amount and viscosity of cervical mucus depend on the predominance of estrogen or progesterone during the menstrual cycle. During embryonic development, cervix arises from the two paramesonephric ducts, also called as Mullerian ducts. These two ducts fuse to form urogenital tract that develops into vagina, cervix, and uterus [21]. Initially, genital ducts namely mesonephric ducts (also called as Wolffian ducts) and paramesonephric ducts are present in the embryo. The absence of *SRY* gene and the anti-Mullerian hormone in females results in further differentiation of Mullerian ducts and no development of Wolffian ducts [22].

The cervix is mainly divided into different regions. Ectocervix is mainly made up of multiple layers of stratified nonkeratinizing squamous epithelium. The squamous epithelium mainly consists of a basement membrane, parabasal layer, intermediate and superficial cell layers (Fig. 13.2). The basement membrane is made up of a layer of basal cells with large nuclei, which further divide and mature to form parabasal cells. The parabasal cells further divide and differentiate into polygonal cells with small nuclei that form the intermediate cell layer. The polygonal cells further mature to form cells of superficial layer. The intermediate and superficial layers contain large amounts of glycogen [23]. Endocervix is the innermost mucosa lining of the cervix that forms the endocervical canal. The endocervical canal is mainly made up of a single layer of columnar epithelial cells. These lining of cells merge with the endometrial epithelium on one end and with the squamous cells of the ectocervix on the other end. The junction at which the squamous cells of ectocervix and columnar cells of endocervix merge is called as squamocolumnar junction or transformation zone and is usually present near the external cervical orifice (Fig. 13.2). Stroma is a dense fibromuscular tissue through which the blood, lymphatic, and nerve supply take place (Fig. 13.2). Blood supply to the cervix is carried out through the internal iliac arteries of uterine artery.

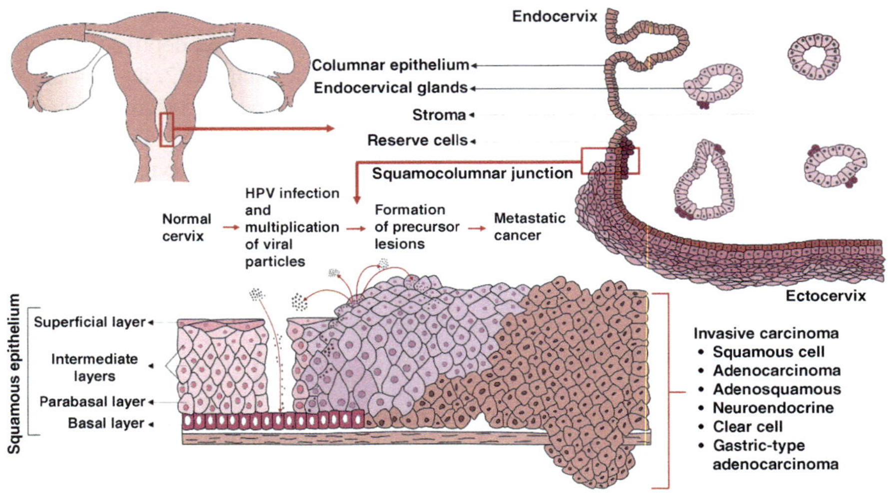

Fig. 13.2 Pathophysiology of cervical cancer. The anatomy of cervix depicting different squamous epithelial layers of ectocervix that develop into histological subtypes of cervical cancer

Cell of Origin: The rate of development of abnormal cells in the squamocolumnar junction is relatively high (Fig. 13.2). The squamous cells of ectocervix are repeatedly destroyed due to vaginal acidity and there is a need to replenish these cells by the columnar cells of the endocervix. The columnar epithelium when exposed to the vaginal acidity results in the formation of subcolumnar epithelial cells called as the reserve cells. These cells multiply and differentiate into a single layer of immature metaplastic squamous cells, which further differentiate into atypical or dysplastic squamous epithelium upon infection with oncogenic HPV types or into normal squamous epithelium that contains glycogen. Chronic HPV infection may result in the formation of precursor lesions called as cervical intraepithelial neoplasia (CINs) and squamous intraepithelial lesions (SILs) [24]. The CINs are further classified into CIN1 (small lesions indicative of HPV infection), CIN2 (heterogenous group of lesions), and CIN3 (high-grade lesions) [25]. SILs are classified into low- and high-grade SILs. CIN1 and low-grade SIL are relatively equal, and high-grade SIL, CIN2, and CIN3 are similar [26]. The HPV usually attacks the basal cells of ectocervix and the replication of HPV occurs in the parabasal differentiating cells of ectocervix (Fig. 13.2) [27]. But these parabasal cells undergo maturation and senescence, and don't have replicative machinery required for the HPV survival. The HPV encodes E6 and E7 proteins that promote proliferation of cells and prevent apoptosis [28]. This results in hundreds to thousands of HPV in a single cell that further infects healthy cells (Fig. 13.2).

Genetics: Hereditary cervical cancers are very rare and associated known familial risk factors include DICER1 syndrome and Peutz-Jeghers syndrome (PJS). *DICER1* gene variations are associated with increased risk for cervical embryonal rhabdomyosarcoma (ERMS) and other sarcomas of the cervix while *STK11* mutations account for 1–3% of cervical adenocarcinomas [29, 30]. The *KRAS*, *ARID1A*, and *PTEN* gene mutations were highly frequent in HPV-negative cervical cancer while HPV-positive cancer possesses several genomic aberrations, mainly in PI3K/MAPK and TGF-beta signaling pathways [31]. Recent genomic studies on 178 primary cervical tumors discovered frequent mutations in *BCAR4* and variants in *MED1*, *ERBB3*, *CASP8*, *HLA-A*, and *TGFBR2* genes [31].

The E6 of HPV interacts with TP53 [32] and E7 interacts with RB1, RBL1, and RBL2 [33, 34] resulting in the degradation of these proteins via ubiquitination that leads to abnormal growth of cells. High-risk E6 decreases the surface expression of E-cadherin by epithelial cells, thereby reducing both the contact between keratinocytes and Langerhans cells (intraepithelial dendritic cells), and the ability to present HPV antigens [35]. *TP53* with a missense polymorphism, R72P was observed to have less binding capacity with E6 of HPV when compared to the wild-type TP53 [36]. A study of 7146 SNPs in 305 genes revealed that SNPs in *FANCA*, *EXO1*, *CYBA*, *XRCC1*, *IRF3*, and *TLR2* were significantly associated with the development of CIN3 and cervical carcinoma [37]. Missense SNPs in *FANCA* (T266A, G501S, and G809A) increase the risk of developing cervical carcinoma from CIN3 while missense SNPs in *IRF3* (S427T) and *XRCC1* (Q399R) were associated with the persistence of HPV infection [37].

Mutation analysis of 79 SCC and 24 AC samples revealed significant frequencies of mutations in *EP300* (16%), *FBXW7* (15%), *PIK3CA* (14%), inactivating mutations in *HLA-B* (9%), *TP53* (9%), E322K mutation in *MAPK1* (8%), *PTEN* (6%), *ERBB2* (5%), *NFE2L2* (4%), and *STK11* (4%) in SCC, and *PIK3CA* (16%), *ELF3* (13%), *KRAS* (8%), and *CBFB* (8%) in AC [38]. Molecular characterization of 228 cervical cancer samples revealed that (i) high frequencies of somatic copy number alterations (SCNAs) were observed in *TERC* and *MECOM* (78%), *TP63* (77%), *MYC* and *PVT1* (41%), *CD274* and *PDCD1LG2* (21%), *BCAR4* (20%), *KLF5* (18%), *EGFR* (17%), *YAP1* and *BIRC2/3* (17%), and *ERBB2* (17%), and (ii) deletions were observed in *FAT1* (36%), *TGFBR2* (36%), *PTEN* (31%), and *SMAD4* (28%) genes [31]. Activating mutations (E542K and E545K) in the helical domain of *PIK3CA* [31] gained through mutagenesis by APOBEC group of cytidine deaminases revealed that the mutagenesis by APOBECs is the primary source of mutations in cervical cancers [39]. Mesothelin (MSLN), a cell-surface druggable glycoprotein is significantly expressed in non-SCC and is associated with poor overall survival (OS) [40]. Loss of HMGCS1, an enzyme in cholesterol metabolism was found to sensitize cervical cancer cells to radiation [41]. Thus, HMGCS1 can be targeted to improve the efficacy of radiotherapy [41].

13.4 Treatment

Cervical cancer can be prevented by HPV vaccination. In a phase 3 trial in 12,167 women (15–26 years of age) who were not infected previously with HPV, the quadrivalent vaccine has reduced the risk of high-grade SILs [42]. Another population-based study in Swedish women in the age group of 10–30 years revealed that the

HPV vaccination (quadrivalent) was associated with the reduced risk of invasive cervical cancer [43]. The surgical interventions to treat cervical cancer include conization in order to preserve fertility or extra fascial hysterectomy in patients with stage IA1 [44], and radical hysterectomy and bilateral pelvic lymphadenectomy in patients with node metastasis [45, 46]. Patients who had undergone open abdominal radical hysterectomy (OARH) had better disease-free survival (DFS) of 96.5% when compared to patients who had undergone minimally invasive radical hysterectomy (MIRH) (DFS: 86%) [47]. In early-stage high-risk cervical cancer, the 4-year PFS (progression-free survival) and OS were significantly higher (PFS: 80%; OS: 81%) in patients receiving concurrent chemotherapy along with pelvic radiation therapy (PRT) than in PRT alone group (PFS: 63%; OS: 71%) [48]. The progression of cervical cancer correlated with the expression of HOTAIR and resulted in poor prognosis [49]. In patients treated with chemoradiation and brachytherapy, increased levels of caspase-8 and CDK9 levels correlated with improved survival whereas elevated levels of pCDK9 predicted poor survival [50].

In a phase 3 trial of pembrolizumab, the PFS and OS at 24 months were higher in patients treated with pembrolizumab and chemotherapy ± bevacizumab (PFS: 10.4 months; OS: 53%) than in placebo group with chemotherapy ± bevacizumab (PFS: 8.2 months; OS: 41.7%) [51]. Among patients with recurrent cancer, the objective response rate (ORR) and OS were longer in patients treated with cemiplimab (ORR: 16.4%; OS: 12.0 months) when compared to patients receiving chemotherapy (ORR: 6.3%; OS: 8.5 months) [52]. Tisotumab vedotin had an ORR of 24% in patients with previously treated recurrent or metastatic cancer [53]. In patients with any of the stage IB to stage IV cervical cancer, the PFS and OS were high in statin-therapy group (PFS and OS: 92.9%) when compared to the control group (PFS: 58.3%; OS: 70.8%) [54]. An analysis of 31 studies in women with HIV as well as SIL or CIN concluded that the early initiation of antiretroviral therapy reduced the progression of SIL and CIN, and invasive cervical cancer incidence [55]. Propofol, an intravenous anesthetic was observed to have in vitro antitumor activity against cervical cancer [56]. Decitabine, a nucleic acid synthesis inhibitor was shown to have immunomodulating and chemosensitizing effects in cervical cancer in vitro [57].

13.5 Conclusion

The growing health burden due to rising cervical cancer incidence and mortality is a major concern globally, especially in Asian countries. Unlike many cancers, cervical cancers are largely preventable by systemic mandatory screening of women aged above 20 years for high-risk subtypes of HPV, diagnosis of CINs, and HPV vaccination programs. Treatment options for early detected patients are many resulting in remarkable improvement in survival rates and decreased mortality. Emerging treatment strategies include immunotherapy address metastatic, chemo/radio-resistant, and recurrent cervical cancer. Genomic studies have revealed potential therapeutic/actionable drug targets and offer new hope in the treatment of cervical cancer.

References

1. Sung H, Ferlay J, Siegel RL, Laversanne M, Soerjomataram I, Jemal A, Bray F. Global cancer statistics 2020: GLOBOCAN estimates of incidence and mortality worldwide for 36 cancers in 185 countries. CA Cancer J Clin. 2021;71(3):209–49.
2. Dyba T, Randi G, Bray F, Martos C, Giusti F, Nicholson N, Gavin A, Flego M, Neamtiu L, Dimitrova N, Carvalho RN. The European cancer burden in 2020: incidence and mortality estimates for 40 countries and 25 major cancers. Eur J Cancer. 2021;157:308–47.
3. Siegel RL, Miller KD, Jemal A. Cancer statistics, 2020. CA Cancer J Clin. 2020 Jan;70(1):7–30.
4. Cohen PA, Jhingran A, Oaknin A, Denny L. Cervical cancer. Lancet. 2019;393(10167):169–82.
5. Jemal A, Ward EM, Johnson CJ, Cronin KA, Ma J, Ryerson AB, Mariotto A, Lake AJ, Wilson R, Sherman RL, Anderson RN. Annual report to the nation on the status of cancer, 1975–2014, featuring survival. JNCI J Natl Cancer Inst. 2017;109(9):djx030.
6. Wohlmuth C, Wohlmuth-Wieser I. Gynecologic malignancies in children and adolescents: how common is the uncommon? J Clin Med. 2021;10(4):722.
7. Johnson CA, James D, Marzan A, Armaos M. Cervical cancer: an overview of pathophysiology and management. Sem Oncol Nurs. 2019;35(2):166–74.
8. De Sanjosé S, Diaz M, Castellsagué X, Clifford G, Bruni L, Muñoz N, Bosch FX. Worldwide prevalence and genotype distribution of cervical human papillomavirus DNA in women with normal cytology: a meta-analysis. Lancet Infect Dis. 2007;7(7):453–9.
9. Bhatla N, Aoki D, Sharma DN, Sankaranarayanan R. Cancer of the cervix uteri. Int J Gynecol Obstet. 2018;143:22–36.
10. Muñoz N, Bosch FX, De Sanjosé S, Herrero R, Castellsagué X, Shah KV, Snijders PJ, Meijer CJ. Epidemiologic classification of human papillomavirus types associated with cervical cancer. N Engl J Med. 2003;348(6):518–27.
11. Li N, Franceschi S, Howell-Jones R, Snijders PJ, Clifford GM. Human papillomavirus type distribution in 30,848 invasive cervical cancers worldwide: variation by geographical region, histological type and year of publication. Int J Cancer. 2011;128(4):927–35.
12. Guan P, Howell-Jones R, Li N, Bruni L, De Sanjosé S, Franceschi S, Clifford GM. Human papillomavirus types in 115,789 HPV-positive women: a meta-analysis from cervical infection to cancer. Int J Cancer. 2012;131(10):2349–59.
13. International Collaboration of Epidemiological Studies of Cervical Cancer. Carcinoma of the cervix and tobacco smoking: collaborative reanalysis of individual data on 13,541 women with carcinoma of the cervix and 23,017 women without carcinoma of the cervix from 23 epidemiological studies. Int J Cancer. 2006;118(6):1481–95.
14. Wuerthner BA, Avila-Wallace M. Cervical cancer: screening, management, and prevention. Nurse Pract. 2016;41(9):18–23.
15. Lie AK, Kristensen G. Human papillomavirus E6/E7 mRNA testing as a predictive marker for cervical carcinoma. Expert Rev Mol Diagn. 2008;8(4):405–15.
16. Al-Shibli K, Mohammed HA, Maurseth R, Fostervold M, Werner S, Sørbye SW. Impact of HPV mRNA types 16, 18, 45 detection on the risk of CIN3+ in young women with normal cervical cytology. PLoS One. 2022;17(11):e0275858.
17. Ries LA, Melbert D, Krapcho M, Mariotto A, Miller BA, Feuer EJ, Clegg L, Horner MJ, Howlader N, Eisner MP, Reichman M. SEER cancer statistics review, vol. 2004. Bethesda, MD: National Cancer Institute; 1975.
18. Small W Jr, Bacon MA, Bajaj A, Chuang LT, Fisher BJ, Harkenrider MM, Jhingran A, Kitchener HC, Mileshkin LR, Viswanathan AN, Gaffney DK. Cervical cancer: a global health crisis. Cancer. 2017;123(13):2404–12.

19. Salvo G, Frumovitz M, Ramalingam P, Bhosale P. Advanced stage (FIGO IVB) neuroendocrine cervical carcinoma presenter. Int J Gynecol Cancer. 2022;32(11):1469.
20. Saleh M, Virarkar M, Javadi S, Elsherif SB, de Castro FS, Bhosale P. Cervical cancer: 2018 revised international federation of gynecology and obstetrics staging system and the role of imaging. Am J Roentgenol. 2020;214(5):1182–95.
21. Kobayashi A, Behringer RR. Developmental genetics of the female reproductive tract in mammals. Nat Rev Genet. 2003;4(12):969–80.
22. Robbins JB, Broadwell C, Chow LC, Parry JP, Sadowski EA. Müllerian duct anomalies: embryological development, classification, and MRI assessment. J Magn Reson Imaging. 2015;41(1):1–2.
23. Henry JS Jr, Latour JP. Glycogen in the squamous epithelium of the cervix uteri. Am J Obstet Gynecol. 1957;74(3):610–5.
24. Schiffman M, Castle PE, Jeronimo J, Rodriguez AC, Wacholder S. Human papillomavirus and cervical cancer. Lancet. 2007;370(9590):890–907.
25. Rodríguez AC, Schiffman M, Herrero R, Hildesheim A, Bratti C, Sherman ME, Solomon D, Guillén D, Alfaro M, Morales J, Hutchinson M. Longitudinal study of human papillomavirus persistence and cervical intraepithelial neoplasia grade 2/3: critical role of duration of infection. J Natl Cancer Inst. 2010;102(5):315–24.
26. Alrajjal A, Pansare V, Choudhury MS, Khan MY, Shidham VB. Squamous intraepithelial lesions (SIL: LSIL, HSIL, ASCUS, ASC-H, LSIL-H) of uterine cervix and bethesda system. Cytojournal. 2021;18.
27. Woodman CB, Collins SI, Young LS. The natural history of cervical HPV infection: unresolved issues. Nat Rev Cancer. 2007;7(1):11–22.
28. Ghittoni R, Accardi R, Hasan U, Gheit T, Sylla B, Tommasino M. The biological properties of E6 and E7 oncoproteins from human papillomaviruses. Virus Genes. 2010;40:1–3.
29. Hirose S, Murakami N, Takahashi K, Kuno I, Takayanagi D, Asami Y, Matsuda M, Shimada Y, Yamano S, Sunami K, Yoshida K. Genomic alterations in STK11 can predict clinical outcomes in cervical cancer patients. Gynecol Oncol. 2020;156(1):203–10.
30. Robertson JC, Jorcyk CL, Oxford JT. DICER1 syndrome: DICER1 mutations in rare cancers. Cancers. 2018;10(5):143.
31. Cancer Genome Atlas Research Network. Integrated genomic and molecular characterization of cervical cancer. Nature. 2017;543(7645):378.
32. Tommasino M, Accardi R, Caldeira S, Dong W, Malanchi I, Smet A, Zehbe I. The role of TP53 in cervical carcinogenesis. Hum Mutat. 2003;21(3):307–12.
33. Boyer SN, Wazer DE, Band V. E7 protein of human papilloma virus-16 induces degradation of retinoblastoma protein through the ubiquitin-proteasome pathway. Cancer Res. 1996;56(20):4620–4.
34. MuÈnger K, Basile JR, Duensing S, Eichten A, Gonzalez SL, Grace M, Zacny VL. Biological activities and molecular targets of the human papillomavirus E7 oncoprotein. Oncogene. 2001;20(54):7888–98.
35. Hubert P, Caberg JH, Gilles C, Bousarghin L, Franzen-Detrooz E, Boniver J, Delvenne P. E-cadherin-dependent adhesion of dendritic and Langerhans cells to keratinocytes is defective in cervical human papillomavirus-associated (pre) neoplastic lesions. J Pathol. 2005;206(3):346–55.
36. Storey A, Thomas M, Kalita A, Harwood C, Gardiol D, Mantovani F, Breuer J, Leigh IM, Matlashewski G, Banks L. Role of a p53 polymorphism in the development of human papilloma-virus-associated cancer. Nature. 1998;393(6682):229–34.
37. Wang SS, Bratti MC, Rodríguez AC, Herrero R, Burk RD, Porras C, González P, Sherman ME, Wacholder S, Lan ZE, Schiffman M. Common variants in immune and DNA repair genes and risk for human papillomavirus persistence and progression to cervical cancer. J Infect Dis. 2009;199(1):20–30.
38. Ojesina AI, Lichtenstein L, Freeman SS, Pedamallu CS, Imaz-Rosshandler I, Pugh TJ, Cherniack AD, Ambrogio L, Cibulskis K, Bertelsen B, Romero-Cordoba S. Landscape of genomic alterations in cervical carcinomas. Nature. 2014;506(7488):371–5.

39. Revathidevi S, Murugan AK, Nakaoka H, Inoue I, Munirajan AK. APOBEC: a molecular driver in cervical cancer pathogenesis. Cancer Lett. 2021;496:104–16.
40. Takamizawa S, Yazaki S, Kojima Y, Yoshida H, Kitadai R, Nishikawa T, Shimoi T, Sudo K, Okuma HS, Tanioka M, Noguchi E. High mesothelin expression is correlated with non-squamous cell histology and poor survival in cervical cancer: a retrospective study. BMC Cancer. 2022;22(1):1–9.
41. Zhang X, Sun C, Wan J, Zhang X, Jia Y, Zhou C. Compartmentalized activities of HMGCS1 control cervical cancer radiosensitivity. Cell Signal. 2023;101:110507.
42. Future II Study Group. Quadrivalent vaccine against human papillomavirus to prevent high-grade cervical lesions. N Engl J Med. 2007;356(19):1915–27.
43. Lei J, Ploner A, Elfström KM, Wang J, Roth A, Fang F, Sundström K, Dillner J, Sparén P. HPV vaccination and the risk of invasive cervical cancer. N Engl J Med. 2020;383(14):1340–8.
44. National Comprehensive Cancer Network. NCCN clinical practice guidelines in oncology: hepatobiliary cancers. Fort Washington: National Comprehensive Cancer Network; 2013.
45. Lee YN, Wang KL, Lin MH, Liu CH, Wang KG, Lan CC, Chuang JT, Chen AC, Wu CC. Radical hysterectomy with pelvic lymph node dissection for treatment of cervical cancer: a clinical review of 954 cases. Gynecol Oncol. 1989;32(2):135–42.
46. Schmeler KM, Frumovitz M, Ramirez PT. Conservative management of early stage cervical cancer: is there a role for less radical surgery? Gynecol Oncol. 2011;120(3):321–5.
47. Ramirez PT, Frumovitz M, Pareja R, Lopez A, Vieira M, Ribeiro R, Buda A, Yan X, Shuzhong Y, Chetty N, Isla D. Minimally invasive versus abdominal radical hysterectomy for cervical cancer. N Engl J Med. 2018;379(20):1895–904.
48. Peters WA III, Liu PY, Barrett RJ, Stock RJ, Monk BJ, Berek JS, Souhami L, Grigsby P, Gordon W Jr, Alberts DS. Concurrent chemotherapy and pelvic radiation therapy compared with pelvic radiation therapy alone as adjuvant therapy after radical surgery in high-risk early-stage cancer of the cervix. Obstet Gynecol Surv. 2000;55(8):491–2.
49. Huang L, Liao LM, Liu AW, Wu JB, Cheng XL, Lin JX, Zheng M. Overexpression of long noncoding RNA HOTAIR predicts a poor prognosis in patients with cervical cancer. Arch Gynecol Obstet. 2014;290:717–23.
50. Fleischmann M, Mandal R, Kostova I, Raab M, Sanhaji M, Hehlgans S, Diefenhardt M, Rödel C, Fokas E, Strebhardt K, Rödel F. Prognostic impact of Caspase-8, CDK9 and Phospho-CDK9 (Thr 186) expression in patients with uterine cervical cancer treated with definitive chemoradiation and brachytherapy. Cancers. 2022;14(22):5500.
51. Colombo N, Dubot C, Lorusso D, Caceres MV, Hasegawa K, Shapira-Frommer R, Tewari KS, Salman P, Hoyos Usta E, Yañez E, Gümüş M. Pembrolizumab for persistent, recurrent, or metastatic cervical cancer. N Engl J Med. 2021;385(20):1856–67.
52. Tewari KS, Monk BJ, Vergote I, Miller A, de Melo AC, Kim HS, Kim YM, Lisyanskaya A, Samouëlian V, Lorusso D, Damian F. Survival with cemiplimab in recurrent cervical cancer. N Engl J Med. 2022;386(6):544–55.
53. Coleman RL, Lorusso D, Gennigens C, González-Martín A, Randall L, Cibula D, Lund B, Woelber L, Pignata S, Forget F, Redondo A. Efficacy and safety of tisotumab vedotin in previously treated recurrent or metastatic cervical cancer (innovaTV 204/GOG-3023/ENGOT-cx6): a multicentre, open-label, single-arm, phase 2 study. Lancet Oncol. 2021;22(5):609–19.
54. Song MK, Shin BS, Ha CS, Park WY. Would lipophilic statin therapy as a prognostic factor improve survival in patients with uterine cervical cancer? Int J Gynecol Cancer. 2017;27(7):1431–7.
55. Kelly H, Weiss HA, Benavente Y, de Sanjose S, Mayaud P, Qiao YL, Feng RM, DeVuyst H, Tenet V, Jaquet A, Konopnicki D. Association of antiretroviral therapy with high-risk human papillomavirus, cervical intraepithelial neoplasia, and invasive cervical cancer in women living with HIV: a systematic review and meta-analysis. Lancet HIV. 2018;5(1):e45–58.
56. Sun N, Zhang W, Liu J, Yang X, Chu Q. Propofol inhibits the progression of cervical cancer by regulating HOTAIR/miR-129-5p/RPL14 axis. Onco Targets Ther. 2021;14:551.
57. Alexandraki A, Strati K. Decitabine treatment induces a viral mimicry response in cervical cancer cells and further sensitizes cells to chemotherapy. Int J Mol Sci. 2022;23(22):14042.

Prostate Cancer

14

Mohd Adnan, Himavarshitha Babbur, Sai Sandeep Annamaraju, Abhayananda Behera, Satya Dattatreya Palanki, Anvesh Karthik Yalavarthy, Bindu Madhava Reddy Aramati, and Rama Krishna Kancha

14.1 Introduction

Epidemiology: In the year 2020, the second most diagnosed cancer was prostate cancer with 1,414,259 new cases accounting to 14.1% of all cancer cases and ranked fifth in mortality with 3,75,304 deaths accounting to 6.8% of all cancer-related deaths globally. In more than half of the world, i.e., 112 out of 185 countries, the most diagnosed cancer was prostate cancer [1]. Incidence rates of PCa were three times higher in transitioned countries than in transitioning countries (37.5 cases/100,000 vs. 11.3 cases/100,000, respectively) [1]. However, the mortality rates were less variable: 8.1 deaths/100,000 in transitioned countries vs. 5.9 deaths/100,000 in transitioning countries [1, 2]. The highest age-standardized incidence rate (ASIR) per a population of 100,000 was found in Northern Europe with 83.4 cases followed by Western Europe with 77.6 cases, the Caribbean with 75.8 cases, Australia/New Zealand with 75.8 cases, Northern America with 73 cases, and Southern Africa with 65.9 cases while the lowest ASIR was found in South Central Asia with 6.3 cases, South-Eastern Asia with 13.5 cases, and Northern Africa with 16.6 cases [1].

The highest all-age-mortality ASIR per a population of 100,000 was found in the Caribbean (28 deaths), middle Africa (25 deaths), and Southern Africa (22 deaths)

M. Adnan · H. Babbur · S. S. Annamaraju · R. K. Kancha (✉)
Molecular Medicine and Therapeutics Laboratory, CPMB, Osmania University, Hyderabad, India
e-mail: ramakancha@osmania.ac.in

A. Behera · B. M. R. Aramati
Department of Animal Biotechnology, School of Life Sciences, University of Hyderabad, Hyderabad, India

S. D. Palanki · A. K. Yalavarthy
Renovo Soumya Cancer Centre, Hyderabad, India

R. K. Kancha (ed.), *Biomedical Aspects of Solid Cancers*,
https://doi.org/10.1007/978-981-97-1802-3_14

while South-Central Asia (3.1 deaths), Eastern Asia (4.7 deaths), and South-Eastern Asia (5.4 deaths) had the lowest death rates [2]. The highest incidence and mortality rates were recorded in Germany (Europe) and Zimbabwe (Africa) [2]. PCa was generally observed in men aged more than 65 years [3]. The overall survival (OS) was found to be 6.39 years in men who were diagnosed at the time of metastases, while patients who had metastases after 6 months of developing castration resistance had an OS of 19.07 years [4]. Globally, among all ages, 5-year prevalence was 126 cases per 100,000 men and the highest incidence was observed in Northern America (735 cases per 100,000) [2]. For all stages combined, the 5-year survival rate was higher in white men as compared to black or Hispanic men [5]. But, the 5-year survival rate was higher in black men as compared to white men for distant stage prostate cancer [5].

Risk Factors: The most common risk factors associated with development of PCa are age, family history, germline mutations (especially *BRCA1* and *BRCA2*), race/ethnicity, and environmental hazards [6]. About 20% of men with PCa (up to an age of 72 years) have a familial history of prostate cancer [6]. Age and other human malignancies are significant risk factors, the incidence peaking between the ages 65 and 75 years. The risk of PCa is nearly 26% in men above the age of 75 years [7]. Despite low incidence, newer data suggest that PCa in younger men may be increasing globally. Since the year 1995, the number of PCa diagnoses have relatively doubled at an age of less than 40 years, with most of the increase was observed in men aged between 30 and 4 years; notably, these men were at a high risk of metastatic disease, and they had a higher death rate compared to older men. Ethnicity plays an important role in PCa. African American men exhibited higher incidence of 54.2 cases per 100,000 when compared to other ethnicities, probably related to an association of genetic and/or dietary factors [7]. Chromosome 8q24 has been reported in PCa cases and was expressed highly in African American men [7]. The risk of PCa increases by 2.5-fold if a person has one first-degree relative with PCa who is younger than 60 years and the risk rises by 5.7-fold if the person has two or more first-degree relatives with PCa who are younger than 60 years [8]. The risk of PCa may further increase with a family history or cancers such as colorectal cancer, ovarian cancer, breast cancer diagnosed at an age less than 50 years, pancreatic cancer, and melanoma, which are likely to be heritable. Germline mutations in *BRCA2* and *ATM* correlate to increased risk of PCa and more aggressive disease features in men.

Screening and Diagnosis: The most common clinical tools for PCa diagnosis were digital rectal exam and test for prostate-specific antigen (PSA) [9–11]. Further tests include transrectal ultrasound (TRUS), multiparametric MRI (mpMRI), dynamic contrast-enhanced magnetic resonance imaging (DCE-MRI), CT or PET/CT scan, and biopsy [9–11]. PSA testing was widely accepted for diagnosing PCa [9, 12–14]. An elevated serum PSA value can also be caused due to benign prostatic hyperplasia, prostatic inflammation/infection, and perianal trauma. Serum PSA above 4.0 ng/mL should validate further tests. Digital rectal examination (DRE) was another method to detect PCa [15, 16]. Imaging tools like transrectal ultrasonography (TRUS) was used to distinguish peripheral zone and central zone cancers [9, 11]. MRI techniques such as mpMRI, DCE-MRI, and diffusion-weighted imaging (DWI) were often used in the diagnosis of PCa and PETCT imaging in conjunction with newer, more sensitive radionuclides may be of value in assessing pelvic lymph node involvement such as GA-68 PSMA-11 [11].

Biomarkers: Biomarkers for the diagnosis and prognosis of PCa which were mostly tissue, blood, and urine based, became successful due to advancements in genomic and proteomic technologies [17]. PSA is a blood-based biomarker that is mostly used for the early detection of PCa [17]. The prostate gland epithelial cells produce PSA, which is a kallikrein-related serine protease [18]. α-Methylacyl coenzyme A racemase (AMACR) was a tissue-based biomarker that was over expressed in PCa and showed 100% specificity and a 97% sensitivity for prostate cancer detection [19]. There are two urine-based biomarkers: prostate cancer antigen 3 (PCA3) is a lncRNA that is highly expressed in more than 95% of primary and metastatic cases [17, 18, 20], and *TMPRSS2-ERG* gene fusions were widely observed in prostate tumors with a specificity of 93% and positive predictive value of 94%; however, this biomarker exhibited a low sensitivity of 37% in urinary sediments [21–23].

14.2 Classification

Different classifications were made based on histological type, Gleason's grading and staging [24–26]. Based on histological types, PCa was classified into adenocarcinoma, neuroendocrine prostate cancer (NEPC), urothelial carcinoma, basal cell carcinoma, lymphoma, and sarcoma (Fig. 14.1) [24]. Adenocarcinoma accounts to more than 95% of all the PCa [24]. Adenocarcinomas include acinar, ductal, mucinous, and signet ring cell carcinomas (Fig. 14.1) [24]. Acinar adenocarcinomas were the most prevalent among these [24]. Nearly 75–85% acinar adenocarcinomas were observed in peripheral zone of prostate while transition zone and central zone account to 10–15% each [24, 27]. Mucinous carcinomas and signet ring cell carcinomas were extremely rare and are aggressive cancers [24]. NEPC were very rare (accounts to <1% of all the PCa's) with an incidence of 35 new cases per 100,000, each year [24, 28, 29]. Based on morphological characteristics, NEPC can be classified into prostatic adenocarcinoma with neuroendocrine differentiation,

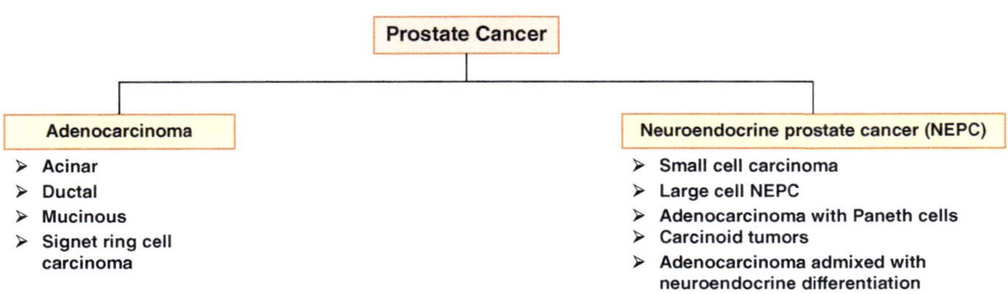

Fig. 14.1 Classification of prostate cancer based on histology

well-differentiated neuroendocrine tumors, small cell and large cell neuroendocrine carcinomas (Fig. 14.1) [30].

Gleason grading was the most crucial prognostic factor to manage PCa [26]. The scoring method was based on PCa cell histology, pattern of growth in the stroma, and differentiation [26]. Five numbers or grades were assigned in the Gleason system that ranges from 1 to 5 depending upon the abnormality of the cells: the grade 1 was assigned to cell type that looks like normal prostate cells while grade 5 was assigned to abnormal cell type that looks very different from normal cells (Fig. 14.2) [25, 29]. The Gleason score was obtained by addition of grades of the two most common cell types within the tumor: grade of the most predominant cell type plus grade of the second most prevalent cell type in the tumor [25, 29]. The score ranges from 2 to 10 [25]. If the tumor had only one histological pattern, then the Gleason score would be 2 $(1 + 1 = 2)$ [25]. If the two most common grades of the cells in the prostate tumor are of grade 2 and grade 4, then the score would be 6 $(2 + 4)$ [25, 31, 32]. A new grade group system is adopted and is based on the Gleason score (GS) and provides more accurate risk stratification. The risk of prostate cancer mortality increases with an increase in the grade group. The 5-year recurrence-free survival rates were 95, 83, 65, 63, and 35%, respectively, for grade group 1, 2, 3, 4, and 5. Tumors are separated into five categories based on the primary and secondary Gleason pattern: Grade 1 with a GS ≤ 6, Grade 2 with GS $3 + 4 = 7$, Grade 3 with GS $4 + 3 = 7$, Grade 4 with GS $= 8$ (including $4 + 4 = 8$, $3 + 5 = 8$, or $5 + 3 = 8$), and Grade 5 with GS 9 to 10 (including $4 + 5$, $5 + 4$, or $5 + 5$).

According to World Health Organization (WHO), prostate tumors were classified into six subtypes (Fig. 14.3). (1) Epithelial tumors: Glandular neoplasms, which are further classified into (1a-1) Acinar adenocarcinomas. (1a-2) Prostatic intraepithelial neoplasia-high grade/high-grade prostatic intraepithelial neoplasia (HGPIN) is a nonobligatory precursor lesion of invasive prostate cancer and refers to the glandular epithelial cell proliferation (Fig. 14.3). (1a-3) intraductal carcinoma is present predominately in periurethral ducts and exhibits similarity with high-grade prostatic intraepithelial neoplasia (HGPIN), but with greater cytological atypia and/

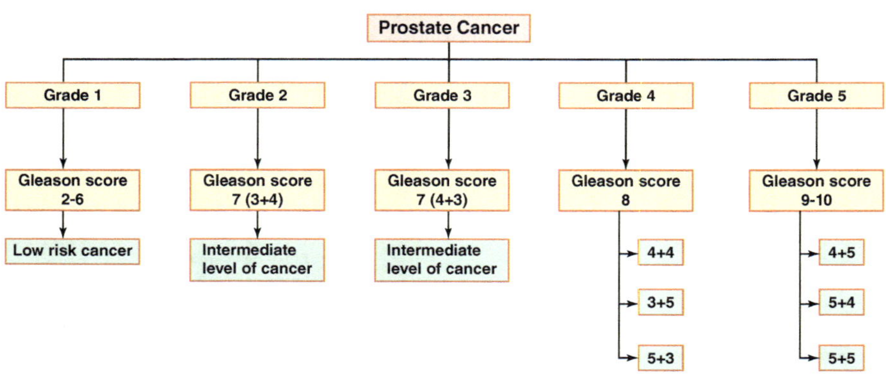

Fig. 14.2 Gleason grading-based classification for prostate cancer

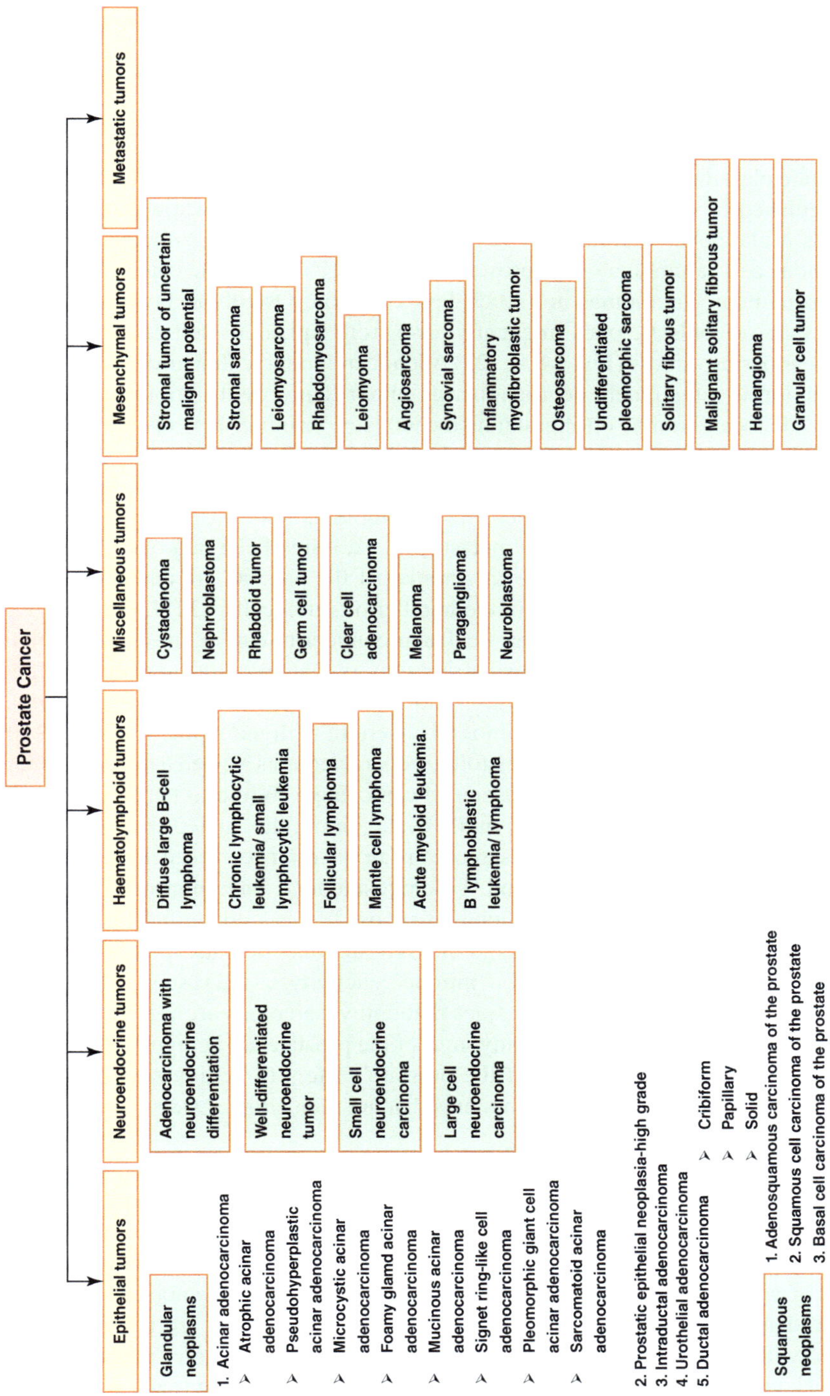

Fig. 14.3 WHO classification for prostate cancer

or enlargement of the glandular architectural atypia; this condition is classed as carcinoma in situ. (1a-4) Ductal adenocarcinoma, which is classified again as cribriform, papillary, and solid. (1a-5) Urothelial carcinoma/transitional cell carcinomas are malignant and occur as primary cancers of the prostate. They usually originate from the prostatic urethra or the prostate ducts. (1b) Squamous neoplasms, which are classified into (1b-1) Adenosquamous carcinoma of the prostate, which is distinguished by the elements of squamous cell carcinoma in variable degrees as well as a glandular or frequently high-grade adenocarcinoma component. (1b-2) Squamous cell carcinoma of the prostate that are <1% of prostate cancer cases, and adenosquamous carcinomas are much less common. Osteolytic bone metastases rather than osteoblastic ones frequently arise from squamous cell carcinomas. (2) Neuroendocrine tumors (Fig. 14.3): (2a) Adenocarcinoma with neuroendocrine differentiation is a malignant neuroendocrine tumor that only differs from acinar or ductal adenocarcinomas on immunohistochemistry staining. It is distinguished by the presence of one of the three neuroendocrine markers chromogranin A, synaptophysin, or CD56. (2b) Well-differentiated neuroendocrine tumor/low-grade neuroendocrine carcinoma of the prostate or carcinoid tumors are low-grade tumors arising from the prostate that may metastasize. (2c) Small cell neuroendocrine carcinoma/small cell neuroendocrine carcinomas of the prostate are characterized by aggressive conduct and a growth in the number of small cells. (2d) Large cell neuroendocrine carcinoma/prostatic large cell neuroendocrine carcinomas are extremely rare and severe high-grade neuroendocrine tumors that are almost never identified on their own and are typically found alongside an adenocarcinoma. (3) Mesenchymal tumors (Fig. 14.3): (3a) Stromal tumor of uncertain malignant potential (STUMP) of the prostate has a wide range of histologic characteristics as well as variable clinical behavior. The macroscopic appearance can change. White to tan to yellow are the different colors, and solid, firm, partly cystic, or multiloculated are the different consistency options. (3b) Leiomyosarcoma is an uncommon mesenchymal smooth muscle cancer of the prostate gland. Leiomyosarcomas have nonspecific macroscopic characteristics. When a tumor is diagnosed, it is frequently big and has a bladder invasion or a capsular breach. Leiomyosarcoma often has spindle cells with nuclear atypia and elevated mitotic activity, microscopically. (3c) Rhabdomyosarcoma/genitourinary tract rhabdomyosarcomas are rare cancers that develop in pelvic organs. (3d) Leiomyomas of the prostate are benign mesenchymal tumors. The term "leiomyomas of the prostate" refers to benign smooth muscle tumors without any glandular components that are seen either inside the prostate or in close proximity to it.

Staging: The AJCC and the UICC classify men with prostate cancer into prognostic stage groups based on TNM factors along with the PSA levels and the histologic grade group of the primary tumor [26]. T determines the local extent of the disease and was classified into T0, T1, T2, T3, and T4 [24]. T0 refers to zero evidence of primary tumor, T1 indicates inapparent tumor, which is not noticeable but can be detected only by PSA levels, T2 refers to tumors that are noticeable and limited within the prostate gland, T3 indicates extra-prostatic tumor invading seminal vesicles, and T4 indicates tumor is anchored or is metastasized to adjacent structures [24]. Nodal staging (N) was classified into Nx indicating nodal status was not evaluated, N0 refers to zero evidence of nodal metastases, and N1 indicates the involvement of regional lymph nodes [24]. Metastasis (M) staging was classified into Mx indicating metastatic disease not assessed, M0 for no metastasis, and M1 for distant metastasis [24].

14.3 Pathophysiology

Anatomy: The human prostate is the largest male accessory gland [33]. The prostate is a walnut-shaped gland that weighs around 20–30 gm [33]. The storage and secretion of a slightly alkaline fluid (constitutes 25% to 35% of total volume of semen) that helps to nourish the sperms and carry them through a slightly acidic vaginal environment constitute the main function of the prostate gland [33, 34]. The prostate lobes include anterior (isthmus), median, posterior, and lateral lobes [33]. Prostate can be divided into peripheral zone (PZ), central zone (CZ), and transition zone (TZ) [33]. PZ constitutes about 70% of glandular tissue of prostate while CZ makes up 20% of glandular tissue of prostate [24, 33]. Only 5% of TZ forms glandular tissue of prostate [35]. Prostate cancer is classified into androgen-dependent and androgen-independent, based on the expression of androgen receptors. Most of the prostate cancers are androgen-dependent. Adenocarcinomas constitute more than 95% of the PCa cases, with the majority having an acinar origin and the rest having ductal origin. Nearly 80% of prostate adenocarcinomas arise from luminal or basal epithelial cells, which constitute about 70% of the prostate tissue.

Cell of Origin: Epithelial cells that include basal, luminal, and neuroendocrine cells, and stem cells make up the prostate gland (Fig. 14.4) [36]. The undifferentiated basal cells were androgen-independent, and the secretory products produced

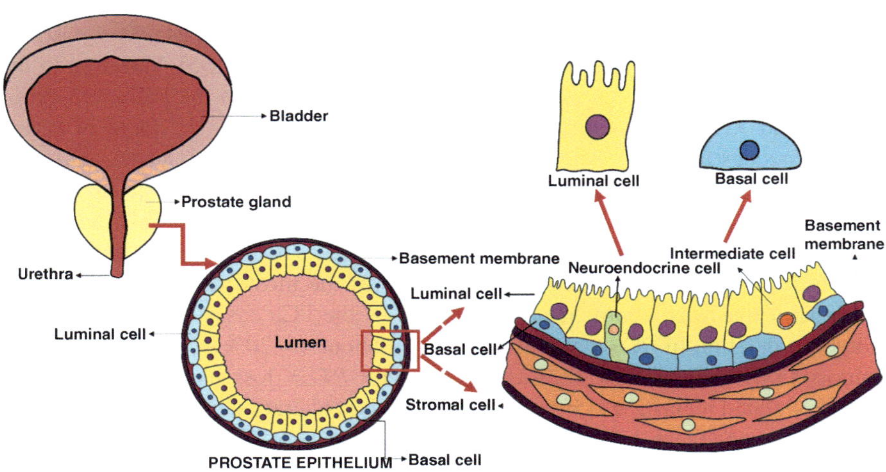

Fig. 14.4 Anatomy and pathophysiology of prostate cancer

by these cells include CD44, p63, p27^{kip}, c-Met, CK5, and CK14 [37–40]. Luminal, also known as the secretory cells are differentiated and androgen-dependent, which in response to androgen, produce PSA and prostatic acid phosphatase [36]. AR was highly expressed in luminal cells [37, 40]. Neuroendocrine cells are androgen-insensitive, differentiated, and express neuroendocrine-specific markers such as chromogranin A and synaptophysin (Fig. 14.4) [41]. Prostate stromal cells express AR, are androgen-responsive, and assist epithelial cell development and maintenance [42].

Both basal and luminal epithelial layers are important in benign and metastatic PCa pathogenesis [43]. The basal compartment was predominated with actively dividing cells, indicating that luminal cells can arise from basal cells in adults [43]. Basal cells promote luminal differentiation when they undergo oncogenic transformation; this transformation can lead to both basal- and luminal-like tumors with luminal phenotype [43–45]. Based on the gene set enrichment analysis, it was suggested that the basal-origin prostate cancer is less likely to be aggressive when compared to luminal-origin prostate cancer [45]. Luminal-like adenocarcinomas constitute about 95% of human prostate tumors and PCa cell lines with this phenotype can show neuroendocrine features following androgen deprivation [46–48].

Cancer stem cells (CSCs) can create their own niche by recruiting bone marrow-derived mesenchymal stem cells (BM-MSCs) [49]. Apart from niche creation, BM-MSCs can also convert normal fibroblasts into cancer-associated fibroblasts resulting in PCa invasion and metastasis [49]. A subpopulation of prostate CSCs could metastasize the bone due to their higher adherence to endothelial cells and osteoblasts [50]. Circulating tumor cells (CTCs) express TOPK, a member of the MAPK family kinases [51]. TOPK inhibition prevents CTC migration both in vitro and in vivo [51]. Furthermore, elevated levels of TOPK were linked to advanced stages of PCa; particularly elevated levels of TOPK were observed in patients with a Gleason score of 8 or above [52, 53]. Changes in macrophages and chemokines also lead to PCa [52, 53].

Molecular Pathology: PCa is a known heritable cancer type [54]. Nearly 30% to 40% of genetic factors can be attributed to PCa familial risk [55]. Variation in the 8q24 region, which is adjacent to the *MYC* oncogene, and in the kallikrein genes (*KLK2* and *KLK3*) of chromosome 19 were associated with the PCa, of which KLK3 encodes for the PSA [55]. *BRCA2* mutation was a strongly penetrant germline variant which increases the risk of PCa by fivefold when compared to men without *BRCA2* mutation [54]. Germline mutation in *HOXB13* was also identified in PCa [56]. The fusion of androgen-regulated gene *TMPRSS2* with members of *ETS* transcription factor family (*ERG, ETV*) was the most common genetic rearrangement that was identified in nearly 50% of the PCa cases [57]. *PTEN* was a common deletion in PCa that was reported in about 15–20% of surgically treated tumors [58]. Patients that were associated with *PTEN* loss had a higher risk of surgery-related metastases [59]. A common genetic alteration namely amplification of the proto-oncogene *MYC* (8q) has a prevalence range of 10–30% in localized PCa and 50% in case of advanced PCa [59]. In response to androgen inhibition, a subset of PCa develops neuroendocrine differentiation [59]. Nearly 70% of castration-resistant neuroendocrine PCa has deletions in the genomic regions of *RB1* gene while only 30% of adenocarcinoma castrate-resistant tumor is *RB1* deficit [59].

14.4 Treatment

Surgery: Prostatectomy is a common surgical procedure in the PCa treatment [31]. There are three methods of prostatectomy: open prostatectomy, laparoscopic prostatectomy, and transurethral resection of the prostate (TURP) [31]. Radical prostatectomy (RP) remains crucial in both localized PCa and high-risk PCa treatment [31, 60]. Generally, prostatectomy involves removal of entire prostate, but in RP, the tissue surrounding the prostate was also removed [31]. The risk of wound infection was nearly 5–9% with these open prostatectomy procedures [61]. Despite the fact that radical perineal prostatectomy was less painful and has a faster recovery, radical retropubic prostatectomy was the most common approach [31]. Laparoscopic methods were better than open prostatectomy as it provides faster recovery along with less blood loss and pain [31]. TURP was commonly used for treating benign prostatic hyperplasia (BPH) [31].

Radiation Therapy: Variety of radiation therapy techniques were used in PCa treatment such as the external beam radiation therapy (EBRT), 3-D conformal radiation therapy (3D-CRT), intensity-modulated radiation therapy (IMRT), stereotactic body radiation therapy (SBRT), proton beam radiation therapy (PBRT), brachytherapy (internal radiation therapy), and the use of radiopharmaceuticals [24]. After receiving the radiation therapy, the median overall survival has increased from 3.3 years to 5.6 years [62]. Early-stage PCa patients were generally treated with EBRT that involves the focusing of radiation beams onto the prostate gland [24]. 3D-CRT uses advanced computers to image the prostate, after which radiation beams were directed at the prostate from various angles, preventing injury to adjacent normal tissues. IMRT was a more advanced version of 3D-CRT therapy in which the beams were not only be targeted at the prostate from various angles, they also can be modified to restrict the amount of radiation that reaches neighboring normal tissues. SBRT was an image-guided approach that delivers higher doses of radiation to a precise area in less time than IMRT (days instead of weeks). PBRT concentrates beams of protons rather than photons of x-rays and this was not widely used as it was expensive and due to lack of clear evidence to prove that it is better than photon treatment. Brachytherapy (internal radiation therapy) uses small radioactive pellets that were set directly into prostate. HDR brachytherapy was used with the combination of EBRT for treating PCa while LDR monotherapy has better outcomes compared to its combination with EBRT [36, 63, 64]. HDR brachytherapy as monotherapy was also being used mainly for all stages of patients [65, 66].

Hormone Therapy: Also known as the androgen deprivation therapy (ADT), it lowers the levels of androgens in the body to obstruct them from fueling the growth of prostate cancer cells. Most of the androgens are produced by the testicles; androgens are also made by adrenal glands and PCa cells as well. Orchiectomy is the surgical removal of testes. Luteinizing hormone-releasing hormone (LHRH) agonists such as goserelin, leuprolide, or triptorelin could be used to lower the amount of testosterone. LHRH antagonists degarelix and relugolix lower testosterone levels more readily and do not cause tumor flare. Abiraterone blocks a protein called CYP17, which aids cells to stop the synthesis of androgens. Abiraterone can be used for advanced, very high-risk prostate cancer, and castration-resistant PCa [67]. AR antagonists such as flutamide or nilutamide can be combined to orchiectomy or an LHRH agonist for complete androgen blockade. Newer antiandrogens enzalutamide, apalutamide, and darolutamide can be put to use for castration-resistant PCa and metastatic castration-sensitive PCa [68].

Cryotherapy: Cryotherapy was performed using argon and helium for freeze and heating cycles respectively, and this procedure is less invasive [69]. For all risk categories, the estimated 5-year BPFS was 91.1%, 78.5%, and 62.2%, respectively [69]. For men of age >75 years, the estimated 5-year BPFS rate for the low-, moderate-, and high-risk groups was 74.9%, 61.4%, and 58%, respectively [70].

Immunotherapy: Immunotherapy assists the immune system of the patient to identify and eliminate cancer cells [71, 72]. Nivolumab plus ipilimumab showed 19 months of median overall survival (OS) in patients who had never undergone chemotherapy and 15.2 months of OS in those who had undergone chemotherapy [71, 72]. PD-1 inhibition has produced positive OS results [72]. When compared to placebo, sipuleucel-T (a cell-based cancer immunotherapy) showed a 4.1-month increase in OS [72]. In patients with metastatic CRPC whose cancer had proceeded through initial docetaxel and hormone therapy, pembrolizumab is suggested as a subsequent systemic therapy.

Targeted Therapy: Apalutamide was an androgen receptor antagonist that was used for the treatment of nonmetastatic CRPC [73]. Upon treatment with apalutamide, a median OS of 73.9 months was observed [74]. PARP inhibitors have displayed positive outcomes in treating PCa [74]. In 2020, FDA approved rucaparib and olaparib for the treatment of CRPC patients with germline mutations in the *BRCA1/2* and *ATM* genes, and somatic mutations in the *HRR* gene [73, 75]. Antiandrogens such abiraterone and enzalutamide were more responsive after receiving γ-secretase inhibitor GSI-1 treatment [73, 76].

14.5 Conclusion

The second most diagnosed cancer among men is prostate cancer. Risk factors for prostate cancer are family history, germline mutations, ethnicity, environmental and occupational hazards. Based on the histology, prostate cancer is classified into adenocarcinoma and neuroendocrine prostate cancer, the majority of them are of the type luminal-like adenocarcinoma. The most common clinical tools for prostate cancer diagnosis are digital rectal exam and PSA testing. Prostatectomy was a common surgical procedure in the prostate cancer treatment; nearly 5–9% of risk of wound infection was associated with these open prostatectomy procedures. Along with surgery, various other treatment procedures are also employed that include radiation therapy, hormone therapy, cryotherapy, immunotherapy, and targeted therapy. Although beneficial therapies have been given to disease-affected males, improving patient outcomes, process improvements such as therapy titration and augmentation, are required to optimize tumor control and reduce normal tissue destruction from the treatment.

References

1. Sung H, Ferlay J, Siegel RL, Laversanne M, Soerjomataram I, Jemal A, Bray F. Global cancer statistics 2020: GLOBOCAN estimates of incidence and mortality worldwide for 36 cancers in 185 countries. CA Cancer J Clin. 2021;71(3):209–49.
2. Gandaglia G, Leni R, Bray F, Fleshner N, Freedland SJ, Kibel A, et al. Epidemiology and prevention of prostate cancer. Eur Urol Oncol. 2021;4(6):877–92.
3. Doja MN, Kaur I, Ahmad T. Age-specific survival in prostate cancer using machine learning. Data Technol Appl. 2020;54(2):215–34.
4. Frees S, Akamatsu S, Bidnur S, Khalaf D, Chavez-Munoz C, Struss W, et al. The impact of time to metastasis on overall survival in patients with prostate cancer. World J Urol. 2018;36(7):1039–46.
5. Siegel DA, O'Neil ME, Richards TB, Dowling NF, Weir HK. Prostate cancer incidence and survival, by stage and race/ethnicity—United States, 2001–2017. Morb Mortal Wkly Rep. 2020;69(41):1473.
6. Han H, Lee HH, Choi K, Moon YJ, Heo JE, Ham WS, et al. Prostate epithelial genes define therapy-relevant prostate cancer molecular subtype. Prostate Cancer Prostatic Dis. 2021;24(4):1080–92.
7. Perdana NR, Mochtar CA, Umbas R, Hamid ARA. The risk factors of prostate cancer and its prevention: a literature review. Acta Med Indones. 2017;48(3):228–38.
8. Hemminki K. Familial risk and familial survival in prostate cancer. World J Urol. 2012;30(2):143–8.
9. De Visschere P, Oosterlinck W, De Meerleer G, Villeirs G. Clinical and imaging tools in the early diagnosis of prostate cancer, a review. J Belg Radiol. 2010;93(2):62.
10. Wu X, Reinikainen P, Kapanen M, Vierikko T, Ryymin P, Kellokumpu-Lehtinen PL. Dynamic contrast-enhanced imaging as a prognostic tool in early diagnosis of prostate cancer: correlation with PSA and clinical stage. Contrast Media Mol Imaging. 2018;2018.
11. Porfyris O, Al-Awon A, Liatsikos E, Kallidonis P. Novel imaging in prostate cancer. Urol Ann. 2020;12(3):205.
12. Makarov DV, Loeb S, Getzenberg RH, Partin AW. Biomarkers for prostate cancer. Annu Rev Med. 2009;60(1):139–51.
13. Catalona WJ, Loeb S. The PSA era is not over for prostate cancer. Eur Urol. 2005;48(4):541–5.
14. Candefjord S, Ramser K, Lindahl OA. Technologies for localization and diagnosis of prostate cancer. J Med Eng Technol. 2009;33(8):585–603.
15. Kijvikai K. Digital rectal examination, serum prostatic specific antigen or transrectal ultrasonography: the best tool to guide the treatment of men with benign prostatic hyperplasia. Curr Opin Urol. 2009;19(1):44–8.
16. Bosch JLHR, Bohnen AM, Groeneveld FPMJ. Validity of digital rectal examination and serum prostate specific antigen in the estimation of prostate volume in community-based men aged 50 to 78 years: the Krimpen study. Eur Urol. 2004;46(6):753–9.
17. Hatakeyama S, Yoneyama T, Tobisawa Y, Ohyama C. Recent progress and perspectives on prostate cancer biomarkers. Int J Clin Oncol. 2017;22(2):214–21.
18. Otero JR, Gomez BG, Juanatey FC, Touijer KA. Prostate cancer biomarkers: an update. Urol Oncol. 2014, April;32(3):252–60.

19. Rubin MA, Zhou M, Dhanasekaran SM, Varambally S, Barrette TR, Sanda MG, et al. α-Methylacyl coenzyme a racemase as a tissue biomarker for prostate cancer. JAMA. 2002;287(13):1662–70.
20. Bussemakers MJ, Van Bokhoven A, Verhaegh GW, Smit FP, Karthaus HF, Schalken JA, et al. Dd3:: A new prostate-specific gene, highly overexpressed in prostate cancer. Cancer Res. 1999;59(23):5975–9.
21. Saini S. PSA and beyond: alternative prostate cancer biomarkers. Cell Oncol. 2016;39(2):97–106.
22. Auprich M, Bjartell A, Chun FKH, de la Taille A, Freedland SJ, Haese A, et al. Contemporary role of prostate cancer antigen 3 in the management of prostate cancer. Eur Urol. 2011;60(5):1045–54.
23. Squire JA, Park PC, Yoshimoto M, Alami J, Williams JL, Evans A, Joshua AM. Prostate cancer as a model system for genetic diversity in tumors. Adv Cancer Res. 2011;112:183–216.
24. Kampel LJ. Dx/Rx: prostate cancer: prostate cancer. Burlington, MA: Jones & Bartlett Publishers; 2012.
25. Epstein JI. The Gleason grading system: a complete guide for pathologists and clinicians. Philadelphia, PA: Wolters Kluwer/Lippincott Williams & Wilkins Health; 2013.
26. Sathianathen NJ, Konety BR, Crook J, Saad F, Lawrentschuk N. Landmarks in prostate cancer. Nat Rev Urol. 2018;15(10):627–42.
27. Byar DP, Mostofi FK, Veterans Administration Cooperative Urological Research Group. Carcinoma of the prostate: prognostic evaluation of certain pathologic features in 208 radical prostatectomies. Cancer. 1972;30(1):5–13.
28. Zhu J, Liang X, Wu D, Chen S, Yang B, Mao W, Shen D. Clinicopathological characteristics and survival outcomes in neuroendocrine prostate cancer: a population-based study. Medicine. 2021;100(15):e25237.
29. Ro JY, Ayala AG, Shen SS. Advances in surgical pathology: prostate cancer, vol. 1. Philadelphia, PA: Lippincott Williams & Wilkins; 2012.
30. Aggarwal R, Zhang T, Small EJ, Armstrong AJ. Neuroendocrine prostate cancer: subtypes, biology, and clinical outcomes. J Natl Compr Cancer Netw. 2014;12(5):719–26.
31. Kaler J, Hussain A, Haque A, Naveed H, Patel S. A comprehensive review of pharmaceutical and surgical interventions of prostate cancer. Cureus. 2020;12(11).
32. Gordetsky J, Epstein J. Grading of prostatic adenocarcinoma: current state and prognostic implications. Diagn Pathol. 2016;11(1):1–8.
33. Lee CH, Akin-Olugbade O, Kirschenbaum A. Overview of prostate anatomy, histology, and pathology. Endocrinol Metab Clin. 2011;40(3):565–75.
34. Romero FR, Romero AW, Filho TB, Kulysz D, Oliveira FC Jr, Filho RT. The prostate exam. Health Educ J. 2012;71(2):239–50.
35. Bhavsar A, Verma S. Anatomic imaging of the prostate. BioMed Res Int. 2014;2014.
36. Karl M. Encyclopedia of Prostate Cancer. 2015.
37. Liu AY, True LD, LaTray L, Nelson PS, Ellis WJ, Vessella RL, et al. Cell–cell interaction in prostate gene regulation and cytodifferentiation. Proc Natl Acad Sci. 1997;94(20):10705–10.
38. Signoretti S, Waltregny D, Dilks J, Isaac B, Lin D, Garraway L, et al. p63 is a prostate basal cell marker and is required for prostate development. Am J Pathol. 2000;157(6):1769–75.
39. Van Leenders GJ, Gage WR, Hicks JL, Van Balken B, Aalders TW, Schalken JA, De Marzo AM. Intermediate cells in human prostate epithelium are enriched in proliferative inflammatory atrophy. Am J Pathol. 2003;162(5):1529–37.
40. Sherwood ER, Theyer G, Steiner G, Berg LA, Kozlowski JM, Lee C. Differential expression of specific cytokeratin polypeptides in the basal and luminal epithelia of the human prostate. Prostate. 1991;18(4):303–14.
41. Palapattu GS, Wu C, Silvers CR, Martin HB, Williams K, Salamone L, et al. Selective expression of CD44, a putative prostate cancer stem cell marker, in neuroendocrine tumor cells of human prostate cancer. Prostate. 2009;69(7):787–98.
42. Berry PA, Maitland NJ, Collins AT. Androgen receptor signalling in prostate: effects of stromal factors on normal and cancer stem cells. Mol Cell Endocrinol. 2008;288(1–2):30–7.

43. Strand DW, Goldstein AS. The many ways to make a luminal cell and a prostate cancer cell. Endocr Relat Cancer. 2015;22(6):T187–97.
44. Choi N, Zhang B, Zhang L, Ittmann M, Xin L. Adult murine prostate basal and luminal cells are self-sustained lineages that can both serve as targets for prostate cancer initiation. Cancer Cell. 2012;21(2):253–65.
45. Wang ZA, Mitrofanova A, Bergren SK, Abate-Shen C, Cardiff RD, Califano A, Shen MM. Lineage analysis of basal epithelial cells reveals their unexpected plasticity and supports a cell-of-origin model for prostate cancer heterogeneity. Nat Cell Biol. 2013;15(3):274–83.
46. Grisanzio C, Signoretti S. p63 in prostate biology and pathology. J Cell Biochem. 2008;103(5):1354–68.
47. Wang ZA, Toivanen R, Bergren SK, Chambon P, Shen MM. Luminal cells are favored as the cell of origin for prostate cancer. Cell Rep. 2014;8(5):1339–46.
48. Burchardt T, Burchardt M, Chen MW, Cao Y, De La Taille ALEXANDRE, Shabsigh A, et al. Transdifferentiation of prostate cancer cells to a neuroendocrine cell phenotype in vitro and in vivo. J Urol. 1999;162(5):1800–5.
49. Wen S, Niu Y, Yeh S, Chang C. BM-MSCs promote prostate cancer progression via the conversion of normal fibroblasts to cancer-associated fibroblasts. Int J Oncol. 2015;47(2):719–27.
50. Santoni M, Piva F, Scarpelli M, Cheng L, Lopez-Beltran A, Massari F, et al. The origin of prostate metastases: emerging insights. Cancer Metastasis Rev. 2015;34(4):765–73.
51. Sun H, Zhang L, Shi C, Hu P, Yan W, Wang Z, et al. TOPK is highly expressed in circulating tumor cells, enabling metastasis of prostate cancer. Oncotarget. 2015;6(14):12392.
52. Wang W, Bergh A, Damber JE. Morphological transition of proliferative inflammatory atrophy to high-grade intraepithelial neoplasia and cancer in human prostate. Prostate. 2009;69(13):1378–86.
53. Nguyen DP, Li J, Yadav SS, Tewari AK. Recent insights into NF-κ B signalling pathways and the link between inflammation and prostate cancer. BJU Int. 2014;114(2):168–76.
54. Faisal FA, Lotan TL. The genomic and molecular pathology of prostate cancer: clinical implications for diagnosis, prognosis, and therapy. Adv Anat Pathol. 2020;27(1):11–9.
55. Eeles R, Goh C, Castro E, Bancroft E, Guy M, Olama AAA, et al. The genetic epidemiology of prostate cancer and its clinical implications. Nat Rev Urol. 2014;11(1):18–31.
56. Ewing CM, Ray AM, Lange EM, Zuhlke KA, Robbins CM, Tembe WD, et al. Germline mutations in HOXB13 and prostate-cancer risk. N Engl J Med. 2012;366(2):141–9.
57. Tomlins SA, Rhodes DR, Perner S, Dhanasekaran SM, Mehra R, Sun XW, et al. Recurrent fusion of TMPRSS2 and ETS transcription factor genes in prostate cancer. Science. 2005;310(5748):644–8.
58. Shaikhibrahim Z, Wernert N. ETS transcription factors and prostate cancer: the role of the family prototype ETS-1. Int J Oncol. 2012;40(6):1748–54.
59. Guedes LB, Tosoian JJ, Hicks J, Ross AE, Lotan TL. PTEN loss in Gleason score 3+ 4= 7 prostate biopsies is associated with nonorgan confined disease at radical prostatectomy. J Urol. 2017;197(4):1054–9.
60. Brannigan RE. Urology, an issue of medical clinics of North America. Vol. 102, No. 2. Elsevier Health Sciences. 2018.
61. Wroński S. Radical perineal prostatectomy–the contemporary resurgence of a genuinely minimally invasive procedure: procedure outline. Comparison of the advantages, disadvantages, and outcomes of different surgical techniques of treating organ-confined prostate cancer (PCa). A literature review with special focus on perineal prostatectomy. Central Eur J Urol. 2012;65(4):188.
62. Yang DD, Butler SS, Muralidhar V, Mahal BA, Martin NE, Mouw KW, et al. Impact of prostate-directed radiation therapy on overall survival for patients with M1a prostate cancer. Int J Radiat Oncol Biol Phys. 2019;105(1):E315–6.
63. Chen YC, Chuang CK, Hsieh ML, Chen WC, Fan KH, Yeh CY, et al. High-dose-rate brachytherapy plus external beam radiotherapy for T1 to T3 prostate cancer: an experience in Taiwan. Urology. 2007;70(1):101–5.

64. Demanes DJ, Brandt D, Schour L, Hill DR. Excellent results from high dose rate brachytherapy and external beam for prostate cancer are not improved by androgen deprivation. Am J Clin Oncol. 2009;32(4):342–7.
65. Demanes DJ, Martinez AA, Ghilezan M, Hill DR, Schour L, Brandt D, Gustafson G. High-dose-rate monotherapy: safe and effective brachytherapy for patients with localized prostate cancer. Int J Radiat Oncol Biol Phys. 2011;81(5):1286–92.
66. Ghilezan M, Martinez A, Gustason G, Krauss D, Antonucci JV, Chen P, et al. High-dose-rate brachytherapy as monotherapy delivered in two fractions within one day for favorable/intermediate-risk prostate cancer: preliminary toxicity data. Int J Radiat Oncol Biol Phys. 2012;83(3):927–32.
67. Rice MA, Malhotra SV, Stoyanova T. Second-generation antiandrogens: from discovery to standard of care in castration resistant prostate cancer. Front Oncol. 2019;9:801.
68. Sochacka-Ćwikła A, Mączyński M, Regiec A. FDA-approved Small molecule compounds as drugs for solid cancers from early 2011 to the end of 2021. Molecules. 2022;27(7):2259.
69. Mercader C, Musquera M, Franco A, Alcaraz A, Ribal MJ. Primary cryotherapy for localized prostate cancer treatment. Aging Male. 2020;23(5):1460–6.
70. Dhar N, Ward JF, Cher ML, Jones JS. Primary full-gland prostate cryoablation in older men (> age of 75 years): results from 860 patients tracked with the COLD registry. BJU Int. 2011;108(4):508–12.
71. Sharma P, Pachynski RK, Narayan V, Fléchon A, Gravis G, Galsky MD, et al. Nivolumab plus ipilimumab for metastatic castration-resistant prostate cancer: preliminary analysis of patients in the CheckMate 650 trial. Cancer Cell. 2020;38(4):489–99.
72. Runcie KD, Dallos MC. Prostate cancer immunotherapy—finally in from the cold? Curr Oncol Rep. 2021;23(8):1–13.
73. Fontana F, Anselmi M, Limonta P. Molecular mechanisms and genetic alterations in prostate cancer: from diagnosis to targeted therapy. Cancer Lett. 2022;534:215619.
74. Smith MR, Saad F, Chowdhury S, Oudard S, Hadaschik BA, Graff JN, et al. Apalutamide and overall survival in prostate cancer. Eur Urol. 2021;79(1):150–8.
75. Teyssonneau D, Margot H, Cabart M, Anonnay M, Sargos P, Vuong NS, et al. Prostate cancer and PARP inhibitors: progress and challenges. J Hematol Oncol. 2021;14(1):1–19.
76. Mohamed AA, Tan SH, Xavier CP, Katta S, Huang W, Ravindranath L, et al. Synergistic activity with NOTCH inhibition and androgen ablation in ERG-positive prostate cancer CellsNOTCH inhibitors synergize with AR-directed therapies. Mol Cancer Res. 2017;15(10):1308–17.

Testicular Cancer

15

Ankitha Anchula, Vaishnavi Gantyala, Apoorva Degala,
Meghana Korikani, Nageswara Rao Amanchi,
and Rama Krishna Kancha

15.1 Introduction

Epidemiology: According to the IARC, 74,458 men were diagnosed with testicular cancer (TC) in the year 2020 and 9334 deaths were recorded worldwide [1]. The overall 5-year survival rate was 95% for the period 2012–2018 [2]. TC is common in men between 15 and 45 years of age [3]. Survival rates range from 99% for localized disease, 96% for local spread to nearby organs or lymph nodes, and 73% for distant metastasis [1]. Globally, the age-standardized rates (ASR) were 137.4, 116.9, 94.9, 66.5, and 27.1 per 100,000 men in Europe, Oceania, North America, South America, and Central America, respectively and are reported to be the least in Asia [4]. The average age is 33 years at the time of first diagnosis [3].

Risk Factors: The major risk factors for TC include cryptorchidism (also called maldescended or undescended testis), which is the failure of testicles to descend into the scrotum before birth [5]. Other risk factors include low sperm count and hypospadias [6]. A high risk of TC is associated with a rare genetic condition called testicular dysgenesis, which frequently coexists with hypospadias and undescended testes [7]. About 2% of men with TC in only one testicle have a possibility of developing cancer in the contralateral testis [2]. Higher levels of estrogen during early pregnancy may permanently alter germ cells leading to TC later in the male children [8]. The factors that are associated with TC are an increase in maternal estrogen levels, extreme nausea, and bleeding/spotting during pregnancy, maternal cigarette smoking, young maternal age, maternal weight, and preterm birth [8]. Viruses such

A. Anchula · V. Gantyala · A. Degala · N. R. Amanchi
Department of Zoology, Osmania University, Hyderabad, India

M. Korikani · R. K. Kancha (✉)
Molecular Medicine and Therapeutics Laboratory, CPMB, Osmania University, Hyderabad, India
e-mail: ramakancha@osmania.ac.in

R. K. Kancha (ed.), *Biomedical Aspects of Solid Cancers*,
https://doi.org/10.1007/978-981-97-1802-3_15

as EBV, CMV, B19, and HIV are associated with the development of TC [9]. Some occupations such as firefighters, air craftworkers, and leather tanners who are exposed to a variety of carcinogenic substances are at an increased risk of developing TC [10, 11]. Long-term consumption of alcohol and the usage of marijuana were found to increase the risk of TC [12].

Diagnosis: Diagnosis of TC is primarily done by performing a physical examination and ultrasonography of the testes [13]. The trans-scrotal ultrasonography is highly effective at differentiating benign cysts from complicated solid tumors. It is accurate at determining whether lesions are extra- or intratesticular [14]. If the ultrasonography results show the presence of a tumor, then initial inguinal orchiectomy is performed where one or both testicles and full spermatic cord are removed [2]. Computed tomography (CT) scan is used for patients with nonspecific symptoms such as retroperitoneal adenopathy with abdominal pain or other generalized symptoms. For primary testicular lesions, a CT scan is not performed. Magnetic resonance imaging accurately determines the local spread of the disease in case of testicular carcinoma [14].

Biomarkers: The primordial germ cells but not the adult germ cell express immunohistochemical markers such as PLAP, OCT3/4, NANOG, SOX2, REX1, AP-2γ, and LIN28 [15]. The diagnosis of germ cell tumors requires the immunoassay of several biochemical markers, such as the lactic dehydrogenase, human chorionic gonadotropin, α-fetoprotein, and LD-1 [15]. Nonseminomatous tumors, yolk sac tumors, and choriocarcinoma syncytiotrophoblast release α-fetoprotein and human chorionic gonadotropin, while seminoma secretes lactic dehydrogenase [15]. According to a recent expression profiling study, GCT cells can be identified by hypomethylation of *CSF1R*, *PTPRC*, and *MMP9* genes [16]. The noninvasive markers for GCNIS that are being expressed in both serum and semen are miR371–373 and miR-302/367 that can also be used in the evaluation of GCT [16].

15.2 Classification

Testicular cancer is classified into two groups: (1) Germ cell tumors (GCT) and (2) stromal tumors (Fig. 15.1). In 2022, the World Health Organization classified TC based on advances in histopathologic, genetic, and molecular studies that have improved knowledge of the GCT pathologenesis [17]. GCTs are further classified into Germ cell neoplasia in situ-related tumors (GCNIS) and Nongerm Cell Neoplasia In situ-related tumors (Fig. 15.1) [18]. GNCIS is usually located in the parenchyma of the testicles, and 4–8 percent of patients develop GNCIS in the contralateral testicles [19]. GCNIS-related tumors are characterized by the presence of chromosome 12p amplification which increases the invasiveness of TGCTs [18]. GCNIS is further classified into seminoma, nonseminoma, and burned-out TGCTs (Fig. 15.1). Testicular tumors in the germinoma category have one type of tumor, i.e., seminoma. Granulomata and tubular morphology are the characteristics of seminomas [17]. Seminomas also affect other extra-gonadal sites including mediastinum and retroperitoneum [20]. Nonseminoma germ cell tumor (NSGCT) can be either pure (with only one histologic subtype) or mixed (with several histologic

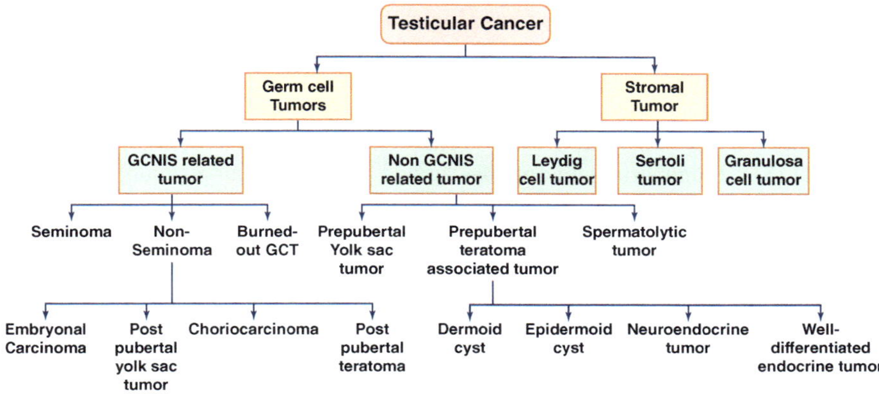

Fig. 15.1 World health organization classification of testicular cancer

subtypes) [21]. Burned-out germ cell tumors arise in extragonadal tissue with spontaneous regression of the intragonadal tumor [22]. The burned-out tumor phenomenon is described as the spontaneous regression of primary germ cell tumors after metastasis that is caused due to an immune response or tumor ischemia. De novo formation of primary testicular GCT in extragonadal tissues is also the reason to develop burned-out GCT [23].

The NSGCT is further classified into four groups. Embryonal carcinoma cells are undifferentiated with amphophilic cytoplasm and pleomorphic nucleus and are frequently seen as mixed germ cell tumors (Fig. 15.1) [24, 25]. These tumors can develop in papillary, glandular-alveolar, tubular, or solid sheet growth patterns, which result in a wide range of microscopic appearances [26]. Postpubertal yolk sac tumors (primitive endodermal tumors/endodermal sinus tumors), seen predominantly in children under the age of 10 years, resemble primitive mesenchyma of the yolk sac, and can be in pure or mixed form of germ cell tumors [27]. Postpubertal yolk sac tumors secrete AFP, hCG, or both and are frequently associated with hematogenous metastasis [21]. Choriocarcinoma is the rarest type of nonseminomatous germ cell tumor and is present as pure or mixed types. Pure choriocarcinoma is the most aggressive and rare form of choriocarcinoma [28, 29]. Choriocarcinomas are composed of both syncytiotrophoblasts and cytotrophoblast cells. They are highly vascular and prone to hemorrhage [25]. Choriocarcinoma exhibits elevated levels of β-HCG, increased metastasis, and rapid progression [30]. Increased levels of HCG cause gynecomastia in males. Postpubertal teratoma is a malignant germ cell tumor made up of several germ cell layers (endoderm, mesoderm, and ectoderm) and has high metastatic potential (metastasizes in 22–37% of cases) [31, 32]. Less than 5% of GCTs in adults are caused by pure teratomas, which are uncommon in postpubertal teratomas [26].

Non-GCNIS-related tumors contain prepubertal yolk sac tumors, prepubertal teratomas, and spermatocytic tumors that are characterized by the absence of chromosome 12p amplification [18]. Although prepubertal yolk sac tumors and postpubertal yolk sac tumors are physiologically and pathogenetically distinct from one another, they share a variety of general histologic characteristics and patterns [33]. Prepubertal yolk sac tumors have lower extra-testicular involvement compared to postpubertal germ cell tumors [33]. Prepubertal teratomas are considered as indolent tumors where the testis shows normal spermatogenesis with no metastatic potential [31]. Prepubertal teratoma has a good prognosis than postpubertal teratomas. Prepubertal teratomas are classified into dermoid cysts, epidermoid cysts, and neuroendocrine tumors [18]. The dermoid cyst is a rare, benign, para-testicular tumor composed of pilosebaceous units [34]. Even though dermoid cyst contains lipogranulomas but lack other germ cell layers [35]. An epidermoid cyst is made up of benign squamous epithelium that contains keratin with a lamellar target appearance [18]. Well-differentiated neuroendocrine tumors are malignancies that arise from neuroendocrine cells throughout the body. These tumors are also called carcinoid tumors; they produce peptides that cause hormonal syndromes [36]. Spermatocytic tumor is a rare GCT originating from mature germ cells. These tumors rarely metastasize and patients have normal serum tumor marker levels [18].

Stromal Tumors: They are derived from the stroma and supporting cells surrounding the germ cells [37]. It includes Leydig cell tumors, Sertoli cell tumors, and granulosa cell tumors (Fig. 15.1) [38]. Leydig cell tumors (LCT), which are sex cord-stromal tumors, are often present in unilateral and are found bilaterally in only 3% of cases. It is a rare tumor in adults that is primarily benign and sometimes malignant [39]. Even though LCTs are the most common subtype of nongerm cell tumors, they only make up to 1–3% of testicular neoplasms [40]. Sertoli cell tumor is a sex cord-stromal neoplasm with Sertoli cell differentiation and they are usually well confined and often lobulated [41]. It does not occur in extra-testicular locations and is mostly described as painless testicular tumor [42]. Granulosa cell tumor: In an adult testicle, granulosa cell tumors are quite uncommon. In the testicle, it often appears as a painless lump. The average age of occurrence is 45 years [43].

Staging: The AJCC tumor-node-metastasis staging is commonly followed for testicular germ cell tumors [3]. TNM staging is a major factor that determines the treatment and prognosis in men with TC. In this classification system, the T stage is determined by pathological studies followed by orchiectomy and refers to the localized spread of the tumor [44]. N stage is determined by the involvement of the number and size of lymph nodes as well as the extra-nodal extension [45]. The presence or absence of distant metastatic disease is indicated by the M stage [44]. It is characterized by visceral metastatic disease and nonregional lymph node involvement. Visceral metastases are caused by testicular cancer spread through a hematogenous route, and CT scans are the most accurate way to detect them in the lungs and other target organs [46]. The four stages of TNM classification are: Stage 0 includes patients with GCNIS cells with a risk of developing testicular germ cell tumors with the need for close surveillance [3]. Stage I cancer is restricted to the testicle, epididymis, and spermatic cord. Although removing the testicle itself is needed to cure the patient but many patients seek further medical care to avoid relapse of the disease [47]. Stage II disease is restricted to retroperitoneal lymph nodes and is further subdivided into stages IIA, IIB, and IIC based on lymph node size. In IIC, the size of nodes can be greater than 5 cm [44]. The stage III, the tumor has progressed to tissues above the diaphragm, including the lungs and the neck/brain. Cancer may also develop in other regions of the body such as the bones or the liver. Chemotherapy is necessary in this situation. Surgery may also be required [47].

15.3 Pathophysiology

The male reproductive system contains a paired organ called the testicles. The testis is oval in structure and compressed laterally, present outside the body in the scrotal sac [48]. The tunica albuginea, which is a thick, fibrous capsule, encloses the testicles. The tunica vaginalis, which contains an inner visceral layer and an exterior parietal layer, envelopes the tunica albuginea [49]. The gubernaculum or caudal genital ligament shortens throughout the development of the fetus which allows the testis to descend into the scrotal cavity. For appropriate spermatogenesis to take place, this process is necessary to reduce the temperature by 1–2 °C in the testis. The blood flow in the testicles also helps to reduce the temperature as the arteries and veins are organized in a spiral pattern [48]. The testis contains three distinct cell types: germ cells, Sertoli cells, and Leydig cells, which develop into mature spermatozoa, provide support, and produce testosterone respectively [45].

The testicles are surrounded by tunica albuginea, which divides testicular tissue into lobules with seminiferous tubules or interstitial tissue [48]. The seminiferous tubules become rete testis at a portion that is not covered by the tunica layers and later into efferent tubules that combine to form a single duct called epididymis [45]. The mature sperms are transported into the anterior region of the epididymis by efferent tubules from the rete testis [48]. The vas deferens passes through the spermatic cord and finally combines with the excretory duct of the seminal vesicle to drain sperm into the ejaculatory duct in the prostate [45]. Numerous blood and lymphatic arteries are encircled in the interstitial compartment, which is composed of interstitial cells and loose connective tissue. The most well-known form of cells in the interstitial tissue that can synthesize several sex steroid hormones from precursor components are known as Leydig cells (Fig. 15.2). The lamina propria surrounds the seminiferous tubules, which are composed of somatic Sertoli cells or various stages of germ cells. Sertoli cells are known as nursery cells because these cells build the blood-testis barrier and secrete the tubular fluids (Fig. 15.2). They also provide the germ cells with hormonal stimulation and a nourishing environment. Several fetal and adult cell markers on the Sertoli cells help in their identification. The Sertoli cells play a significant role in releasing matured sperm into the tubular lumen [48].

Cell of Origin: Testicular cancer in adolescents and young adults has a common precursor cell known as the germ cell neoplasm in situ (GCNIS). GCNIS is a primordial germ cell (PGC), also known as the gonocyte, as it is an embryonic germ cell that failed to mature into a spermatogonium during the process of development [16]. The GCNIS cells that are located on the basal lamina have a considerable amount of cytoplasm. The nucleus can be large and spherical or irregular in shape

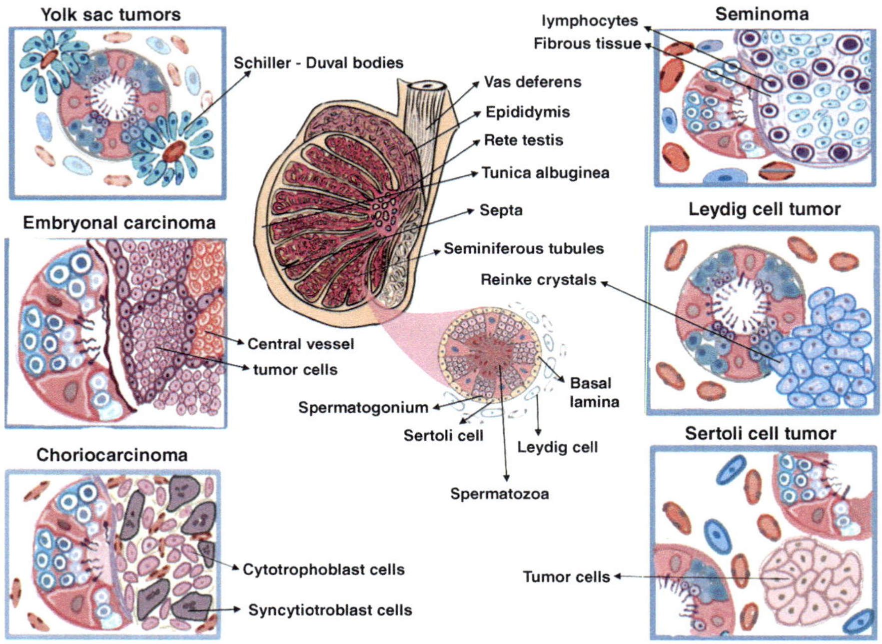

Fig. 15.2 Subtypes of testicular cancer and their cells of origin

containing tetraploid DNA with one or two nucleoli. The germ cells do not differentiate until puberty; during puberty, Sertoli and Leydig cells produce growth signals and hormones for inducing GCNISs to proliferate. Nonseminoma is derived from an earlier PGC and pure seminoma is derived from a later gonadal stem cell or the gonocyte (Fig. 15.2). Therefore, nonseminomas do not develop from seminomas and have a distinct cell of origin. Nonseminomas may express embryonal, extraembryonic, somatic germ cell (seminoma) components, whereas pure seminomas express only the germ cell phenotype [3, 50].

Genetics: TGCT is a cancer with high heritability with about 50 susceptibility genes [51]. The first genetic marker to be discovered for TGCT is a gain of chromosome 12 and the formation of an isochromosome (12p) in nearly 80% of cases [52]. According to The Cancer Genome Atlas, somatic mutations in the genes *KIT*, *KRAS*, and *NRAS* are frequent in TCs [53]. Testicular seminoma arises as a result of mutations in these three genes along with that of the *CDC27* gene [54]. The pathogenetic variations in GCNIS-related TGCTs set them apart from GCNIS-unrelated TGCTs. Aneuploidy or triploidy, including the gain of chromosomes X, 7, 8, 12p, and 21 as well as loss of chromosomes Y, 1p, 11, 13, and 18 are linked to GCNIS-related GCTs [55]. In rare cases, mutations in *KIT*, *K-RAS*, and *TP53* genes were observed for GCNIS-related GCTs [55]. Seminomas are typically hypertriploid, while nonseminomas are typically hypotriploid. The most common mutation, isochromosome 12p, can be found in both seminomas and nonseminomas [56]. The *KIT* gene expression is low in spermatogonia, but it is high in all GCNIS, the majority of seminomas, and certain nonseminomas. The tumor cell proliferation is thought to be triggered briefly by autocrine and paracrine stimulation when KIT is produced by malignant cells. In about 2% of nonseminoma tumors and 19% of seminoma tumors, the *KIT* gene is altered [56]. GCNIS-unrelated GCTs, on the other hand, express diploidy or aneuploidy with a gain of chromosomes 1q, 12, 20q and deletion of chromosomes 1p, 4, and 6p [55]. With clearly defined chromosomal gains and losses, yolk sac tumors are always aneuploid [57]. These are related to the gain on chromosome 1, loss on chromosome 6q, and gain on a portion of 12p (particularly 12p13) [57]. Genes *STELLA*, *NANOG*, and *GDF3* are speculated to be involved in yolk sac tumors [57]. In contrast to other TGCTs, spermatocytic tumors have a gain of chromosome 9 and in rare instances, mutations in the genes *H-RAS* and *FGFR3* [55].

15.4 Treatment

Radical inguinal orchiectomy is the primary treatment for testicular cancers [58]. After the affected testis is removed, histological analyses and staging assist in deciding on the next course of treatment, which may involve surgery, radiation, active monitoring, surveillance, dissection of the retroperitoneal lymph node, chemotherapy, or a combination of these treatments [59]. Treatment of GCNIS for stage 0 is surveillance with ultrasonography, orchiectomy, and radiotherapy [3]. For clinical stage I seminoma, patients who refused to engage in surveillance, primary radiation of 20–30 Gy to the ipsilateral pelvis and retroperitoneum is the recommended course of treatment [3]. This treatment has a 1% recurrence rate, but its widespread use is now restricted due to its longer-term cardiovascular side effects [3]. After orchiectomy, if the rising of tumor markers occur without evidence of metastasis on imaging, patients further undergo systemic chemotherapy [60].

Patients with stage I nonseminoma can be treated with adjuvant chemotherapy, nerve-sparing retroperitoneal lymph node dissection (NS-RPLND), and surveillance [61]. Patients with stage I nonseminoma at high risk and those with remaining retroperitoneal masses less than 1 cm after adjuvant chemotherapy and systemic chemotherapy may benefit from retroperitoneal lymph node removal [61, 62]. The probability of recurrence was extremely low in patients with histologically advanced teratomas that had not yet invaded the blood vessels [61]. In most cases, PEB (cisplatin, etoposide, and bleomycin) is administered twice to high-risk patients with vascular invasion [61]. Radiotherapy is the treatment of choice for patients in clinical stages IIA and IIB, with a relapse-free survival rate of 90 to 95% [60]. Induction chemotherapy with three cycles of BEP or four cycles of EP (etoposide and cisplatin) is becoming more popular for treating clinical stage IIA and IIB seminoma. From the para-aortic area to the ipsilateral iliac region, the standard radiation field should be expanded [3]. Chemotherapy using BEP, EP, or cisplatin-based chemotherapy regimens like VIP (etoposide, ifosfamide, cisplatin) or VeIP (vinblastine, ifosfamide, cisplatin) is the usual therapeutic option for advanced malignancies in stages IIC and III [3]. The IGCCCG included serum levels of hCG, AFP, and LDH in their approach for classifying diseases with high, moderate, and low prognosis risk [63].

15.5 Conclusion

Nearly 95% of cases of testicular cancer are curable, making it a highly treatable disease. The major risk factors include cryptorchidism followed by hypospadias, low sperm count, testicular dysgenesis, viruses, occupational exposure, and long-term consumption of drugs. WHO classified testicular cancer into germ cell tumors and stromal tumors. GCT is further classified into germ cell-related neoplasia in situ characterized by chromosome 12p amplification associated with aneuploidy or triploidy, and nonrelated germ cell neoplasia in situ that lacks 12p amplification and exhibits diploidy or aneuploidy. Based on TNM staging, treatment and diagnosis of TC are determined. Fertility and quality of life are key topics to address in testicular cancer patients, in addition to early detection, diagnosis, and therapy, which are all critical aspects of treating the condition. There is a need for individualized monitoring of testicular cancer-risk patients based on age, risk factors, infertility, and dysgenesis syndrome. This aids in determining whether patients require more attention or testicular biopsies. Men who underwent surgery for testicular cancer have experienced minimal impact on their health status than the men treated with chemotherapy or radiotherapy as part of their treatment.

References

1. Giona S. The epidemiology of testicular cancer. Exon Publications. 2022:107–16.
2. Cheng L, Albers P, Berney DM, Feldman DR, Daugaard G, Gilligan T, Looijenga LH. Testicular cancer. Nat Rev Dis Primers. 2018;4(1):29.
3. Gaddam SJ, Chesnut GT. Testicle cancer. In: StatPearls [Internet]. Treasure Island, FL: StatPearls Publishing; 2022.
4. Kusler KA, Poynter JN. International testicular cancer incidence rates in children, adolescents and young adults. Cancer Epidemiol. 2018;56:106–11.
5. Toppari J, Rodprasert W, Virtanen HE. Cryptorchidism–disease or symptom? Ann d'endocrinol. 2014;75(2):72–6.
6. Skakkebaek NE, Rajpert-De Meyts E, Buck Louis GM, Toppari J, Andersson AM, Eisenberg ML, Jensen TK, Jørgensen N, Swan SH, Sapra KJ, Ziebe S. Male reproductive disorders and fertility trends: influences of environment and genetic susceptibility. Physiol Rev. 2016;96(1):55–97.
7. Skakkebaek NE, De Meyts ER, Main KM. Testicular dysgenesis syndrome: an increasingly common developmental disorder with environmental aspects. APMIS. 2001;109(S103):S22–30.
8. Sonke GS, Chang S, Strom SS, Sweeney AM, Annegers JF, Sigurdson AJ. Prenatal and perinatal risk factors and testicular cancer: a hospital-based case-control study. Oncol Res. 2006;16(8):383–7.
9. Farmanfarma KK, Mahdavifar N, Mohammadian-Hafshejani A, Salehiniya H. Testicular cancer in the world: an epidemiological review. J Canc Res. 2018;5(4):1–5.

10. Reece AS, Hulse GK. State trends of cannabis liberalization as a causal driver of increasing testicular cancer rates across the USA. Int J Environ Res Public Health. 2022;19(19):12759.
11. Garner MJ, Turner MC, Ghadirian P, Krewski D. Epidemiology of testicular cancer: an overview. Int J Cancer. 2005;116(3):331–9.
12. McGlynn KA, Trabert B. Adolescent and adult risk factors for testicular cancer. Nat Rev Urol. 2012;9(6):339–49.
13. Winter C, Albers P. Testicular germ cell tumors: pathogenesis, diagnosis and treatment. Nat Rev Endocrinol. 2011;7(1):43–53.
14. Marko J, Wolfman DJ, Aubin AL, Sesterhenn IA. Testicular seminoma and its mimics: from the radiologic pathology archives. Radiographics. 2017;37(4):1085–98.
15. Boccellino M, Vanacore D, Zappavigna S, Cavaliere C, Rossetti S, D'Aniello C, Chieffi P, Amler E, Buonerba C, Di Lorenzo G, Di Franco R. Testicular cancer from diagnosis to epigenetic factors. Oncotarget. 2017;8(61):104654.
16. Baroni T, Arato I, Mancuso F, Calafiore R, Luca G. On the origin of testicular germ cell tumors: from gonocytes to testicular cancer. Front Endocrinol. 2019;10:343.
17. Berney DM, Cree I, Rao V, Moch H, Srigley JR, Tsuzuki T, Amin MB, Comperat EM, Hartmann A, Menon S, Netto GJ. An introduction to the WHO 5th edition 2022 classification of testicular tumours. Histopathology. 2022;81(4):459–66.
18. Katabathina VS, Vargas-Zapata D, Monge RA, Nazarullah A, Ganeshan D, Tammisetti V, Prasad SR. Testicular germ cell tumors: classification, pathologic features, imaging findings, and management. Radiographics. 2021;41(6):1698–716.
19. Gupta M, Cheaib JG, Patel HD, Sharma R, Zhang A, Bass EB, Pierorazio PM. Diagnosis and management of intratubular germ cell neoplasia in situ: a systematic review. J Urol. 2020;204(1):33–41.
20. Lamichhane A, Mukkamalla SK. Seminoma. In: StatPearls [Internet]. Treasure Island, FL: StatPearls Publishing; 2022.
21. Smith ZL, Werntz RP, Eggener SE. Testicular cancer: epidemiology, diagnosis, and management. Med Clin. 2018;102(2):251–64.
22. Balalaa N, Salman M, Hassen W. Burned-out testicular tumor: a case report. Case Rep Oncol. 2011;4(1):12–5.
23. Shahrokh S, Hebert M, Jeong W, Guo S. Burned-out testicular germ cell tumor presenting as retroperitoneal lymphadenopathy in a patient with cryptorchidism: a case report & review of literature. Cureus. 2022;14(7):e26776.
24. Iczkowski KA. Germ cell neoplasms of the testis: update for 2022. Sem Diagn Pathol. 2023;40(1):2–21.
25. Nauman M, Leslie SW. Nonseminomatous testicular tumors. [Updated 12 August 2021]. In: StatPearls. Treasure Island, FL: StatPearls Publishing. p. 2022.
26. Howitt BE, Berney DM. Tumors of the testis: morphologic features and molecular alterations. Surg Pathol Clin. 2015;8(4):687–716.
27. Ml K, Kumar A. Yolk sac tumors. 2020.
28. Nassri R, Muftah M, Nassri A, Alkhasawneh A, Corak J. Pure testicular choriocarcinoma with dermatological, brain, and gastrointestinal metastases. Cureus. 2018;10(8).
29. Yun J, Lee SW, Lim SH, Kim SH, Kim CK, Park SK. Successful treatment of a high-risk nonseminomatous germ cell tumor using etoposide, methotrexate, actinomycin D, cyclophosphamide, and vincristine: a case report. World J Clin Cases. 2020;8(21):5334.
30. Sindhu II, Noor N, Mansoor R. Choriocarcinoma syndrome: a rare presentation of testicular germ cell tumour. J Pak Med Assoc. 2021;71(8):2090–2.
31. Farci F, Shamsudeen S. Testicular teratoma. 2021.
32. Ameli F, Panahi P, Soleimani V. Burned-out post pubertal teratoma presenting as a liver metastases in a 34-year-old male. Iran J Pathol. 2021;16(2):232.
33. Williamson SR, Delahunt B, Magi-Galluzzi C, Algaba F, Egevad L, Ulbright TM, Tickoo SK, Srigley JR, Epstein JI, Berney DM. Members of the ISUP testicular tumour panel. The World Health Organization 2016 classification of testicular germ cell tumours: a review and

update from the International Society of Urological Pathology Testis Consultation Panel. Histopathology. 2017;70(3):335–46.
34. Betancourt-Torres M, Figueroa-Diaz L, Rodriguez-Mojica W. Paratesticular dermoid cyst mimicking a Torsed supernumerary testis: a case report. Am J Case Rep. 2020;21:e923752–1.
35. Sangüesa C, Veiga D, Llavador M, Serrano A. Testicular tumours in children: an approach to diagnosis and management with pathologic correlation. Insights Imaging. 2020;11:1–4.
36. Amine MM, Mohamed B, Mourad H, Majed H, Slim C, Mehdi B, Hela M, Nouri R, Rim K, Tahya B, Nabil MM. Neuroendocrine testicular tumors: a systematic review and meta-analysis. Curr Urol. 2017;10(1):15–25.
37. Friedlander TW, Small E. Testicular cancer. In: Abeloff's clinical oncology. Elsevier; 2020. p. 1442–67.
38. Zhu P, Duan Y, Ao Q, Wang G. Microcystic stromal tumor of testicle: first case report and literature review. Cancer Res Treat. 2018;50(4):1452–7.
39. Kong Q, Yu Y, Tian T, Zhang H, Sun M, Liu R, Liu Y. Leydig cell tumor of a testis with azoospermia: a case report and literature review. Medicine. 2020;99(36):e22085.
40. Ruf CG, Sanatgar N, Isbarn H, Ruf B, Simon J, Fankhauser CD, Dieckmann KP. Leydig-cell tumour of the testis: retrospective analysis of clinical and therapeutic features in 204 cases. World J Urol. 2020;38:2857–62.
41. Ross J. Testicular tumors. 2010. https://doi.org/10.1016/B978-1-4160-3204-5.00052-9.
42. Levin HS. Neoplasms of the testis. In: Genitourinary pathology. Churchill Livingstone; 2007. p. 534–622.
43. Song Z, Vaughn DJ, Bing Z. Adult type granulosa cell tumor in adult testis: report of a case and review of the literature. Rare Tumors. 2011;3(4):117–9.
44. Coursey Moreno C, Small WC, Camacho JC, Master V, Kokabi N, Lewis M, Hartman M, Mittal PK. Testicular tumors: what radiologists need to know—differential diagnosis, staging, and management. Radiographics. 2015;35(2):400–15.
45. Magers MJ, Idrees MT. Updates in staging and reporting of testicular cancer. Surg Pathol Clin. 2018;11(4):813–24.
46. Brunereau L, Bruyère F, Linassier C, Baulieu JL. The role of imaging in staging and monitoring testicular cancer. Diagn Interv Imaging. 2012;93(4):310–8.
47. Vasdev N, Moon A, Thorpe AC. Classification, epidemiology and therapies for testicular germ cell tumours. Int J Dev Biol. 2013;57(2-3-4):133–9.
48. Fietz D, Bergmann M. Functional anatomy and histology of the testis. Endocrinology of the testis and male reproduction. Cham: Springer International Publishing; 2017. p. 313–41.
49. Kundra V. Testicular cancer. Sem Roentgenol. 2004;39(3):437–50.
50. Som A, Wen S, Tu SM. Stem cell origin of testicular seminoma. Clin Genitourin Cancer. 2013;11(4):489–94.
51. Das MK, Kleppa L, Haugen TB. Functions of genes related to testicular germ cell tumour development. Andrology. 2019;7(4):527–35.
52. Kiliccioglu I, Konaç E, Sozen S. Genomic evaluation of testicular germ cell tumors and its role in treatment planning. Bull Urooncol. 2018;17.
53. Mealey NE, O'Sullivan DE, Peters CE, Heng DY, Brenner DR. Mutational signatures among young-onset testicular cancers. BMC Med Genet. 2021;14(1):1–9.
54. Mo L, Yu Z, Lv Y, Cheng J, Yan H, Lu W, Su C, Ling Q, Mo Z. Single-cell RNA sequencing of metastatic testicular seminoma reveals the cellular and molecular characteristics of metastatic cell lineage. Front Oncol. 2022;12.
55. Ronchi A, Pagliuca F, Franco R. Testicular germ cell tumors: the changing role of the pathologist. Ann Transl Med. 2019;7(Suppl 6):S204.
56. Buljubašić R, Buljubašić M, Bojanac AK, Ulamec M, Vlahović M, Ježek D, Bulić-Jakuš F, Sinčić N. Epigenetics and testicular germ cell tumors. Gene. 2018;661:22–33.
57. Looijenga LH, Kao CS, Idrees MT. Predicting gonadal germ cell cancer in people with disorders of sex development; insights from developmental biology. Int J Mol Sci. 2019;20(20):5017.
58. Shaw J. Diagnosis and treatment of testicular cancer. Am Fam Physician. 2008;77(4):469–74.

59. Krege S. Diagnostik, Therapie und Nachsorge beim Hodentumor. Der Urol Ausg A. 2017;56(12):1623–36.
60. Chovanec M, Cheng L. Advances in diagnosis and treatment of testicular cancer. BMJ. 2022:379.
61. Kopp HG, Kuczyk M, Classen J, Stenzl A, Kanz L, Mayer F, Bamberg M, Hartmann JT. Advances in the treatment of testicular cancer. Drugs. 2006;66:641–59.
62. Hu B, Daneshmand S. Retroperitoneal lymph node dissection as primary treatment for metastatic seminoma. Adv Urol. 2018;2018.
63. Ehrlich Y, Margel D, Lubin MA, Baniel J. Advances in the treatment of testicular cancer. Transl Androl Urol. 2015;4(3):381.

Brain Cancer

16

Salwa Hareem, Vigneswar Reddy Ashireddygari,
Prasad Tammineni, and Rama Krishna Kancha

16.1 Introduction

Epidemiology: Central nervous system (CNS) cancers affect a staggering percentage of the population across all ages accounting to 1.6% of global incidence of all cancers [1]. CNS cancer ranks tenth in terms of mortality [1]. Eastern Asia has the highest cases and fatality rate, followed by South-Central Asia and Northern America. According to GLOBOCAN, males show higher global incidence (168,346 cases; cumulative risk: 0.40) and mortality rates (138,277 deaths; cumulative risk 0.34) than females (incidence: 139,756 cases; cumulative risk 0.31; mortality: 113,052 deaths; cumulative risk 0.26). In the United States, the median age of diagnosis and death are 59 and 66, respectively and the age-adjusted rate of incidence was 7.08 per 100,000 during 2013–2017 [2]. Malignant tumors constitute 29.7% and nonmalignant tumors comprise 70.3% of all the brain and CNS cancers [3]. The frequencies of nonmalignant tumors also vary by type: nonmalignant meningioma (37.9%) and nonmalignant glioma (1.0%) [3]. Besides the incidence, it is found that primary brain malignancies are more frequent in the frontal region (24.3%) followed by the temporal (17.5%), parietal (10.4%), and occipital (2.6%) areas making up to 54.8% of the total [3].

Risk Factors: The risk factors for brain tumors include environmental and genetic disorders or synchronous chronic diseases [4]. Ionizing radiation is a risk factor whose exposure might be occupational or resulting from medical operations such as the radiotherapy [4]. Meningiomas are the most prevalent tumors associated with

S. Hareem · R. K. Kancha (✉)
Molecular Medicine and Therapeutics Laboratory, CPMB, Osmania University, Hyderabad, India
e-mail: ramakancha@osmania.ac.in

V. R. Ashireddygari · P. Tammineni
Department of Animal Biology, School of Life Sciences, University of Hyderabad, Hyderabad, India

R. K. Kancha (ed.), *Biomedical Aspects of Solid Cancers*,
https://doi.org/10.1007/978-981-97-1802-3_16

prior brain irradiation, the others being glioblastomas and low-grade gliomas [5]. Children appear to be more susceptible to radiation-induced carcinogenic effects. Allergic and atopic disorders such as asthma and allergic rhinitis reduce the risk of several neoplasms such as the gliomas and the meningiomas [4]. For example, a 40% reduced risk of gliomas was associated with allergies [6]. Levels of IgE in blood, a potential marker for allergies, are lower in patients with gliomas. Regular statin use has been linked to a 25% reduction in the risk of glioma [7]. Based on multiple prospective studies for various malignancies, a person's height is recognized as a risk factor for glioma; a 20% increase in the glioma risk was observed per 10 cm increase in height [7]. Most glioma cases lack a family history; however, it is important to note that nearly 5% of gliomas are familial.

Diagnosis: Diagnosis of a brain tumor involves the use of an MRI, CT scan, biopsy, blood tests, and lumbar puncture. Headache is a presenting symptom in up to 50% of patients [8]. Optic disc swelling is linked to headaches in 15–25% of individuals [8]. Up to 40% of patients presenting with brain metastases experience localized symptoms such as paralysis or numbness, while 15–20% of patients experience seizures [8]. MRI and CT scans are the most commonly used imaging tests for brain malignancies (CAT scan, CT scan) [8]. MRS and fMRI are two more procedures that are frequently used for research and sometimes surgical planning. Positron emission test (PET) can identify minute abnormalities in blood flow and oxygen consumption, which are common in brain malignancies.

Mutation in *IDH1* or *IDH2* and *TP53* genes and overexpression of *PDGFA* and *PDGFB* genes are the most common molecular markers for WHO grade 2 astrocytoma [9]. IDH1-R132H protein may be detected with high accuracy using mutation-specific antibodies [10, 11]. Loss of 9p and 19q, as well as an *RB1* mutation, contributes to astrocytoma (WHO grade 3); further loss of 10q leads to astrocytoma (WHO grade 4) [9, 12]. 1p and 19q co-deletion were found in up to 80% of grade 2 and around 60% of grade 3 oligodendrogliomas [13, 14]. The most common techniques used for 1p/19q testing are loss of heterozygosity or fluorescent in situ hybridization analyses [12, 15, 16]. In primary glioblastomas, the *EGFR* gene amplification or overexpression affects approximately 40% of these tumors [17, 18]. Analysis of *EGFRvIII* gene can be done by RT-PCR [12]. The GFAP and miRNA-21 are the only circulating diagnostic markers for glioblastoma patients [19].

16.2 Classification

Initial categorization of brain and CNS cancers was based on histological features, including marked mitotic activity, florid microvascular proliferation, and necrosis: grade I refers to benign, grade II to semi-benign, grade III to less malignant, and grade IV to highly malignant tumors. However, with the advent of genomic data, the WHO integrated histological–molecular features into classification (Fig. 16.1) [20]. Recently, the fifth edition of WHO classification (2021) incorporated molecular markers of clinicopathologic importance for the purpose of most accurate

Cancers of CNS

- **1. GLIOMAS, GLIONEURAL & NEURONAL TUMORS**
  - **Adult-type diffuse gliomas**
    Astrocytoma, IDH-mutant, oligodendroglioma, IDH-mutant, and 1p/19q-codeleted, glioblastoma, IDH-wildtype.
  - **Pediatric-type diffuse low-grade gliomas**
    Diffuse astrocytoma MYB- or MYBL1-altered, angiocentric glioma, polymorphous low-grade neuroepithelial tumor of the young, diffuse low-grade glioma, MAPK pathway-altered.
  - **Pediatric-type diffuse high-grade gliomas**
    Diffuse midline glioma, H3 K27-altered, diffuse hemispheric glioma, H3 G34-mutan, diffuse pediatric-type high-grade glioma, H3-wildtype and IDH-wildtype, infant-type hemisphericglioma.
  - **Circumscribed astrocytic gliomas**
    Pilocytic astrocytoma, high-grade astrocytoma with piloid features, pleomorphic xanthoastrocytoma, subependymal giant cell astrocytoma, chordoid glioma astroblastoma, MN1-altered.
  - **Ependymal tumors**
    Supratentorial ependymoma, supratentorial ependymoma, ZFTA fusion-positive, supratentorial ependymoma, YAP1 fusion-positive, posterior fossa ependymoma, Posterior fossal ependymoma, group PFA, posterior fossa ependymoma, group PFB, spinal ependymoma, spinal ependymoma, MYCN-amplified, myxopapillary ependymoma, subependymoma.
  - **Glioneuronal and neuronal tumors**
    Ganglioglioma, desmoplastic infantile ganglioglioma / desmoplastic infantile astrocytoma, dysembryoplastic neuroepithelial tumor, diffuse glioneuronal tumor with oligodendroglioma-like features and nuclear clusters, papillary glioneuronal tumor, rosette-forming glioneuronal tumor, myxoid glioneuronal tumor, diffuse leptomeningeal glioneuronal tumor, gangliocytoma multinodular and vacuolating neuronal tumor, dysplastic cerebellar gangliocytoma (Lhermitte-Duclos disease), central neurocytoma, extraventricular neurocytoma, cerebellar liponeurocytoma.
- **2. CHOROID PLEXUS TUMORS**
  Choroid plexus papilloma, atypical choroid plexus papilloma, choroid plexus carcinoma.
- **3. HISTIOCYTIC TUMORS**
  erdheim-chester disease, rosai-Dorfman disease, Juvenile xanthogranuloma, langerhans cell, histiocytic sarcoma.
- **4. HEMATOLYMPHOID TUMORS**
  Lymphomas (CNS lymphomas ,miscellaneous lymphomas).
- **5. MELANOCYTIC TUMORS**
  Diffuse meningeal melanocytic neoplasms (meningeal melanocytosis and meningeal melanomatosis), circumscribed meningeal melanocytic neoplasms (meningeal melanocytoma and meningeal melanoma).
- **6. PINEAL TUMORS**
  Pineocytoma Pineal, parenchymal tumor of intermediate differentiation, pineoblastoma Papillary tumor of the pineal region, desmoplastic myxoid tumor of the pineal region, SMARCB1-mutant.
- **7. MENINGIOMAS**
- **8. MESENCHYMAL, NON-MENINGIOTHELIAL**
  Soft tissue tumors (fibroblastic and myofibroblastic tumors, vascular tumors, skeletal muscle tumors, uncertain differentiation), chondro-osseous tumors, notochordal tumors.
- **9. CRANIAL AND PARASPINAL NERVE TUMORS**
  Schwannoma, neurofibroma, perineurioma hybrid nerve sheath tumor, malignant melanotic nerve sheath tumor, malignant peripheral nerve sheath tumor, paraganglioma.
- **10. EMBRYONAL TUMORS**
  Medulloblastoma (medulloblastomas molecularly defined, medulloblastomas histologically defined), other CNS embryonal tumors (atypical teratoid/rhabdoid tumor, cribriform neuroepithelial tumor, embryonal tumor with multilayered rosettes, CNS neuroblastoma FOXR2-activated, CNS tumor with BCOR internal tandem duplication, CNS embryonal tumor.
- **11. GERM CELL TUMORS**
  Mature teratoma, immature teratoma, teratoma with somatic-type malignancy, germinoma, embryonal carcinoma, yolk sac tumor choriocarcinoma, mixed germ cell tumor.
- **12. TUMORS OF THE SELLAR REGION**
  Adamantinomatous craniopharyngioma, papillary craniopharyngioma, pituicytoma, granular cell tumor of the sellar region, and spindle cell oncocytoma, pituitary adenoma/PitNET, Pituitary blastoma.
- **13. Metastases to the CNS**

Fig. 16.1 Classification of central nervous system cancers

classification (Fig. 16.1) [21]. Some of the salient features of WHO's fifth edition (WHO CNS5) are:

(a) The categorization of gliomas, glioneuronal tumors, and neuronal tumors has been expanded to 14 new types. Importantly, the CNS5 distinguishes diffuse gliomas as "adult-type" and "pediatric-type" as prognostically and physiologically diverse tumors (Fig. 16.1) [21].
(b) Based on the histological and molecular changes, adult common diffuse gliomas were updated to three major categories: IDH-mutant astrocytoma, IDH-mutant and 1p/19q-co-deleted oligodendroglioma, and IDH-wild-type glioblastoma (Fig. 16.1) [21].
(c) Meningioma is classified as a single type, with 15 subgroups reflecting its wide morphological diversity. It is currently stressed that regardless of the underlying subtype, the criteria for identifying atypical or grade 2 and 3 anaplastic meningioma should be the same [21].
(d) "Melanotic schwannoma" is an aggressive cancer with distinct genetic foundations that differentiate it from all other nerve sheath tumors and is renamed as malignant melanotic nerve sheath tumor [21].
(e) In nonmeningothelial mesenchymal tumors, the word "hemangiopericytoma" has been phased out, and the tumor is now known simply as a Solitary fibrous tumor.
(f) Tumors such as adamantinomatous craniopharyngioma and papillary craniopharyngioma were categorized as different tumor entities [21–23].
(g) The WHO endocrine group recommended the new term pituitary neuroendocrine tumor (PitNET) [21, 24]. Finally, Pituitary blastoma was included in the WHO CNS5 [21].

16.3 Pathophysiology

Anatomy: Meninges are three membranes that wrap and separate the brain from the walls of the skull. Dura mater, arachnoid mater, and pia mater are the outer, middle, and inner membrane coverings of the meninges [25]. Meningiomas arise from the cap cells of the arachnoid layer and are usually benign [26]. In adults, they account for more than 30% of the CNS cancers [27]. The cerebrospinal fluid (CSF) fills the spaces of pia mater and arachnoid mater that serves as a cushion [25]. In the CNS, CSF replaces the lymph [25]. The brain's ventricular system comprises four CSF-filled cavities [28]. The brain almost floats in the CSF, preventing exerting any weight on the neck [25]. CSF is found in the ventricle system and the subarachnoid area of the brain as well as the spinal cord [25]. Ependymal cells line the ventricular system [29]. CSF is primarily produced by choroid plexuses (CPs) that are specialized, highly vascularized ependymal structures [30]. Choroid plexus tumors (CPT) arise from the epithelium and contribute to 10–20% of pediatric (less than 1 year of age) brain cancers [31, 32]. Anatomically, CPT tumors are located in supratentorial (32%), fourth ventricular (57%), and supra-infratentorial regions (11%) [33].

Ependymomas, which account for 10% and 25% of primary CNS and spinal cord cancers, respectively, arise from the lining of the cerebral ventricles or the spinal cord central canal [34].

Cerebrum, cerebellum, and brainstem are the three major regions of the brain [35]. The cerebral hemispheres are two enormous masses that are virtually similar and present side by side [36]. The corpus callosum is a large, flat, densely myelinated axon bundle that unites the brain hemispheres [36]. Gyri (convolutions and ridges), which are divided by sulcus (slightly deeper groove) or fissure (exceedingly deep groove), are present on the surface of cerebral hemisphere [37]. Central, lateral, and parietooccipital sulci along with the two imaginary lines on the lateral surface of the brain, divide the cerebrum into frontal, parietal, temporal, and occipital lobes [36]. Diffuse gliomas (DGs) can occur in any part of the brain; however, they are most common in the frontal (25.9%) and temporal lobes (19.8%) (Fig. 16.2) [38]. Supratentorial, particularly in the frontal lobe, is a common location for diffuse astrocytomas (DAs) (Fig. 16.2). Oligoastrocytomas (OAs) can occur anywhere in the brain's central hemisphere, but the most prevalent sites are the frontal and temporal lobes (Fig. 16.2). Oligodendrogliomas (ODGs) affect the cerebral hemispheres and are more localized in the frontal, occipital, and parietal lobes [39]. Glioblastomas (GBMs) are more frequent in cerebral hemispheres followed by the temporal and parietal lobes (Fig. 16.2) [40].

The cerebellum is divided into two massive bilateral lobes known as cerebellar hemispheres [41]. A midline worm-like part, the vermis, connects these two lobes [42]. Medulloblastoma represents 30% of pediatric brain cancers and 7–8% of all

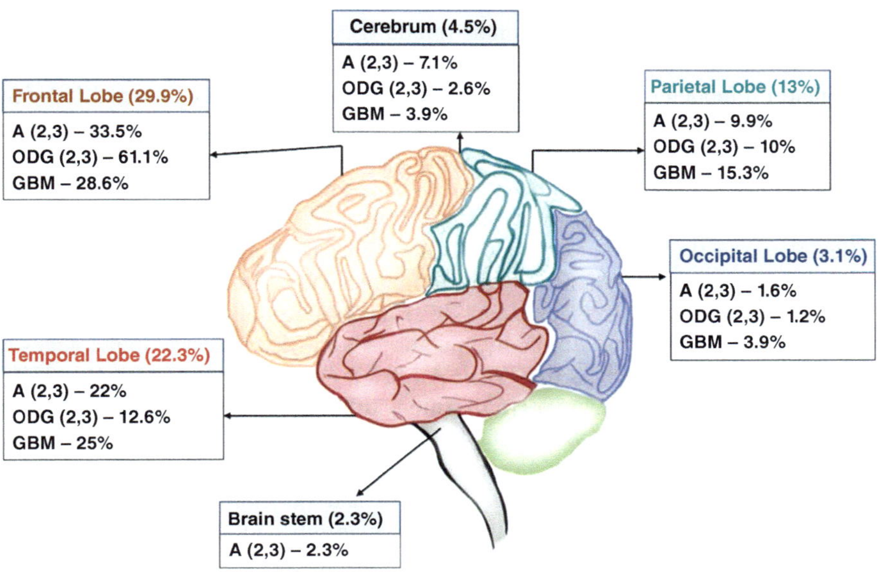

Fig. 16.2 Based on anatomy and histology, the distribution of malignant gliomas and adult diffuse-type diffuse gliomas

brain malignancies [43]. It begins in the cerebellum and can spread via CSF into the spine [44]. The cavity of the fourth ventricle separates the cerebellum from the pons and the medulla [42]. The cerebellum is connected to the brainstem by three bundles (superior, middle, and inferior) of fibers known as cerebellar peduncles [41]. The brainstem comprises a diencephalon followed by the midbrain, pons, and medulla oblongata. The diencephalon constitutes the epithalamus, subthalamus, hypothalamus, and thalamus [45]. Langerhans cell histiocytic tumor (LCH) is a histiocytic tumor most typically found in the hypothalamus [46]. The midbrain connects the pons and the diencephalon. The medulla oblongata is the most inferior portion of the midbrain, connecting the pons to the spinal cord. It meets the spinal cord at the foramen magnum.

Cell of Origin: Cells of the CNS are of two types: neuroectodermal origin that includes neurons, astrocytes, oligodendrocytes, and ependymocytes, and mesenchymal origin that contributes to the formation of meninges, adipose tissue, and microglia [47]. Astrocytes are the predominant type of glial cells with fibrous cells present in the white matter and protoplasmic cells present in the gray matter [48–50]. Oligodendrocytes extend from the brain into the proximal segments of cranial nerves [29, 47].

Gliomas, Glioneural, and Neuronal Tumors: Adult-type diffuse gliomas (DGs) account for about one-fourth of primary brain cancers and about three-quarters of malignant brain cancers with a slightly higher incidence observed in males than in females (male:female ratio, 1.29:1) [51]. These tumors are more common and may occur at any age. Men are marginally more likely to develop astrocytomas (grade II) than women in the range of 30–40 years of age [51]. In astrocytic and oligodendroglial gliomas, more than 70% of patients have mutated *IDH1,* or less commonly, *IDH2* mutations [52]. In astrocytomas (grade II), *IDH* mutation (70%), activating *TERT* mutation (4%), loss-of-function *TP53* (94%), *ATRX* (86%), and SWI/SNF chromatin remodeler *SMARCA4* (6%) mutations are frequently reported [53–55]. Astrocytomas have the propensity to grow into higher-grade gliomas over 4–5 years [56]. The most frequent mutations in astrocytoma (grade III) are *MGMT* promoter methylation (54.7%) and *ATRX loss* (40%) [57]. Astrocytoma (grade III) has a poor prognosis with a 5-year survival rate of 27.9% [58]. Oligodendroglioma (ODG) cases were mostly reported between 40 and 60 years of age and the frequency is slightly higher in males when compared to females [51]. Mutations in ODG include that of *TERT* promoter (96%), *IDH* (70%), 1p/19q co-deletion, *CIC* (62%), and *FUBP1* (29%) [54, 55]. Additionally, mutations were also observed in the genes of PI3K-AKT pathway such as the *PIK3CA* (20%), *PIK3R1* (9%), *NOTCH1* (31%), *ZBTB20* (9%), and *ARID1A* (6%) [55]. Among diffuse gliomas, ODGs have the best prognosis, with a 10-year OS rate of 64%. ODG-grade III accounts for about 2% of DGs [51]. ODG is characterized by the mutations in *IDH* (100%), *CIC* (50–70%), *FUBP1* (30%), loss of *CDKN2A* (35–50%), and deletions in chromosome 10 (19–25%) [59]. ODG has a better prognosis than other grade III cancers, with a 10-year OS rate of 38.9% [59–61]. GBMs contribute to 45–50% of all malignant brain tumors, are more frequent in males than females, and have a 2-year OS rate of 15.2% [40]. Majority of genetic alterations include the amplification of *EGFR*

(~40%), *BRAF* (5%), *PTEN* (~30%), and *NF1* (15–18%) apart from the disruption in p53 (87%) and retinoblastoma (Rb) (78%) pathways.

Choroid Plexus Tumors: Anatomically, most CPT tumors are located either in the lateral ventricles (32%) or in the fourth ventricle (57%) [33]. Copy-number alterations that were frequently observed are gains of chromosomes 12q (77%), 12p (72%), and 7 (72%), and loss of 21q (34%), 10 (23%), and 13q (19%) [33]. Choroid plexus carcinomas (CPC) are most common in children and are linked to Li-Fraumeni syndrome with *TP53* gene germline mutations [62]. Somatic *TP53* mutations were found in 36–60% of CPCs and have poor prognosis [62, 63].

Histiocytic Tumors: In CNS5, histiocytic tumors were further classified into Langerhans cell (LCH), Juvenile xanthogranuloma (JXG), Erdheim-Chester disease (ECD), Rosai-Dorfman disease (RDD), and histiocytic sarcoma [26]. LCH is the most frequent of the histiocytic tumors, with a median incidence age of 12 years [50]. JXG predominantly affects young children, whereas ECD primarily affects adults. RDD can affect people of all ages including children and adults [50]. The rarest subtype, histiocytic sarcoma is seen in both juvenile and adult populations, located in the hypothalamus, optic chiasm, and infundibulum and has mutations frequently either in *BRAF* (V600E) or *MAP2K1* genes [50]. The most frequent mutations were found in *KRAS* and *MAP2K1,* accounting for 33% of tumors [64]. ECD is a condition that often manifests in the middle age with a median age of onset of 53 years. ECD is characterized by mutations in *BRAF, ARAF, N/KRAS, MAP2K1,* and *PIK3CA* genes, and fusions involving *ALK* and *NTRK1* genes [65].

Hematolymphoid Tumors: In the new CNS5 classification, CNS and miscellaneous lymphomas were kept under one type of lymphoma [26]. Primary central nervous system lymphomas (PCNSL) make up to 4% of all extra-nodal lymphomas as well as intracranial neoplasms [66]. Only 10–15% of the PCNSLs affect the infratentorial region of the brain [50]. The majority of tumors are deep and near the lateral ventricles [50]. PCNSL occurs more frequently in immunocompetent patients than immunocompromised patients [67]. Importantly, PCNSLs were generally identified with either single-nucleotide variants (SNVs) or coSNVs of MYD88L265P and CD79B, which are engaged in upregulating the NF-kB signaling pathway [67]. CNAs include loss of chromosomal regions that harbor *HLA-B, HLA-C, TNFAIP3, PTPRK, PRDM1,* and *CDKN2A* genes and gain of chromosomal regions that harbor *STAT6, MDM2, CDK4, JAK2, PD-L1,* and *PD-L2* genes [68, 69].

Melanocytic Tumors: The number of leptomeningeal melanocytes are higher in people with dark skin [70]. Melanocytes are abundantly located in the brainstem as well as the base of the brain [70]. According to CNS5, melanocytic tumors were further divided into diffuse and circumscribed meningeal melanocytic neoplasms [26]. Diffuse meningeal melanocytic neoplasms developed from melanocytes are highly related to activating somatic mutations in codon 61 of *NRAS* and BRAF (V600E) [58, 71]. Meningeal melanocytoma is a well-differentiated circumscribed tumor that differs from highly aggressive melanoma [72, 73]. They are rare low-grade tumors and are prevalent in adults but can appear at any age from 9 to 73 years [74]. Melanocytomas are characterized by *GNAQ* or *GNA11* hotspot mutations, commonly involving codon 209 [75]. Additionally, mutations in *SF3B1* and *EIF1AX* genes are also reported [76].

Pineal Tumors: Pinealocytes are the primary cells in the pineal gland, which is situated between the brain's two hemispheres [77]. The essential role of pinealocytes is to secrete melatonin, which is vital for regulating circadian rhythms [77]. The pineal gland constitutes 95% of pinealocytes and 5% of astrocytes [78]. Pineal neoplasms are rare tumors primarily affecting children, accounts for 3–11% of pediatric and 1% of adult brain cancers [79]. Loss of function mutations in *DICER1*, *DROSHA*, and *DGCR8* are frequent in the PB [80]. Indeed, PB is the most prevalent CNS tumor in those with germline *DICER1* mutations [81].

Meningiomas: Meningiomas account for 37.6% of all CNS cancers and almost 50% of all benign brain cancers [8, 82]. The WHO classification lists 15 subtypes of meningioma [26]. The most common abnormalities are deletions in chromosomal 22q and mutations in the *NF2* gene [83]. Initial events are deletion of chromosomes 1p and 10 [84]. Homozygous deletion of *CDKN2A/B* is an indication of an aggressive fate [85]. WHO grade 1 meningiomas that are of *NF2* wild-type genotype contain mutations in *AKT1* (20%), *SMO* (11%), *KLF4* (28%), *PIK3CA* (7%), and *TRAF7* (40%) [86–91]. Meningiomas with WHO grade 2 meningiomas have *SMARCE1* mutations (97%) [89]. Mutations in the promoter of *TERT* gene were identified as a risk factor for recurrence [74, 92]. Similarly, regardless of histological criteria for anaplasia, meningiomas with mutation in the promoter of *TERT* gene and/or deletion of *CDKN2A/B* are assigned to WHO grade III [8].

Mesenchymal, Nonmeningothelial: They are classified as soft tissue tumors, chondro-osseous tumors, and notochordal tumors [26]. The fibroblastic neoplasm accounts for fewer than 1% of all CNS tumors with *NAB2-STAT6* gene fusion and immunoexpression of *STAT6* gene [93, 94]. Mutations in the *TERT* promoter and *TP53* were found in aggressive, solitary fibrous tumors [95]. An inflammatory myofibroblastic tumor (IMT) is most commonly found in the lung, retroperitoneum, and pelvis. However, a few cases are reported in the dura and leptomeninges of CNS [96–99]. In IMT, the prevalence of *ALK* immune-expression and *ALK* fusions is around 30% [96]. Vascular tumors comprise hemangiomas and hemangioblastomas [100]. Hemangiomas are benign vascular neoplasms with mutations in *KRAS, BRAF, KRIT, CCM2,* and *PDCD10* genes [100]. Additionally, somatic mutations in certain genes were found [101]. Hemangioblastomas are rare WHO grade 1 tumor that account for fewer than 2% of all brain tumors [100]. The cerebellum is the most common location [102]. Hemangioblastoma has a good prognosis, especially in resected sporadic cases [100]. Tumors of uncertain differentiation are mesenchymal neoplasms characterized by the fusion of *EWSR1* to *CREB1, ATF1,* or *CREM* genes [100]. Mesenchymal chondrosarcoma is a rare, intracranial, and well-defined malignant tumor that primarily affects our skeletal system [103]. It usually affects between 20 to 40 years of age [104]. It was previously thought to be a bone neoplasm, but now CNS is the most prevalent location of extraosseous mesenchymal chondrosarcoma [18].

Cranial and Paraspinal Nerve Tumors: In recent WHO classification of brain and CNS cancer, these tumors are further classified into schwannoma, neurofibroma, malignant melanotic nerve sheath tumor, perineurioma hybrid nerve sheath tumor, paraganglioma, and malignant peripheral nerve sheath tumor [26]. Most schwannomas develop from the dorsal nerve root, whereas neurofibromas develop from the ventral nerve root [105]. The genetic hallmark of schwannomas in both sporadic familial types is a mutation in the *NF2* gene apart from mutations in *ARID1A*, *ARID1B*, *DDR1* genes and *SH3PXD2A-HTRA1* fusion gene [106]. Subsets of schwannomas have recurrent mutations in [107]. Schwannomatosis is sporadic in the majority of cases (75–85%), with roughly 15–25% being hereditary [106]. In most cases, the germline mutations that cause schwannomatosis are present in *SMARCB1* or *LZTR1* genes [108, 109]. Neurofibroma is a benign tumor formed from neoplastic schwann cells. The only recurring defect in neurofibromas is the loss of function mutation in the *NF1* gene [110]. The nerve sheath has three layers endoneurium, perineum, and epineurium [111]. Perineuriomas are benign tumors made up of malignant perineurial cells. Most intraneural perineuriomas contain *TRAF7* mutations, while a significant fraction has *NF2*/chromosome 22 abnormalities [112]. The known molecular genetic alterations are deletions of *NF1* or *NF2* loci and are mutually exclusive to each other [113]. Few subsets of benign nerve sheath tumors are challenging to define and categorize because they have characteristics of more than one known subtype [114]. These tumors are called hybrid nerve sheath tumors [114].

Embryonal Tumors: Medulloblastomas are embryonal tumors of the posterior fossa that contribute to 20% of all pediatric CNS malignancies and include WNT-activated medulloblastoma, SHH-activated (*TP53*-wild type & mutant), and non-WNT/non-SHH, groups 3 and 4 [100, 115, 116]. WNT-activated medulloblastomas frequently carry *CTNNB1* exon 3 activating mutations, while *APC* mutations are found in rare cases [117–119]. Approximately 85% of WNT-activated medulloblastomas have monosomy 6. Mutations in the *PTCH1* gene and *SUFO* or *SMO* gene are common in childhood and adults, respectively [118, 119]. Group 3 and group 4 medulloblastomas primarily affect youngsters and adolescents, respectively. Embryonal tumor with multilayered rosettes (ETMR) is a high-grade cancer that most commonly affects children below 2 years of age [100]. It is distinguished by the amplification or fusion of the chromosome 19 microRNA cluster (C19MC) to the *TTYH1* gene. ETMRs are associated with predominant chromosomal abnormalities, including chromosome 2 gains, 7q or 11q gains, and 6q loss, in addition to C19MC mutations.

Germ Cell Tumors: Germ cells are pluripotent, are formed in the embryo's yolk sac and are generally headed for the ovaries or testes but might move to other places also [120]. Germinomas, choriocarcinomas, teratomas, embryonal carcinomas, yolk sac tumors, and mixed germ cell tumors are the six forms of germ cell cancers [121–123]. Germinomas are the most prevalent pineal tumors, accounting for up to 50% of all pineal tumors [120, 124]. Germinomas are not encapsulated tumors and hence can penetrate adjacent brain regions and spread along the brain surface via the CSF. Pineal choriocarcinomas are rare malignant nongerminomatous GCTs that account for less than 5% of all pineal tumors [122]. Intracranial teratomas are developed in the pineal gland and the third ventricle [125]. Male predominance in pineal teratomas ranges from 2:1 to 8:1, with an OS rate of 90–100% [119].

Tumors of the Sellar Region: Craniopharyngiomas are circumscribed epithelial tumors of WHO grade I that most typically originate in the suprasellar area. Craniopharyngioma accounts for 5–10% of all pediatric and 1.2–4.6% of adult brain cancers [3]. The frequency is highest in children aged 0–19 years and a second peak occurs at 40–79 years [126]. Craniopharyngioma is classified into adamantinomatous (the most common) and papillary types [127]. The beta-catenin gene *CTNNB1* is mutated in the majority of adamantinomatous craniopharyngiomas [126]. *BRAF-V600E* mutations were found in about 95% of papillary craniopharyngioma cases [128].

16.4 Treatment

Surgical resection is considered as the first line of therapy for meningiomas [129]. It offers a complete cure for a low-grade tumor [130]. It decreases cerebral pressure caused by the tumor [131]. Radiation therapy is given 5 days/week and up to 6 weeks [130]. External radiation therapy includes stereotaxic radiosurgery (SRS), fractionated stereotaxic radiotherapy (FSR), and whole brain radiotherapy (WBR) [132]. SRS benefits smaller lesions with 5-year PFS rate ranging between 86% and 100% [133]. FSR alone or combined with surgery is frequently suggested for aggressive meningiomas [129]. A residual meningeal tumor is associated with a 5-year rate of recurrence of more than 60% in high-grade meningiomas [134]. Clinical investigations reveal that adjuvant FSR in treating WHO intermediate and high-risk grade meningioma shows a 94% and 59% PFS, respectively [135, 136]. The standard treatment for gliomas is maximal resection, concurrent radiation, and chemotherapy with temozolomide (TMZ) [137]. The FDA has approved bevacizumab, tumor-treating fields (TTF), and TMZ for treating glioblastoma [138]. In a phase II clinical trial of glioblastoma patients, the safety and anticancer efficacy of bevacizumab alone or together with irinotecan were demonstrated [139, 140]. It is found that glioma patients have higher CTLA-4 expression and are linked to glioma progression [141, 142]. The immune checkpoint inhibitors targeting the PD1, PDL1, and CTLA4 have evidenced dramatic success against a wide range of solid brain tumors [143, 144]. In high-grade meningiomas, VEGF levels are ten times higher than in low-grade meningiomas [145]. The Vasogenic edema in meningiomas is also linked with tumor VEGF expression levels [146]. In high-grade meningiomas, inhibition of mTOR is associated with reduced tumor proliferation [147, 148]. Everolimus, an mTOR inhibitor, was given in combination with octreotide and bevacizumab to suppress the mTOR pathway [149, 150]. Vismodegib, an inhibitor of Hedgehog signaling pathway, was given to meningioma patients with mutations in *SMO* or *PTCH1* genes [129].

16.5 Conclusion

CNS cancers represent 1.6% of all cancer cases globally in 2020 and ranked tenth in terms of mortality. Malignant tumors constituted 29.7% of all primary brain cancers, while nonmalignant tumors made up the remaining 70.3%. Ionizing radiation is associated with the development of brain tumors. Diagnosis of a brain tumor typically involves a range of tests, including MRI and CT scans, blood tests, lumbar puncture, and biopsy. Current research focuses on immunotherapy, targeted medications, and innovative methods of radiotherapy for the treatment of CNS cancers. Many immunotherapies and targeted medicines have been observed to be ineffective, despite the positive effects seen in early-phase clinical studies. Nevertheless, contradictory research results emphasize the importance of conducting further studies prior to implementing clinical trials.

References

1. Sung H, Ferlay J, Siegel RL, Laversanne M, Soerjomataram I, Jemal A, Bray F. Global cancer statistics 2020: GLOBOCAN estimates of incidence and mortality worldwide for 36 cancers in 185 countries. CA Cancer J Clin. 2021;71(3):209–49.
2. Ostrom QT, Patil N, Cioffi G, Waite K, Kruchko C, Barnholtz-Sloan JS. CBTRUS statistical report: primary brain and other central nervous system tumors diagnosed in the United States in 2013–2017. Neuro Oncol. 2020;22(Supplement_1):iv1–96.
3. Ostrom QT, Gittleman H, Stetson L, Virk S, Barnholtz-Sloan JS. Epidemiology of intracranial gliomas. Intrac Gliomas I Surg. 2018;30:1–1.
4. Siedlecki Z, Szafrańska M, Główczewska-Siedlecka E, Śniegocki M. Brain tumors risk factors-current state of knowledge review. J Educ Health Sport. 2021;11(9):101–7.
5. Davis F, Il'yasova D, Rankin K, McCarthy B, Bigner DD. Medical diagnostic radiation exposures and risk of gliomas. Radiat Res. 2011;175(6):790–6.
6. Linos E, Raine T, Alonso A, Michaud D. Atopy and risk of brain tumors: a meta-analysis. J Natl Cancer Inst. 2007;99(20):1544–50.
7. Ostrom QT, Adel Fahmideh M, Cote DJ, Muskens IS, Schraw JM, Scheurer ME, Bondy ML. Risk factors for childhood and adult primary brain tumors. Neuro Oncol. 2019;21(11):1357–75.
8. Singh AA, Rennert RC, Carey A, Riccardo S, Ahluwalia MS, Lakshmi N, Peters S, Arvold ND, Harsh GR, Steeg PS, Chang SD. metastases (primer). Nat Rev Dis Primers. 2019;5(1).
9. Westphal M, Lamszus K. Circulating biomarkers for gliomas. Nat Rev Neurol. 2015;11(10):556–66.
10. Sabit H, Nakada M, Furuta T, Watanabe T, Hayashi Y, Sato H, Kato Y, Hamada JI. Characterizing invading glioma cells based on IDH1-R132H and Ki-67 immunofluorescence. Brain Tumor Pathol. 2014;31:242–6.
11. Capper D, Weißert S, Balss J, Habel A, Meyer J, Jäger D, Ackermann U, Tessmer C, Korshunov A, Zentgraf H, Hartmann C. Characterization of R132H mutation-specific IDH1 antibody binding in brain tumors. Brain Pathol. 2010;20(1):245–54.
12. Riemenschneider MJ, Jeuken JW, Wesseling P, Reifenberger G. Molecular diagnostics of gliomas: state of the art. Acta Neuropathol. 2010;120:567–84.
13. Jeuken JW, Deimling AV, Wesseling P. Molecular pathogenesis of oligodendroglial tumors. J Neuro-Oncol. 2004;70:161–81.

14. Louis DN, Ohgaki H, Wiestler OD, Cavenee WK, Burger PC, Jouvet A, Scheithauer BW, Kleihues P. The 2007 WHO classification of tumours of the central nervous system. Acta Neuropathol. 2007;114:97–109.
15. Hatanpaa KJ, Burger PC, Eshleman JR, Murphy KM, Berg KD. Molecular diagnosis of oligodendroglioma in paraffin sections. Lab Investig. 2003;83(3):419–28.
16. Reifenberger G, Louis DN. Oligodendroglioma: toward molecular definitions in diagnostic neuro-oncology. J Neuropathol Exp Neurol. 2003;62(2):111–26.
17. Yip S, Iafrate AJ, Louis DN. Molecular diagnostic testing in malignant gliomas: a practical update on predictive markers. J Neuropathol Exp Neurol. 2008;67(1):1–5.
18. Kristensen BW, Priesterbach-Ackley LP, Petersen JK, Wesseling P. Molecular pathology of tumors of the central nervous system. Ann Oncol. 2019;30(8):1265–78.
19. Ilhan-Mutlu A, Wagner L, Preusser M. Circulating biomarkers of CNS tumors: an update. Biomark Med. 2013;7(2):267–85.
20. Wesseling P, Capper DW. WHO 2016 classification of gliomas. Neuropathol Appl Neurobiol. 2018;44(2):139–50.
21. Louis DN, Perry A, Wesseling P, Brat DJ, Cree IA, Figarella-Branger D, Hawkins C, Ng HK, Pfister SM, Reifenberger G, Soffietti R. The 2021 WHO classification of tumors of the central nervous system: a summary. Neuro Oncol. 2021;23(8):1231–51.
22. Müller HL, Merchant TE, Warmuth-Metz M, Martinez-Barbera JP, Puget S. Craniopharyngioma. Nat Rev Dis Primers. 2019;5(1):75.
23. Hölsken A, Sill M, Merkle J, Schweizer L, Buchfelder M, Flitsch J, Fahlbusch R, Metzler M, Kool M, Pfister SM, von Deimling A. Adamantinomatous and papillary craniopharyngiomas are characterized by distinct epigenomic as well as mutational and transcriptomic profiles. Acta Neuropathol Commun. 2016;4(1):1–3.
24. Rindi G, Klimstra DS, Abedi-Ardekani B, Asa SL, Bosman FT, Brambilla E, Busam KJ, de Krijger RR, Dietel M, El-Naggar AK, Fernandez-Cuesta L. A common classification framework for neuroendocrine neoplasms: an International Agency for Research on Cancer (IARC) and World Health Organization (WHO) expert consensus proposal. Mod Pathol. 2018;31(12):1770–86.
25. BD Chaurasia's Human anatomy. Volume 3. Head Neck and Brain 6th Edition.
26. Marosi C, Hassler M, Roessler K, Reni M, Sant M, Mazza E, Vecht C. Meningioma. Crit Rev Oncol Hematol. 2008;67(2):153–71.
27. Fathi AR, Roelcke U. Meningioma. Curr Neurol Neurosci Rep. 2013;13:1–8.
28. Mortazavi MM, Adeeb N, Griessenauer CJ, Sheikh H, Shahidi S, Tubbs RI, Tubbs RS. The ventricular system of the brain: a comprehensive review of its history, anatomy, histology, embryology, and surgical considerations. Childs Nerv Syst. 2014;30:19–35.
29. Kovacs GG. Cellular reactions of the central nervous system. Handb Clin Neurol. 2018;145:13–23.
30. Redzic ZB, Segal MB. The structure of the choroid plexus and the physiology of the choroid plexus epithelium. Adv Drug Deliv Rev. 2004;56(12):1695–716.
31. Ostrom QT, Bauchet L, Davis FG, Deltour I, Fisher JL, Langer CE, Pekmezci M, Schwartzbaum JA, Turner MC, Walsh KM, Wrensch MR. The epidemiology of glioma in adults: a "state of the science" review. Neuro Oncol. 2014;16(7):896–913.
32. Rickert CH, Paulus W. Tumors of the choroid plexus. Microsc Res Tech. 2001;52(1):104–11.
33. Thomas C, Soschinski P, Zwaig M, Oikonomopoulos S, Okonechnikov K, Pajtler KW, Sill M, Schweizer L, Koch A, Neumann J, Schüller U. The genetic landscape of choroid plexus tumors in children and adults. Neuro Oncol. 2021;23(4):650–60.
34. Wu J, Armstrong TS, Gilbert MR. Biology and management of ependymomas. Neuro Oncol. 2016;18(7):902–13.
35. Nowinski WL. Introduction to brain anatomy. Biomechanics of the. Brain. 2011:5–40.
36. Gupta D, Barachant A, Gordon AM, Ferre C, Kuo HC, Carmel JB, Friel KM. Effect of sensory and motor connectivity on hand function in pediatric hemiplegia. Ann Neurol. 2017;82(5):766–80.

37. Moini J, Avgeropoulos N, Samsam M. Epidemiology of brain and spinal tumors. New York, NY: Academic Press; 2021.
38. Ostrom QT, Gittleman H, Fulop J, Liu M, Blanda R, Kromer C, Wolinsky Y, Kruchko C, Barnholtz-Sloan JS. CBTRUS statistical report: primary brain and central nervous system tumors diagnosed in the United States in 2008-2012. Neuro Oncol. 2015;17(suppl_4):iv1–62.
39. Larjavaara S, Mäntylä R, Salminen T, Haapasalo H, Raitanen J, Jääskeläinen J, Auvinen A. Incidence of gliomas by anatomic location. Neuro Oncol. 2007;9(3):319–25.
40. Aldape K, Zadeh G, Mansouri S, Reifenberger G, von Deimling A. Glioblastoma: pathology, molecular mechanisms and markers. Acta Neuropathol. 2015;129:829–48.
41. Driscoll P. Gray's anatomy, 39th Edition. Emerg Med J. 2006;23(6):492. /pmc/articles/PMC2564372/
42. Singh R. Cerebellum: its anatomy, functions and diseases. In: Neurodegenerative diseases-molecular mechanisms and current therapeutic approaches. IntechOpen; 2020.
43. DeWitt JC, Mock A, Louis DN. The 2016 WHO classification of central nervous system tumors: what neurologists need to know. Curr Opin Neurol. 2017;30(6):643–9.
44. Quinlan A, Rizzolo D. Understanding medulloblastoma. JAAPA. 2017;30(10):30–6.
45. Fernández-Gil MA, Palacios-Bote R, Leo-Barahona M, Mora-Encinas JP. Anatomy of the brainstem: a gaze into the stem of life. Sem Ultrasound CT MRI. 2010;31(3):196–219.
46. Paulus W, Perry A. Lymphomas and histiocytic tumors. In: Practical surgical neuropathology: a diagnostic approach. Elsevier; 2018. p. 405–22.
47. Garman RH. Histology of the central nervous system. Toxicol Pathol. 2011;39(1):22–35.
48. Agulhon C, Petravicz J, McMullen AB, Sweger EJ, Minton SK, Taves SR, et al. What is the role of astrocyte calcium in neurophysiology? Neuron. 2008;59(6):932–46.
49. Yeh TH, Lee DY, Gianino SM, Gutmann DH. Microarray analyses reveal regional astrocyte heterogeneity with implications for neurofibromatosis type 1 (NF1)-regulated glial proliferation. Glia. 2009;57(11):1239–49.
50. Hewett JA. Determinants of regional and local diversity within the astroglial lineage of the normal central nervous system. J Neurochem. 2009;110(6):1717–36.
51. Ostrom QT, de Blank PM, Kruchko C, Petersen CM, Liao P, Finlay JL, Stearns DS, Wolff JE, Wolinsky Y, Letterio JJ, Barnholtz-Sloan JS. Alex's lemonade stand foundation infant and childhood primary brain and central nervous system tumors diagnosed in the United States in 2007–2011. Neuro Oncol. 2015;16(suppl_10):x1–36.
52. Onizuka H, Masui K, Komori T. Diffuse gliomas to date and beyond 2016 WHO classification of tumours of the central nervous system. Int J Clin Oncol. 2020;25:997–1003.
53. Louis DN, Perry A, Reifenberger G, Von Deimling A, Figarella-Branger D, Cavenee WK, Ohgaki H, Wiestler OD, Kleihues P, Ellison DW. The 2016 World Health Organization classification of tumors of the central nervous system: a summary. Acta Neuropathol. 2016;131:803–20.
54. Kondo T. Molecular mechanisms involved in gliomagenesis. Brain Tumor Pathol. 2017;34:1–7.
55. Appin CL, Brat DJ. Biomarker-driven diagnosis of diffuse gliomas. Mol Asp Med. 2015;45:87–96.
56. Bourne TD, Schiff D. Update on molecular findings, management and outcome in low-grade gliomas. Nat Rev Neurol. 2010;6(12):695–701.
57. Grimm SA, Chamberlain MC. Anaplastic astrocytoma. CNS Oncol. 2016;5(3):145–57.
58. Pedersen M, Küsters-Vandevelde HV, Viros A, Groenen PJ, Sanchez-Laorden B, Gilhuis JH, van Engen-van Grunsven IA, Renier W, Schieving J, Niculescu-Duvaz I, Springer CJ. Primary melanoma of the CNS in children is driven by congenital expression of oncogenic NRAS in melanocytes oncogenic NRAS induces CNS melanoma in children. Cancer Discov. 2013;3(4):458–69.
59. van den Bent MJ, Brandes AA, Rampling R, Kouwenhoven MC, Kros JM, Carpentier AF, Clement PM, Frenay M, Campone M, Baurain JF, Armand JP. Randomized phase II trial of erlotinib versus temozolomide or carmustine in recurrent glioblastoma: EORTC brain tumor group study 26034. J Clin Oncol. 2009;27(8):1268.

60. van den Bent MJ, Brandes AA, Taphoorn MJ, Kros JM, Kouwenhoven MC, Delattre JY, Bernsen HJ, Frenay M, Tijssen CC, Grisold W, Sipos L. Adjuvant procarbazine, lomustine, and vincristine chemotherapy in newly diagnosed anaplastic oligodendroglioma: long-term follow-up of EORTC brain tumor group study 26951. J Clin Oncol. 2013;31(3):344–50.
61. Cairncross G, Wang M, Shaw E, Jenkins R, Brachman D, Buckner J, Fink K, Souhami L, Laperriere N, Curran W, Mehta M. Phase III trial of chemoradiotherapy for anaplastic oligodendroglioma: long-term results of RTOG 9402. J Clin Oncol. 2013;31(3):337.
62. Tabori U, Shlien A, Baskin B, Levitt S, Ray P, Alon N, Hawkins C, Bouffet E, Pienkowska M, Lafay-Cousin L, Gozali A. TP53 alterations determine clinical subgroups and survival of patients with choroid plexus tumors. J Clin Oncol. 2010;28(12):1995–2001.
63. Merino DM, Shlien A, Villani A, Pienkowska M, Mack S, Ramaswamy V, Shih D, Tatevossian R, Novokmet A, Choufani S, Dvir R. Molecular characterization of choroid plexus tumors reveals novel clinically relevant subgroups genomic profiling of choroid plexus tumors. Clin Cancer Res. 2015;21(1):184–92.
64. Garces S, Medeiros LJ, Patel KP, Li S, Pina-Oviedo S, Li J, Garces JC, Khoury JD, Yin CC. Mutually exclusive recurrent KRAS and MAP2K1 mutations in Rosai–Dorfman disease. Mod Pathol. 2017;30(10):1367–77.
65. Diamond EL, Subbiah V, Lockhart C, Blay JY, Faris JE, Puzanov I, Chau I, Raje NS, Wolf JS, Erinjeri J, Torrisi J. Vemurafenib in patients with Erdheim-Chester disease (ECD) and Langerhans cell histiocytosis (LCH) harboring BRAFV600 mutations: a cohort of the histology-independent VE-basket study. Blood. 2016;128(22):480.
66. Nakamura T, Yamashita S, Fukumura K, Nakabayashi J, Tanaka K, Tamura K, Tateishi K, Kinoshita M, Fukushima S, Takami H, Fukuoka K. Genome-wide DNA methylation profiling identifies primary central nervous system lymphoma as a distinct entity different from systemic diffuse large B-cell lymphoma. Acta Neuropathol. 2017;133:321–4.
67. Tateishi K, Miyake Y, Nakamura T, Yamamoto T. Primary central nervous system lymphoma: clinicopathological and genomic insights for therapeutic development. Brain Tumor Pathol. 2021;38(3):173–82.
68. Chapuy B, Roemer MG, Stewart C, Tan Y, Abo RP, Zhang L, Dunford AJ, Meredith DM, Thorner AR, Jordanova ES, Liu G. Targetable genetic features of primary testicular and primary central nervous system lymphomas. Blood J Am Soc Hematol. 2016;127(7):869–81.
69. Nayyar N, White MD, Gill CM, Lastrapes M, Bertalan M, Kaplan A, D'Andrea MR, Bihun I, Kaneb A, Dietrich J, Ferry JA. MYD88 L265P mutation and CDKN2A loss are early mutational events in primary central nervous system diffuse large B-cell lymphomas. Blood Adv. 2019;3(3):375–83.
70. Brat DJ, Perry A. Melanocytic neoplasms of the central nervous system. In: Practical surgical neuropathology: a diagnostic approach. Elsevier; 2018. p. 443–51.
71. Salgado CM, Basu D, Nikiforova M, Hamilton RL, Gehris R, Jakacki R, Panigrahy A, Yatsenko S, Reyes-Múgica M. Amplification of mutated NRAS leading to congenital melanoma in neurocutaneous melanocytosis. Melanoma Res. 2015;25(5):453–60.
72. Brat DJ, Giannini C, Scheithauer BW, Burger PC. Primary melanocytic neoplasms of the central nervous system. Am J Surg Pathol. 1999;23(7):745.
73. Liubinas SV, Maartens N, Drummond KJ. Primary melanocytic neoplasms of the central nervous system. J Clin Neurosci. 2010;17(10):1227–32.
74. Schmidt M, Mock A, Jungk C, Sahm F, Ull AT, Warta R, Lamszus K, Gousias K, Ketter R, Roesch S, Rapp C. Transcriptomic analysis of aggressive meningiomas identifies PTTG1 and LEPR as prognostic biomarkers independent of WHO grade. Oncotarget. 2016;7(12):14551.
75. Koelsche C, Hovestadt V, Jones DT, Capper D, Sturm D, Sahm F, Schrimpf D, Adeberg S, Böhmer K, Hagenlocher C, Mechtersheimer G. Melanotic tumors of the nervous system are characterized by distinct mutational, chromosomal and epigenomic profiles. Brain Pathol. 2015;25(2):202–8.
76. Küsters-Vandevelde HV, Creytens D, Grunsven AC, Jeunink M, Winnepenninckx V, Groenen PJ, Küsters B, Wesseling P, Blokx WA, Prinsen CF. SF3B1 and EIF1AX mutations occur in

primary leptomeningeal melanocytic neoplasms; yet another similarity to uveal melanomas. Acta Neuropathol Commun. 2016;4(1):1–1.
77. Miller SC, Pandi PS, Esquifino AI, Cardinali DP, Maestroni GJ. The role of melatonin in immuno-enhancement: potential application in cancer. Int J Exp Pathol. 2006;87(2):81–7.
78. Favero G, Bonomini F, Rezzani R. Pineal gland tumors: a review. Cancers. 2021;13(7):1547.
79. Carr C, O'Neill BE, Hochhalter CB, Strong MJ, Ware ML. Biomarkers of pineal region tumors: a review. Ochsner J. 2019;19(1):26–31.
80. Liu AP, Priesterbach-Ackley LP, Orr BA, Li BK, Gudenas B, Reddingius RE, Suñol M, Lavarino CE, Olaciregui NG, Santa-María López V, Fisher MJ. WNT-activated embryonal tumors of the pineal region: ectopic medulloblastomas or a novel pineoblastoma subgroup? Acta Neuropathol. 2020;140:595–7.
81. Liu AP, Li BK, Pfaff E, Gudenas B, Vasiljevic A, Orr BA, Dufour C, Snuderl M, Karajannis MA, Rosenblum MK, Hwang EI. Clinical and molecular heterogeneity of pineal parenchymal tumors: a consensus study. Acta Neuropathol. 2021;141:771–85.
82. Alruwaili AA, De Jesus O. Meningioma. In: StatPearls [Internet]. Treasure Island, FL: StatPearls Publishing; 2022.
83. Goldbrunner R, Stavrinou P, Jenkinson MD, Sahm F, Mawrin C, Weber DC, Preusser M, Minniti G, Lund-Johansen M, Lefranc F, Houdart E. EANO guideline on the diagnosis and management of meningiomas. Neuro Oncol. 2021;23(11):1821–34.
84. Spille DC, Adeli A, Sporns PB, Heß K, Streckert EM, Brokinkel C, Mawrin C, Paulus W, Stummer W, Brokinkel B. Predicting the risk of postoperative recurrence and high-grade histology in patients with intracranial meningiomas using routine preoperative MRI. Neurosurg Rev. 2021;44:1109–17.
85. Mawrin C, Perry A. Pathological classification and molecular genetics of meningiomas. J Neuro-Oncol. 2010;99:379–91.
86. Clark VE, Erson-Omay EZ, Serin A, Yin J, Cotney J, Özduman K, Avşar T, Li J, Murray PB, Henegariu O, Yilmaz S. Genomic analysis of non-NF2 meningiomas reveals mutations in TRAF7, KLF4, AKT1, and SMO. Science. 2013;339(6123):1077–80.
87. Brastianos PK, Horowitz PM, Santagata S, Jones RT, McKenna A, Getz G, Ligon KL, Palescandolo E, Van Hummelen P, Ducar MD, Raza A. Genomic sequencing of meningiomas identifies oncogenic SMO and AKT1 mutations. Nat Genet. 2013;45(3):285–9.
88. Williams SR, Juratli TA, Castro BA, Lazaro TT, Gill CM, Nayyar N, Strickland MR, Babinski M, Johnstone SE, Frosch MP, Silverman IM. Genomic analysis of posterior fossa meningioma demonstrates frequent AKT1 E17K mutations in foramen magnum meningiomas. J Neurol Surg B Skull Base. 2019;80(06):562–7.
89. Gupte TP, Li C, Jin L, Yalcin K, Youngblood MW, Miyagishima DF, Mishra-Gorur K, Zhao AY, Antonios J, Huttner A, McGuone D. Clinical and genomic factors associated with seizures in meningiomas. J Neurosurg. 2020;135(3):835–44.
90. Williams EA, Santagata S, Wakimoto H, Shankar GM, Barker FG, Sharaf R, et al. Distinct genomic subclasses of high-grade/progressive meningiomas: NF2-associated, NF2-exclusive, and NF2-agnostic. Acta Neuropathol Commun. 2020;8(1):1–10.
91. Abedalthagafi M, Bi WL, Aizer AA, Merrill PH, Brewster R, Agarwalla PK, Listewnik ML, Dias-Santagata D, Thorner AR, Van Hummelen P, Brastianos PK. Oncogenic PI3K mutations are as common as AKT1 and SMO mutations in meningioma. Neuro Oncol. 2016;18(5):649–55.
92. Mirian C, Duun-Henriksen AK, Juratli T, Sahm F, Spiegl-Kreinecker S, Peyre M, Biczok A, Tonn JC, Goutagny S, Bertero L, Maier AD. Poor prognosis associated with TERT gene alterations in meningioma is independent of the WHO classification: an individual patient data meta-analysis. J Neurol Neurosurg Psychiatry. 2020;91(4):378–87.
93. Chmielecki J, Crago AM, Rosenberg M, O'Connor R, Walker SR, Ambrogio L, Auclair D, McKenna A, Heinrich MC, Frank DA, Meyerson M. Whole-exome sequencing identifies a recurrent NAB2-STAT6 fusion in solitary fibrous tumors. Nat Genet. 2013;45(2):131–2.
94. Schweizer L, Koelsche C, Sahm F, Piro RM, Capper D, Reuss DE, Pusch S, Habel A, Meyer J, Göck T, Jones DT. Meningeal hemangiopericytoma and solitary fibrous tumors carry the

NAB2-STAT6 fusion and can be diagnosed by nuclear expression of STAT6 protein. Acta Neuropathol. 2013;125:651–8.
95. Park HK, Yu DB, Sung M, Oh E, Kim M, Song JY, Lee MS, Jung K, Noh KW, An S, Song K. Molecular changes in solitary fibrous tumor progression. J Mol Med. 2019;97:1413–25.
96. Michailidou K, Hall P, Gonzalez-Neira A, Ghoussaini M, Dennis J, Milne RL, Schmidt MK, Chang-Claude J, Bojesen SE, Bolla MK, Wang Q. Large-scale genotyping identifies 41 new loci associated with breast cancer risk. Nat Genet. 2013;45(4):353–61.
97. Jeon YK, Chang KH, Suh YL, Jung HW, Park SH. Inflammatory myofibroblastic tumor of the central nervous system: clinicopathologic analysis of 10 cases. J Neuropathol Exp Neurol. 2005;64(3):254–9.
98. Tan AR, Swain SM. Therapeutic strategies for triple-negative breast cancer. Cancer J. 2008;14(6):343–51.
99. Vidrine DW, Berry JF, Garbuzov A, Falcon C, Tubbs RS, Bui CJ. DCTN1-ALK gene fusion in inflammatory myofibroblastic tumor (IMT) of the CNS. Childs Nerv Syst. 2021;37(7):2147–51.
100. Meredith DM, Alexandrescu S. Embryonal and non-meningothelial mesenchymal tumors of the central nervous system–advances in diagnosis and prognostication. Brain Pathol. 2022;32(4):e13059.
101. Goss JA, Huang AY, Smith E, Konczyk DJ, Smits PJ, Sudduth CL, Stapleton C, Patel A, Alexandrescu S, Warman ML, Greene AK. Somatic mutations in intracranial arteriovenous malformations. PLoS One. 2019;14(12):e0226852.
102. Bisceglia M, Muscarella LA, Galliani CA, Zidar N, Ben-Dor D, Pasquinelli G, La Torre A, Sparaneo A, Fanburg-Smith JC, Lamovec J, Michal M. Extraneuraxial hemangioblastoma: clinicopathologic features and review of the literature. Adv Anat Pathol. 2018;25(3):197–215.
103. Tanvir I, Riaz S, Khan HA, Loya A, Shahid K. Mesenchymal chondrosarcoma arising in the central nervous system: a diagnostic pitfall. Int J Head Neck Surg. 2013;4(03):152–5.
104. Naumann S, Krallman PA, Unni KK, Fidler ME, Neff JR, Bridge JA. Translocation der (13; 21)(q10; q10) in skeletal and extraskeletal mesenchymal chondrosarcoma. Mod Pathol. 2002;15(5):572–6.
105. Moses ZB, Barzilai O, O'Toole JE. Benign intradural and paraspinal nerve sheath tumors: advanced surgical techniques. Neurosurg Clin. 2020;31(2):221–9.
106. Belakhoua SM, Rodriguez FJ. Diagnostic pathology of tumors of peripheral nerve. Neurosurgery. 2021;88(3):443–56.
107. Agnihotri S, Jalali S, Wilson MR, Danesh A, Li M, Klironomos G, Krieger JR, Mansouri A, Khan O, Mamatjan Y, Landon-Brace N. The genomic landscape of schwannoma. Nat Genet. 2016;48(11):1339–48.
108. Sestini R, Bacci C, Provenzano A, Genuardi M, Papi L. Evidence of a four-hit mechanism involving SMARCB1 and NF2 in schwannomatosis-associated schwannomas. Hum Mutat. 2008;29(2):227–31.
109. Piotrowski A, Xie J, Liu YF, Poplawski AB, Gomes AR, Madanecki P, Fu C, Crowley MR, Crossman DK, Armstrong L, Babovic-Vuksanovic D. Germline loss-of-function mutations in LZTR1 predispose to an inherited disorder of multiple schwannomas. Nat Genet. 2014;46(2):182–7.
110. Pemov A, Li H, Patidar R, Hansen NF, Sindiri S, Hartley SW, Wei JS, Elkahloun A, Chandrasekharappa SC, Boland JF, Bass S. The primacy of NF1 loss as the driver of tumorigenesis in neurofibromatosis type 1-associated plexiform neurofibromas. Oncogene. 2017;36(22):3168–77.
111. Guedes F, Brown RS, Torrão-Junior FJ, Barbosa DA, Ravanini GD, Amorim RM. Pediatric peripheral nerve tumors: clinical and surgical aspects. Childs Nerv Syst. 2019;35:2289–97.
112. Klein CJ, Wu Y, Jentoft ME, Mer G, Spinner RJ, Dyck PJ, Dyck PJ, Mauermann ML. Genomic analysis reveals frequent TRAF7 mutations in intraneural perineuriomas. Ann Neurol. 2017;81(2):316–21.

113. Carter JM, Wu Y, Blessing MM, Folpe AL, Thorland EC, Spinner RJ, Jentoft ME, Wang C, Baheti S, Niu Z, Mauermann ML. Recurrent genomic alterations in soft tissue perineuriomas. Am J Surg Pathol. 2018;42(12):1708–14.
114. Hornick JL, Bundock EA, Fletcher CD. Hybrid schwannoma/perineurioma: clinicopathologic analysis of 42 distinctive benign nerve sheath tumors. Am J Surg Pathol. 2009;33(10):1554–61.
115. Ostrom QT, Gittleman H, Truitt G, Boscia A, Kruchko C, Barnholtz-Sloan JS. CBTRUS statistical report: primary brain and other central nervous system tumors diagnosed in the United States in 2011–2015. Neuro Oncol. 2018;20(suppl_4):iv1–86.
116. Taylor MD, Northcott PA, Korshunov A, Remke M, Cho YJ, Clifford SC, Eberhart CG, Parsons DW, Rutkowski S, Gajjar A, Ellison DW. Molecular subgroups of medulloblastoma: the current consensus. Acta Neuropathol. 2012;123:465–72.
117. Colafati GS, Voicu IP, Carducci C, Miele E, Carai A, Di Loreto S, Marrazzo A, Cacchione A, Cecinati V, Tornesello A, Mastronuzzi A. MRI features as a helpful tool to predict the molecular subgroups of medulloblastoma: state of the art. Ther Adv Neurol Disord. 2018;11:1756286418775375.
118. Ellison DW, Dalton J, Kocak M, Nicholson SL, Fraga C, Neale G, Kenney AM, Brat DJ, Perry A, Yong WH, Taylor RE. Medulloblastoma: clinicopathological correlates of SHH, WNT, and non-SHH/WNT molecular subgroups. Acta Neuropathol. 2011;121:381–96.
119. Choque-Velasquez J, Resendiz-Nieves J, Jahromi BR, Colasanti R, Raj R, Vehviläinen J, Tynninen O, Collan J, Niemelä M, Hernesniemi J. Extent of resection and long-term survival of pineal region tumors in Helsinki neurosurgery. World Neurosurg. 2019;131:e379–91.
120. Villano JL, Propp JM, Porter KR, Stewart AK, Valyi-Nagy T, Li X, Engelhard HH, McCarthy BJ. Malignant pineal germ-cell tumors: an analysis of cases from three tumor registries. Neuro Oncol. 2008;10(2):121–30.
121. Nagasawa DT, Lagman C, Sun M, Yew A, Chung LK, Lee SJ, Bui TT, Ooi YC, Robison RA, Zada G, Yang I. Pineal germ cell tumors: two cases with review of histopathologies and biomarkers. J Clin Neurosci. 2017;38:23–31.
122. Smirniotopoulos JG, Rushing EJ, Mena H. Pineal region masses: differential diagnosis. Radiographics. 1992;12(3):577–96.
123. Liang L, Korogi Y, Sugahara T, Ikushima I, Shigematsu Y, Okuda T, Takahashi M, Kochi M, Ushio Y. MRI of intracranial germ-cell tumours. Neuroradiology. 2002;44:382–8.
124. Nomura K. Epidemiology of germ cell tumors in Asia of pineal region tumor. J Neuro-Oncol. 2001;54:211–7.
125. Peterson CM, Buckley C, Holley S, Menias CO. Teratomas: a multimodality review. Curr Probl Diagn Radiol. 2012;41(6):210–9.
126. Schwetye KE, Dahiya SM. Sellar tumors. Surg Pathol Clin. 2020;13(2):305–29.
127. Larkin SJ, Preda V, Karavitaki N, Grossman A, Ansorge O. BRAF V600E mutations are characteristic for papillary craniopharyngioma and may coexist with CTNNB1-mutated adamantinomatous craniopharyngioma. Acta Neuropathol. 2014;127:927–9.
128. Bi WL, Larsen AG, Dunn IF. Genomic alterations in sporadic pituitary tumors. Curr Neurol Neurosci Rep. 2018;18:1–6.
129. Patel B, Desai R, Pugazenthi S, Butt OH, Huang J, Kim AH. Corrigendum: Identification and management of aggressive meningiomas, vol. 12. Front Oncol; 2022. p. 1107271.
130. Shah V, Kochar P. Brain cancer: implication to disease, therapeutic strategies and tumor targeted drug delivery approaches. Recent Pat Anticancer Drug Discov. 2018;13(1):70–85.
131. McFaline-Figueroa JR, Lee EQ. Brain tumors. Am J Med. 2018;131(8):874–82.
132. Borgelt B, Gelber R, Kramer S, Brady LW, Chang CH, Davis LW, Perez CA, Hendrickson FR. The palliation of brain metastases: final results of the first two studies by the radiation therapy oncology group. Int J Radiat Oncol Biol Phys. 1980;6(1):1–9.
133. Rogers L, Barani I, Chamberlain M, Kaley TJ, McDermott M, Raizer J, Schiff D, Weber DC, Wen PY, Vogelbaum MA. Meningiomas: knowledge base, treatment outcomes, and uncertainties. A RANO review. J Neurosurg. 2015;122(1):4–23.

134. Jääskeläinen J, Haltia M, Servo A. Atypical and anaplastic meningiomas: radiology, surgery, radiotherapy, and outcome. Surg Neurol. 1986;25(3):233–42.
135. Rogers L, Zhang P, Vogelbaum MA, Perry A, Ashby LS, Modi JM, Alleman AM, Galvin J, Brachman D, Jenrette JM, De Groot J. Intermediate-risk meningioma: initial outcomes from NRG oncology RTOG 0539. J Neurosurg. 2017;129(1):35–47.
136. Rogers CL, Won M, Vogelbaum MA, Perry A, Ashby LS, Modi JM, Alleman AM, Galvin J, Fogh SE, Youssef E, Deb N. High-risk meningioma: initial outcomes from NRG oncology/RTOG 0539. Int J Rad Oncol Biol Phys. 2020;106(4):790–9.
137. Xu S, Tang L, Li X, Fan F, Liu Z. Immunotherapy for glioma: current management and future application. Cancer Lett. 2020;476:1–2.
138. Stupp R, Taillibert S, Kanner AA, Kesari S, Steinberg DM, Toms SA, Taylor LP, Lieberman F, Silvani A, Fink KL, Barnett GH. Maintenance therapy with tumor-treating fields plus temozolomide vs temozolomide alone for glioblastoma: a randomized clinical trial. JAMA. 2015;314(23):2535–43.
139. Friedman HS, Prados MD, Wen PY, Mikkelsen T, Schiff D, Abrey LE, Yung WA, Paleologos N, Nicholas MK, Jensen R, Vredenburgh J. Bevacizumab alone and in combination with irinotecan in recurrent glioblastoma. J Clin Oncol. 2009;27(28):4733–40.
140. Cohen MH, Shen YL, Keegan P, Pazdur R. FDA drug approval summary: bevacizumab (Avastin®) as treatment of recurrent glioblastoma multiforme. Oncologist. 2009;14(11):1131–8.
141. Fong B, Jin R, Wang X, Safaee M, Lisiero DN, Yang I, Li G, Liau LM, Prins RM. Monitoring of regulatory T cell frequencies and expression of CTLA-4 on T cells, before and after DC vaccination, can predict survival in GBM patients. PLoS One. 2012;7(4):e32614.
142. Learn CA, Fecci PE, Schmittling RJ, Xie W, Karikari I, Mitchell DA, Archer GE, Wei Z, Dressman H, Sampson JH. Profiling of CD4+, CD8+, and CD4+ CD25+ CD45RO+ FoxP3+ T cells in patients with malignant glioma reveals differential expression of the immunologic transcriptome compared with T cells from healthy volunteers. Clin Cancer Res. 2006;12(24):7306–15.
143. Larkin J, Chiarion-Sileni V, Gonzalez R, Grob JJ, Cowey CL, Lao CD, Schadendorf D, Dummer R, Smylie M, Rutkowski P, Ferrucci PF. Combined nivolumab and ipilimumab or monotherapy in untreated melanoma. N Engl J Med. 2015;373(1):23–34.
144. Haanen JB, Robert C. Immune checkpoint inhibitors. Immuno Oncol. 2015;42:55–66.
145. Lamszus K, Lengler U, Schmidt NO, Stavrou D, Ergün S, Westphal M. Vascular endothelial growth factor, hepatocyte growth factor/scatter factor, basic fibroblast growth factor, and placenta growth factor in human meningiomas and their relation to angiogenesis and malignancy. Neurosurgery. 2000;46(4):938–48.
146. Goldman CK, Bharara S, Palmer CA, Vitek J, Tsai JC, Weiss HL, Gillespie GY. Brain edema in meningiomas is associated with increased vascular endothelial growth factor expression. Neurosurgery. 1997;40(6):1269–77.
147. Graillon T, Romano D, Defilles C, Lisbonis C, Saveanu A, Figarella-Branger D, Roche PH, Fuentes S, Chinot O, Dufour H, Barlier A. Pasireotide is more effective than octreotide, alone or combined with everolimus on human meningioma in vitro. Oncotarget. 2017;8(33):55361.
148. Graillon T, Defilles C, Mohamed A, Lisbonis C, Germanetti AL, Chinot O, Figarella-Branger D, Roche PH, Adetchessi T, Fuentes S, Metellus P. Combined treatment by octreotide and everolimus: octreotide enhances inhibitory effect of everolimus in aggressive meningiomas. J Neuro-Oncol. 2015:124:33–43.
149. Jour Cardona AF, Ruiz-Patiño A, Zatarain-Barrón ZL, Hakim F, Jiménez E, Mejía JA, Ramón JF, Useche N, Bermúdez S, Pineda D, Cifuentes H. Systemic management of malignant meningiomas: a comparative survival and molecular marker analysis between Octreotide in combination with Everolimus and Sunitinib. PLoS One. 2019;14(6):e0217340.
150. Shih KC, Chowdhary S, Rosenblatt P, Weir AB, Shepard GC, Williams JT, Shastry M, Burris HA, Hainsworth JD. A phase II trial of bevacizumab and everolimus as treatment for patients with refractory, progressive intracranial meningioma. J Neuro-Oncol. 2016;129:281–8.

Head and Neck Cancer

17

Manasa Desai, Dorababu Patchva,
Anvesh Karthik Yalavarthy, Satya Dattatreya Palanki,
and Rama Krishna Kancha

17.1 Introduction

Epidemiology: Head and neck cancer (HNC) is a group of cancers that ranks seventh in the world with 890,000 new cases and 450,000 deaths [1, 2]. The incidences for the cancers of lip and oral cavity cancer, nasopharynx, larynx, oropharynx, and hypopharynx are 377,713 (2%), 133,354 (0.7%), 184,615 (1%), 98,412 (0.5%), 84,254 (0.4%) and the mortality rates are 177,757 (1.8%), 80,008 (0.8%), 99,840 (1%), 48,143 (0.5%), 38,599 (0.4%), respectively [1, 3]. In the United States, the percentage of HPV-positive oropharyngeal malignancies increased from 16.3% in the 1980s to more than 72.7% in the 2000s [2]. Men (16.9 new cases per 100,000) were more likely than women (6.2 new cases per 100,000) to be diagnosed with these cancers [3]. Laryngeal cancer is a rare disease with an annual incidence of 3.1 per 100,000 [3]. Men are more likely than women to get laryngeal cancer, with a rate of 4.1 in men and 0.9 in women per 100,000 [3]. The malignancies of the salivary glands are rare, with a frequency of 1.3 per 100,000 [3]. Adenocarcinomas of the parotid, the largest salivary gland, are the most common tumors.

Risk Factors: Tobacco use, alcohol intake, exposure to contaminants in the environment, poor dental health, and infection with HPV and EBV are all risk factors [4, 5]. Concurrent use of cigarettes and alcohol has traditionally been associated with a higher risk than either nicotine or alcohol alone [3, 6]. Tobacco and alcohol use are

M. Desai · R. K. Kancha (✉)
Molecular Medicine and Therapeutics Laboratory, CPMB, Osmania University, Hyderabad, India
e-mail: ramakancha@osmania.ac.in

D. Patchva
Apollo Institute of Medical Sciences and Research, Hyderabad, India

A. K. Yalavarthy · S. D. Palanki
Renovo Soumya Cancer Centre, Hyderabad, India

R. K. Kancha (ed.), *Biomedical Aspects of Solid Cancers*,
https://doi.org/10.1007/978-981-97-1802-3_17

the most common causes of laryngeal cancer [3]. Occupational exposures, particularly woodworking, formaldehyde, asbestos, textile dust, metal industries and canning, farming cocoa, chocolate production, and sugar confectionery have all been linked to the development of sinonasal malignancies [3]. Some sinonasal malignancies, notably nonkeratinizing squamous cell tumors, have been found to include HPV-DNA [7]. Fanconi anemia patients have a several hundredfold increased risk of HNSCC, mainly oral malignancies [4, 8].

Diagnosis: For early detection of cancers, multidisciplinary treatment decisions, the implementation of coordinated care pathways, and increased access to imaging, positron emission tomography (PET), and radiotherapy treatment are recommended [9]. For patients with NPC, EBV DNA is an independent predictive biomarker. In locally advanced oropharyngeal malignancies, HPV positivity is an established predictive indicator of a favorable outcome, and multiple studies have indicated a significantly lower risk of death (40–80%) or relapse (60–70%) in HPV-positive patients compared to HPV-negative patients [10, 11].

17.2 Classification

For nasopharyngeal carcinoma, Tx refers to primary tumor that cannot be assessed. T0 refers to EBV-positive cervical node(s) involvement and no tumor was found. T1 refers to extension till nasopharynx, oropharynx, or nasal cavity but not parapharyngeal. T2 refers to involvement of adjacent soft tissue and parapharyngeal extension. T3 refers to extension to paranasal sinuses and bony structures. T4 refers to extensive soft tissue involvement. Nx refers to the lymph nodes in the region that cannot be examined. N0 refers to no evidence of regional lymph node metastases. N1 refers to retropharyngeal lymph nodes, unilateral, bilateral, above the caudal border of the cricoid cartilage and greater than or equal to 6 cm. N2 refers to above the caudal border of the cricoid cartilage, bilateral metastases in lymph node(s) with a maximum diameter of 6 cm. N3a refers to >6 cm and/or below the cricoid cartilage's caudal margin. M0 and M1 refer to no distant metastasis and distant metastasis respectively [12].

According to TNM classification for oropharyngeal cancers, Tx refers to primary tumor that cannot be assessed. Tis refers to in situ carcinoma. T0 refers to tumor that cannot be identified. T1 refers to tumor with a maximum size of 2 cm. T2 refers to tumor with a diameter of more than 2 cm but less than 4 cm. T3 refers to tumor with a diameter greater than 4 cm or an expansion to the lingual surface of the epiglottis. T4 refers to the tumor that has invaded other parts of the oropharynx sites. Nx refers to the lymph nodes in the region that cannot be examined. N0 refers to no lymph node metastases in the region. N1 refers to metastases to one or more ipsilateral lymph nodes, none larger than 6 cm in diameter. For HPV-positive oropharyngeal cancer, N2 refers to metastases to contralateral or bilateral lymph nodes, none of which are larger than 6 cm in diameter. For HPV-negative oropharyngeal cancer, N2a refers to metastasis to a single ipsilateral node with a maximum dimension of >3 cm but less than 6 cm and no extra-nodal extension. N2b refers to metastases to many ipsilateral lymph nodes, none of which are larger than 6 cm in diameter and have no extra-nodal extension. N2c refers to metastases to bilateral or contralateral lymph nodes, none larger than 6 cm in diameter, and no extra-nodal spread. N3 refers to metastases to one or more lymph nodes, with a maximum size of >6 cm for HPV-positive oropharyngeal cancer. For HPV-negative oropharyngeal cancer, N3a refers to metastasis to a lymph node with a maximum diameter of >6 cm and no extra-nodal extension. N3b refers to one or more lymph nodes have been affected with clinically obvious extra-nodal expansion. M0 and M1 refer to no distant metastasis and distant metastasis, respectively [2].

Staging: The staging differs according to anatomical location. Early phases, in general (I and II) include tumors that aren't large and don't have a lot of lymph nodes. Stages III and IV are the most advanced. Tumors that have progressed locally and invasion of nearby structures or a rise in the number of lymph nodes involved, Stage IV also includes distant metastatic spread [2]. For nasopharyngeal carcinoma (NPC), stage 1 refers to T1 N0 M0, stage 2 refers to T2 N0–1 M0, T0–1 N1 M0, stage 3 refers to T3 N0–2 M0, T0–2 N2 M0, stage 4a refers to T4a or N3 M0, and stage 4b refers to M1 (any T, any N) [12].

17.3 Pathophysiology

Oropharynx: Majority of oropharyngeal cancers are squamous cell cancers (SCC) (Fig. 17.1). There are five layers in the oropharynx: mucosa, submucosa, pharyngobasilar fascia, constrictor muscle, and buccopharyngeal fascia. It is generally divided into four distinct components in clinical oncology: the base of the tongue, the soft palate, the palatine tonsillar fossa, and the pharyngeal wall [13]. HPV-positive squamous cell carcinomas have better clinical outcomes than HPV-negative cancers. High-risk HPV such as HPV16 is found in most SCCs.

Nasopharynx: The nasopharynx is a tube that connects the base of the skull to the lower border of the soft palate (Fig. 17.1). The nasopharynx epithelium is approximately 60% stratified. The WHO classification recognizes three subtypes of nasopharyngeal carcinoma (NPC): Keratinizing squamous cell carcinoma, which is more common in older adults (type 1), Nonkeratinizing carcinoma (type 2), and Undifferentiated carcinoma (type 3) [14, 15]. The majority of childhood and adolescent cases are type 3, while a few are type 2 cases [16]. EBV infection is closely linked to NPC.

Genetics: About 50% of HNSCC cases harbor *TP53* gene mutations [17, 18]. Loss-of-function mechanisms of p53 include silencing of ATM and ubiquitination by E6 of HPV16 [6, 10, 19]. EGFR is overexpressed in the vast majority of HNSCC cancers [6, 20, 21]. STAT3 is constitutively active in HNSCC, as evidenced by higher levels of tyrosine phosphorylated STAT3 in tumors [6]. C-Met activating mutations were also found in HNSCC [6, 22]. HGF is produced primarily by stromal fibroblasts and contributes to oncogenic signaling in tumor cells [6, 23, 24]. IGF-1R has been shown to be overexpressed in HNSCC [6, 25]. Additionally, increased expression of phosphorylated AKT, EGFR, and VEGF was observed in

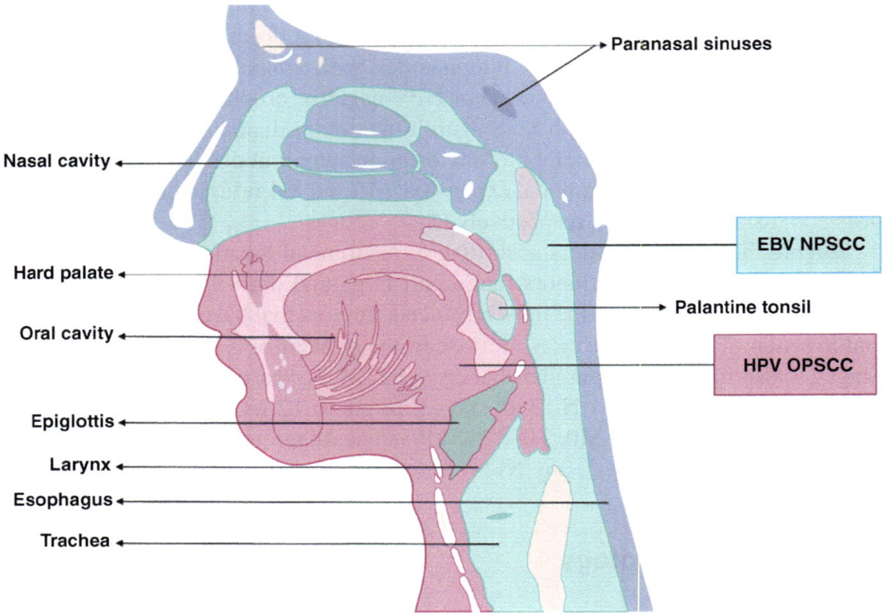

Fig. 17.1 Anatomy and pathophysiology of head and neck cancer. EBV Epstein-Barr virus, NPC (nasopharyngeal carcinoma); HPV (human papilloma virus); OPSCC (oropharyngeal squamous cell carcinoma)

HNSCC [6, 26–29]. The overexpression of EGFR is linked to the poor survival of the NPC [30, 31].

17.4 Treatment

Chemotherapy, radiation, and surgery are the most commonly used treatment modalities for HNSCC, and they are frequently used in combination. Radiation is used either alone or as an adjuvant in the treatment of early-stage cancer. Chemotherapy is usually given in conjunction with radiation to patients in advanced stages of disease, either as a primary strategy or after surgical resection [6, 32]. Concurrent cisplatin treatment and radiotherapy is the preferred treatment for NPC. Targeted therapies such as the cetuximab are used in tandem with chemotherapy and/or radiation. To date, most research has been focused on the various mechanisms of EGFR inhibitors and antiangiogenic agents [33]. NPC is not amenable to surgery for local control due to its anatomical position. The usual surgical procedure is a biopsy of the involved lymph node. The primary nasopharyngeal tumor is rarely biopsied [15]. NPC is particularly susceptible to RT and chemotherapy; depending on the stage of the disease, the conventional treatment is RT with or without chemotherapy. For locoregionally progressed and nonmetastatic NPC, CRT is the usual treatment [34].

17.5 Conclusion

All the malignancies from nose region to the esophagus are grouped into head and neck cancer, where squamous cells are particularly affected. Incidence is increasing in men more than women on account of a variety of risk factors such as viral, environmental, and genetic factors. EPV was shown to cause nasopharyngeal carcinoma while HPV was reported to cause oropharyngeal carcinoma. It is one of the well-studied cancers, with a number of biomarkers to differentiate type and subtypes of cancer, and subsequent targeted therapy. Surgery and radiotherapy are the common prescribed treatments. Chemotherapy is prescribed for advanced stages of cancer. Despite the advanced research, cosmetic and functional defects seem to be inevitable for the latter stages of cancer. With cetuximab being the only molecular target approved so far, there is scope to develop further targeted therapies.

References

1. Sung H, Ferlay J, Siegel RL, Laversanne M, Soerjomataram I, Jemal A, Bray F. Global cancer statistics 2020: GLOBOCAN estimates of incidence and mortality worldwide for 36 cancers in 185 countries. CA Cancer J Clin. 2021;71(3):209–49.
2. Chow LQ. Head and neck cancer. N Engl J Med. 2020;382(1):60–72.
3. Cohen N, Fedewa S, Chen AY. Epidemiology and demographics of the head and neck cancer population. Oral Maxillofac Surg Clin. 2018;30(4):381–95.
4. Johnson DE, Burtness B, Leemans CR, Lui VW, Bauman JE, Grandis JR. Head and neck squamous cell carcinoma. Nat Rev Dis Primers. 2020;6(1):92.
5. Rosenquist K. Risk factors in oral and oropharyngeal squamous cell carcinoma: a population-based case-control study in southern Sweden. Swed Dent J Suppl. 2005;179:1–66.
6. Klein JD, Grandis JR. The molecular pathogenesis of head and neck cancer. Cancer Biol Ther. 2010;9(1):1–7.
7. Thavaraj S. Human papillomavirus-associated neoplasms of the sinonasal tract and nasopharynx. Sem Diagn Pathol. 2016;33(2):104–11.
8. Velleuer E, Dietrich R. Fanconi anemia: young patients at high risk for squamous cell carcinoma. Mol Cell Pediatr. 2014;1(1):1–6.
9. Jéhannin-Ligier K, Dejardin O, Lapôtre-Ledoux B, Bara S, Coureau G, Grosclaude P, Marrer E, Molinié F, Trétarre B, Velten M, Woronoff AS. Oral cancer characteristics in France: descriptive epidemiology for early detection. J Stomatol Oral Maxillofac Surg. 2017;118(2):84–9.
10. Chung CH, Gillison ML. Human papillomavirus in head and neck cancer: its role in pathogenesis and clinical implications. Clin Cancer Res. 2009;15(22):6758–62.
11. Ang KK, Harris J, Wheeler R, Weber R, Rosenthal DI, Nguyen-Tân PF, Westra WH, Chung CH, Jordan RC, Lu C, Kim H. Human papillomavirus and survival of patients with oropharyngeal cancer. N Engl J Med. 2010;363(1):24–35.
12. Chen YP, Chan AT, Le QT, Blanchard P, Sun Y, Ma J. Nasopharyngeal carcinoma. Lancet. 2019;394(10192):64–80.

13. Fossum CC, Chintakuntlawar AV, Price DL, Garcia JJ. Characterization of the oropharynx: anatomy, histology, immunology, squamous cell carcinoma and surgical resection. Histopathology. 2017;70(7):1021–9.
14. Shanmugaratnam K, Sobin LH. The World Health Organization histological classification of tumours of the upper respiratory tract and ear. A commentary on the second edition. Cancer. 1993;71(8):2689–97.
15. Brennan B. Nasopharyngeal carcinoma. Orphanet J Rare Dis. 2006;1(1):1–5.
16. Smith MA, Ries LG, Gurney JG, Bondy ML, Plon SE, Malkin D, Look AT, Kirsch IR, Thiele CJ, Kastan MB, Sondel PM. In: Pizzo PA, Poplack GD, editors. Principles and practice of pediatric oncology; 2002.
17. Brachman DG, Graves D, Vokes E, Beckett M, Haraf D, Montag A, Dunphy E, Mick R, Yandell D, Weichselbaum RR. Occurrence of p53 gene deletions and human papilloma virus infection in human head and neck cancer. Cancer Res. 1992;52(17):4832–6.
18. Hoffmann TK, Sonkoly E, Hauser U, van Lierop A, Whiteside TL, Klussmann JP, Hafner D, Schuler P, Friebe-Hoffmann U, Scheckenbach K, Erjala K. Alterations in the p53 pathway and their association with radio-and chemosensitivity in head and neck squamous cell carcinoma. Oral Oncol. 2008;44(12):1100–9.
19. Bolt J, Vo QN, Kim WJ, McWhorter AJ, Thomson J, Hagensee ME, Friedlander P, Brown KD, Gilbert J. The ATM/p53 pathway is commonly targeted for inactivation in squamous cell carcinoma of the head and neck (SCCHN) by multiple molecular mechanisms. Oral Oncol. 2005;41(10):1013–20.
20. Grandis JR, Zeng Q, Tweardy DJ. Retinoic acid normalizes the increased gene transcription rate of TGF–α and EGFR in head and neck cancer cell lines. Nat Med. 1996;2(2):237–40.
21. Kalyankrishna S, Grandis JR. Epidermal growth factor receptor biology in head and neck cancer. J Clin Oncol. 2006;24(17):2666–72.
22. Ma PC, Maulik G, Christensen J, Salgia R. C-met: structure, functions and potential for therapeutic inhibition. Cancer Metastasis Rev. 2003;22:309–25.
23. Dong G, Lee TL, Yeh NT, Geoghegan J, Waes CV, Chen Z. Metastatic squamous cell carcinoma cells that overexpress c-met exhibit enhanced angiogenesis factor expression, scattering and metastasis in response to hepatocyte growth factor. Oncogene. 2004;23(37):6199–208.
24. Knowles LM, Stabile LP, Egloff AM, Rothstein ME, Thomas SM, Gubish CT, Lerner EC, Seethala RR, Suzuki S, Quesnelle KM, Morgan S. HGF and c-met participate in paracrine tumorigenic pathways in head and neck squamous cell cancer. Clin Cancer Res. 2009;15(11):3740–50.
25. Barnes CJ, Ohshiro K, Rayala SK, El-Naggar AK, Kumar R. Insulin-like growth factor receptor as a therapeutic target in head and neck cancer. Clin Cancer Res. 2007;13(14):4291–9.
26. Molinolo AA, Hewitt SM, Amornphimoltham P, Keelawat S, Rangdaeng S, Meneses García A, Raimondi AR, Jufe R, Itoiz M, Gao Y, Saranath D. Dissecting the Akt/mammalian target of rapamycin signaling network: emerging results from the head and neck cancer tissue array initiative. Clin Cancer Res. 2007;13(17):4964–73.
27. Leong JL, Loh KS, Putti TC, Goh BC, Tan LK. Epidermal growth factor receptor in undifferentiated carcinoma of the nasopharynx. Laryngoscope. 2004;114(1):153–7.
28. Chang KP, Chang YT, Wu CC, Liu YL, Chen MC, Tsang NM, Hsu CL, Chang YS, Yu JS. Multiplexed immunobead-based profiling of cytokine markers for detection of nasopharyngeal carcinoma and prognosis of patient survival. Head Neck. 2011;33(6):886–97.
29. Abubakar MB, Gan SH. Genetics of nasopharyngeal carcinoma and molecular signaling pathways. In: An evidence-based approach to the Management of Nasopharyngeal Cancer. Academic Press; 2020. p. 31–66.
30. Ma X, Huang J, Wu X, Li X, Zhang J, Xue L, Li P, Liu L. Epidermal growth factor receptor could play a prognostic role to predict the outcome of nasopharyngeal carcinoma: a meta-analysis. Cancer Biomark. 2014;14(4):267–77.
31. Ooft ML, Braunius WW, Heus P, Stegeman I, Van Diest PJ, Grolman W, Zuur CI, Willems SM. Prognostic significance of the EGFR pathway in nasopharyngeal carcinoma: a systematic review and meta-analysis. Biomark Med. 2015;9(10):997–1010.

32. Cognetti DM, Weber RS, Lai SY. Head and neck cancer: an evolving treatment paradigm. Cancer. 2008;113(S7):1911–32.
33. Bernier J, Vermorken JB, Koch WM. Adjuvant therapy in patients with resected poor-risk head and neck cancer. J Clin Oncol. 2006;24(17):2629–35.
34. Anderson G, Ebadi M, Vo K, Novak J, Govindarajan A, Amini A. An updated review on head and neck cancer treatment with radiation therapy. Cancers. 2021;13(19):4912.

Eye Cancer

18

Keerthi Reddy, Meghana Korikani,
Rajaram Mohan Roy Karnati, and Rama Krishna Kancha

18.1 Introduction

Epidemiology: Globally eye cancer has very low incidence rates [1]; over all incidence of eye cancer is less than 1% with 850 new cases per year. For the year 2020, the estimated number of new cases in the United States were 3400 cases (males: 1890 cases; females: 1510 cases) and the estimated mortality was 390 deaths (males: 210 deaths; females: 180 deaths). Eye cancer was slightly more predominant in males (53%) when compared to the females (47%). Based on the anatomic site, retinoblastoma and uveal melanoma are the most frequent types of eye cancer [2]. Retinoblastoma contributes to nearly 4% of all the pediatric cancers [3]. Incidence rate in children was 1 in 15,000–18,000 per year worldwide [3]. Global incidence of the retinoblastoma is 9000 new cases per year [4]. Each year, about 300 new retinoblastoma cases are reported in the United States [3]. The incidence of retinoblastoma is equal in boys and girls. The 5-year survival rate of retinoblastoma was 96% in children [3]. For retinoblastoma, the median age of diagnosis was 15 and 24 months for hereditary and sporadic forms, respectively [3]. The incidence rate was higher in the regions of Southeast Asia and South America [3]. The other common type of intraocular cancer is Uveal melanoma (UM), which is usually seen in adults [2]. Uveal melanoma occurs in the uveal tract accounting to 85% of all ocular melanomas [5]. The incidence rate was 4.3% in the United States (male: 4.9%; female: 3.7%) [5]. The incidence rate differs for different ethnic groups, mostly

K. Reddy · M. Korikani · R. K. Kancha (✉)
Molecular Medicine and Therapeutics Laboratory, CPMB, Osmania University, Hyderabad, India
e-mail: ramakancha@osmania.ac.in

R. M. R. Karnati
Department of Animal Biotechnology, School of Life Sciences, University of Hyderabad, Hyderabad, India

R. K. Kancha (ed.), *Biomedical Aspects of Solid Cancers*,
https://doi.org/10.1007/978-981-97-1802-3_18

occurring in non-Hispanic whites (6.02%) followed by Hispanics (1.67%), Asians (0.38%), and Afro-Americans (0.31%) [5]. The median age of Uveal melanoma (UM) diagnosis in the US and Europe is 59–62 years [6]. The mean age-adjusted annual incidence of UM is 5.1 cases per million [6]. UM has an annual incidence of 5 per million; 650 new cases of UM were diagnosed and treated every year [7]. In the age group of above 65 years, UM was more common in males and whites when compared to females and blacks, respectively [2].

Risk Factors: The occurrence of retinoblastoma is mainly influenced by both genetic and environmental factors [8]. *RB1* gene is the main genetic risk factor and low folate (vit B9) intake was the prominent environmental risk factor for the retinoblastoma [8]. The major risk factors for the UM incidence are race, eye color, age, gender, family history, exposure to radiation, choroidal nerve, and somatic mutations [6, 9]. White population is at higher risk than the black population [2]. The incidence ratio of UM in black to white patients was approximately 1:15–1:50 [6]. The incidence rate increases with age; peak age for the incidence was 70 years whereas, in children it was rare [5]. Higher incidence rates were seen in people with light colored skin and eyes, which may be linked to having less melanin resulting in reduced protection from the UV light. UM is higher in males when compared to the incidence in females [6]. Hereditary cancer syndrome is an uncommon condition caused by a mutation in *BAP1* gene that poses an increased risk for UM [6]. The major risk factors for development of basal cell carcinoma (an eye lid cancer) were UV and ionizing radiations, and immune dysfunction [1].

Diagnosis: Eye cancer can be diagnosed by high-frequency ultrasound, computed tomography (CT), fluorescein angiography, and magnetic resonance imaging (MRI) [1]. Different parts of eye have different types of eye cancer; in retina, the tumor size and vitreous status can be detected by ultrasound scanning [1]. Based on the symptoms and rate of progression, diagnosis of uveal melanoma differs for iris, choroid, and ciliary body, which mostly includes CT, ultrasound, MRI, and invasive biopsy [2]. Highly reflective intratumoral calcification which was the diagnosis of retinoblastoma can also be detected by ultrasound [1]. For choroidal melanoma, many office-based imaging techniques are involved for monitoring of the surface and margins of tumors (fundus photography). To detect vasculopathy, cystoid macular edema and fluorescein angiography (FA) can be used [1]. Fundus auto fluorescence (FAF) is used for detecting orange pigment lipofuscin [1]. Ultrasound is used to detect the size of the tumor, internal reflectivity, and extrascleral extensions [1]. MRI and CT are used in the detection of extrascleral extensions and for detecting the stage of the cancer, positron emission tomography/computed tomography (PET-CT) can be used [1].

18.2 Classification

Different classifications for eye cancer were made based on the anatomy and the staging. Eye cancer can be distinguished based on the area of their occurrence as (a) intraocular cancers that arise from the eyeball, (b) orbital cancers that include eye sockets, and (c) adnexal cancers that arise from accessory regions (Fig. 18.1) [2].

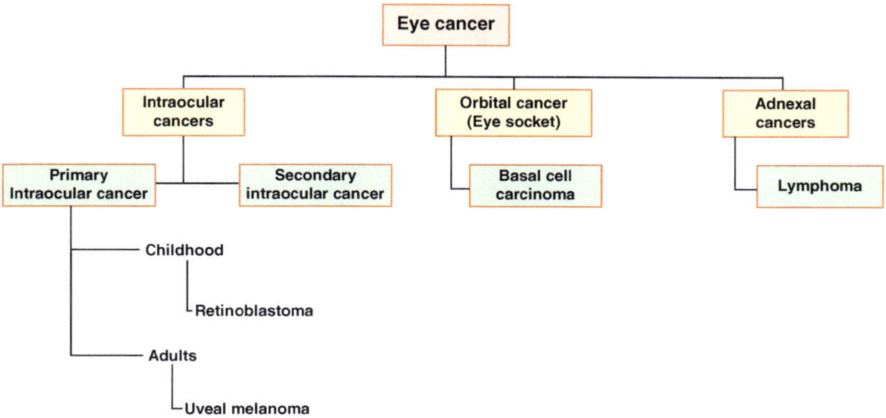

Fig. 18.1 Classification of eye cancer based on the anatomy

Intraocular cancers are further classified as primary that develops in the eye ball of which the frequent type is retinoblastoma and secondary that is metastasized to the eyeball from other parts of the body such as breast and lung tumors (Fig. 18.1) [2]. Retinoblastoma is a primary intraocular cancer and occurs as unilateral (only in one eye) and bilateral (in both eyes) [2]. Bilateral is a heritable form (25%) of eye cancer caused by heritable mutations in the *RB1* gene within a retinal cell, whereas the unilateral retinoblastoma is nonheritable and most common type which accounts for 75% of all the cases [2]. UM is the most frequent intraocular tumor seen in adults that usually develops in three regions: choroid (90%), ciliary body (6–7%), and iris (3–4%) [2]. Ocular adnexal cancer (OAC) occurs in eye lids, lacrimal apparatus, conjunctiva, and orbital soft tissue (Fig. 18.1) [1]. Basal cell carcinoma (BCC) accounts for 90% of eye lid cancers, commonly seen in males [1].

Eye cancer is also classified according to the TNM system, T refers to the tumor size, N refers to the spreading of cancer to nearby lymph nodes, and M refers to the spread of cancer to distant sites [10]. Based on the size of the tumor, uveal melanoma was classified as T1 (small), T2 (medium-sized), T3(large), and T4 (very large) [1]. According to the International Classification for Intraocular Retinoblastoma (ICRB), based on the staging, retinoblastoma is classified into A to E groups [10]. Group A refers to tumors that are retinal, located outside the macula and smaller than 3 mm in size. Group B tumors are located in macula and are >3 mm in size while group C and group D tumors are localized and diffuse vitreous seeds respectively [11]. Group E tumors cover more than 50% of neovascular glaucoma and are reported as unsalvageable [1]. The recent (8th) edition of the TNM added a new trait for retinoblastoma; H refers to heritable trait [12]. According to the AJCC staging of retinoblastoma, size of tumor is stated as Tx (unknown evidence of tumor), T0 (no evidence of tumor), Tis (carcinoma in situ), T1 (intraretinal tumor with subretinal fluid of tumor <5 mm), T1a (with <3 mm tumor), T1b (with >3 mm tumor), T2 (tumor with detachment of retina and vitreous seeds), T2a (with subretinal fluid >5 mm), T2b (vitreous seeding), T3 (advanced tumor), T3a (prephthisis bulbi), T3b (tumor invades other regions of the eye), T3c (intraocular pressure), T3d (with vitreous hemorrhage), T3e (with orbital cellulitis), T4 (with extraocular tumor includes optic nerve and orbit), T4a (with condense of optic nerve), and T4b (tumor with abnormal protrusion of eyes) [1]. NX (cannot assess lymph nodes), N0 (lymph node noninvolvement), and N1 (involvement of preauricular, submandibular, and cervical lymph nodes) [1]. M0 refers to no symptoms of distant metastasis, M1 refers to distant metastasis with no microscopic confirmation, whereas M1a indicates distant site (like bone marrow, liver), and M1b indicates involvement in the CNS [1]. HX refers to no evidence of *RB1* gene mutation, H0 refers to no germline mutation is identified on genetic testing, and H1 refers to an individual with inherited retinoblastoma (*RB1* gene mutation) [1].

According to the AJCC classification of UM based on the TNM: TX (cannot assess primary tumor), T0 (no evidence of primary tumor), T1 (tumor base <9–12 mm with thickness <3–6 mm), T1a (no involvement of ciliary body), T1b (with an involvement of ciliary body), T1c (no involvement of ciliary body but with extraocular extensions <5 mm), T1d (involvement of ciliary body and with extraocular extensions <5 mm), T2 (Tumor base 15–18 mm to <9 mm with thickness <3 mm to 6.1–9 mm), T2a (without involvement of ciliary body and extraocular extension), T2b (no involvement of ciliary body), T2c (no involvement of ciliary body but with extraocular extensions of <5 mm), T2d (involvement of ciliary body and with extraocular extensions of <5 mm), T3 (tumor base 3.1 to 18 mm with thickness of 9.1 to 12 mm), T3a (no involvement of ciliary body and extraocular extension), T3b (no involvement of ciliary body), T3c (no involvement of ciliary body but with extraocular extensions of <5 mm), T3d (involvement of ciliary body and with extraocular extensions of <5 mm of diameter), T4 (tumor base 12.1 to >18 mm and thickness >15 mm to any thickness), T4a (no involvement of ciliary body and extraocular extension), T4b (no involvement of ciliary body), T4c (no involvement of ciliary body and with extraocular extensions and <5 mm in diameter), T4d (involvement of ciliary body and extraocular extensions of <5 mm in diameter), T4e (any size category with extraocular extensions of >5 mm in diameter.

18.3 Pathophysiology

Eye is composed of two connected portions: (a) an anterior segment that consists of cornea, iris, and lens, and (b) a posterior segment that consists of the vitreous, retina, choroid, ciliary bodies, and sclera (Fig. 18.2) [13]. Eye is covered by three layers: outer layer consists of cornea and sclera, middle layer consists of the iris, ciliary body, and choroid, and the innermost retina layer (Fig. 18.2) [14]. The five layers of cornea include an epithelium (made of superficial cells, wing cells, and basal cells), Bowman's membrane (acellular zone of 10–15 mm), lamellar stroma (contains keratocytes surrounded by the extracellular matrix that contains proteoglycans), Descemet's membrane (secreted by endothelial cells), and endothelium (consists of a single layer of cuboidal cells) [15, 16]. The iris of the middle layer is lined by a

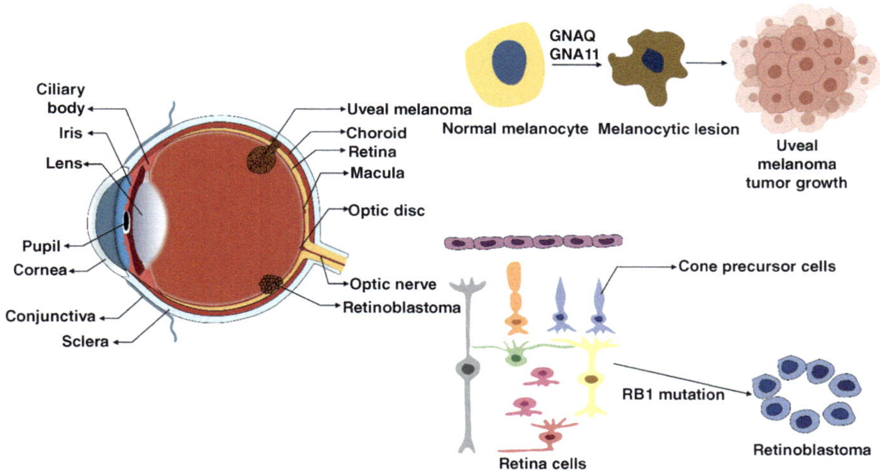

Fig. 18.2 Pathophysiology and cell of origin of eye cancers

pigmented epithelium and consists of a fibrovascular tissue into which the sphincter and dilator pupillae muscles are inserted [13]. Choroid is composed of a dense network of blood vessels and spreads from the margins of the optic nerve to the pars plana, where it continues to anterior and becomes the ciliary body [15, 17]. The outer most layer of the choroid is suprachoroidal. The innermost layer is called the Bruch's membrane (the complex five laminar structures) [17]. Ciliary body is composed of ciliary muscles, which regulate the accommodation of lens; the vitreous is separated from the posterior segment by ciliary bodies [13]. The vertebrate retina develops from the optic cup, of which the inner wall becomes the neural retina that contains six types of neurons, and the outer wall develops into retinal pigment epithelium [16].

UM tumors are derived from the melanocytes which can arise in the iris, ciliary bodies, and the choroid (Fig. 18.2) [18]. Majority of the uveal melanoma arises from the choroid layer; the tumors show vertical growth displacing or rupturing Bruch's membrane. Choroidal melanoma varies in pigmentation from darkly pigmented to amelanotic [13]. The retinoblastoma arises from the retina and destroys the neurosensory retina [18]. Extraocular retinoblastoma spreads from surrounding of the eye to beyond the eye and even may spread to the central nervous system [19]. Endophytic retinoblastoma originates from inner layers of the retina [18]. Exophytic retinoblastoma which arises from the outer retinal layer, causes retinal detachment [18].

Genetics: Mutations in the *CDKN2A* (familial/sporadic) or deletion of genes such as *LZTS1*, *CDKN2A*, *PTEN*, and *BAP1* lead to the uveal melanoma [20]. Amplifications of genes *NSB1, MYC, DDEF1(ASAP1), CCND1, MDM2, BCL-2* on the chromosome 8q21, 8q24, 8q24, 11q13, 12q15, and 18q21, respectively, lead to the UM [20]. Hypermethylation (epigenetic modifications) of *CDKN2A, RASSF1,* and *hTERT* genes are also responsible for the UM pathogenesis [20]. The common chromosomal aberrations in the UM are loss of chromosomes 1p, 3, 6q, 8p and gain of the chromosomes 1q, 6q, and 8q. Mutations in *GNAQ* and *GNA11* genes cause uveal melanoma [21]. Retinoblastoma develops if both the copies of the *RB1* gene are lost/inactivated. Retinoblastoma arises familially and sporadically [18]. About a quarter of sporadic cases are due to germline mutations [18].

18.4 Treatment

Retinoblastoma and uveal melanoma have similar treatment options; the main aim of the retinoblastoma is to save the vision and life of children [22]. The treatment options include surgery (enucleation, orbital exenteration, exo-resection, and endo-resection), radiotherapy (brachytherapy, charged particle therapy (CPT), stereotactic external beam irradiation (SEBI), and transpupillary thermotherapy), focal therapy (photocoagulation, laser, and Cryotherapy), and chemotherapy (Chemoreduction, intra-arterial, and intravitreal) [22].

Surgery: The surgical procedure in which the effected eye and portion of optic nerve are removed is called as enucleation [23]. Based on the treatment, enucleation is of two types: primary enucleation and secondary enucleation [23]. The unilateral intraocular retinoblastoma can be treated by the primary enucleation [22]. Secondary enucleation is preferred when all other treatments have failed and presence of phthisical (wasting, shrinking, and nonfunctioning) in the eye after high-dose chemotherapy [23]. Enucleation is also best treatment option for the uveal melanoma and it is preferred for large tumors which are at high risk for radioactive complications [24]. Orbital exenteration is mostly preferred when the tumor extends into the orbit [25]. All the contents of the orbit are removed and external beam radiation is commonly used as an adjuvant in this resection [25]. Exo-resection and endo-resection are suitable for tumors (uveal melanoma) that are larger than 8 mm in thickness [26]. In exo-resection, tumors are removed by the scleral opening. In endo-resection, tumors are removed by a vitreous cutter that passes through the retina.

Radiation Therapy: Radiation therapy is used for patients who failed on chemotherapy [27]. The recommended dose for the radiation therapy was 40Gy to 45Gy, in 180-cGy to 200-cGy fractions [27]. The major forms of the radiation therapy for eye cancer are brachytherapy, external beam therapy, charged particle therapy (CPT), stereotactic external beam irradiation (SEBI), and transpupillary thermotherapy [25]. Brachytherapy is used for the treatment of small tumors [27]. Brachytherapy is delivered in the form of plaques, applicators, and interstitial implants [28]. The implants of the radioactive material are placed as episcleral plaques to deliver high-dose radiation [27]. The radioactive materials used in brachytherapy are ^{125}I, ^{106}Ru, and ^{113}Pd [27]. Radioactive gold and cobalt are also used in the brachytherapy [27]. In charged particle therapy, helium, proton, and carbon charged particles are used in the treatment of UM [25]. In stereotactic external beam radiation therapy, the radiation is delivered in small fractions over a period of time in the form of gamma knife, stereotactic knife, and cyber knife [28]. Transpupillary thermotherapy is the process of delivering an infrared laser beam into an intraocular tumor to cause cell necrosis [25].

Focal Therapy: Small retinoblastoma tumors can be treated with focal therapy alone, while for large tumors focal therapy will be combined with chemotherapy [22]. Focal therapy includes photocoagulation or laser thermotherapy, chemo-thermotherapy, and cryotherapy [29]. Photocoagulation is application of temperature above 60 °C that results in the protein coagulation and cell death by delivering argon laser [30]. In Chemo-thermotherapy method, thermotherapy is used simultaneously with chemotherapy; heat can be delivered by using a diode or YAG laser at a temperature between 42 °C and 60 °C [31]. Before 1–2 h of chemo-thermotherapy, carboplatin will be given intravenously [32]. Cryotherapy involves the freezing the tumor using direct ophthalmoscopy [33].

Chemotherapy: The chemotherapy treatment includes chemoreduction, intravitreal, and intra-arterial chemotherapy, which are common for both uveal melanoma and retinoblastoma [34]. Chemoreduction technique involves the combination of both chemotherapeutic agents and localized treatments (laser photo coagulation, thermotherapy, cryotherapy or plaque radiotherapy) [34]. The regimes that are used in chemoreduction include alkylating agents, DNA topoisomerase II inhibitors, and vinca alkaloids [34]. In this treatment, the intravenous chemotherapy is administrated for several cycles [34]. In intra-arterial chemotherapy, the agents such as melphalan, topotecan, and carboplatin are directly administered to the eye [34]. The exposure to radiation in the eye is minimum during this treatment [35]. The intravenous chemotherapy is used for the treatment of extraocular retinoblastoma [36]. In this treatment, the chemotherapeutic agents such as vincristine, etoposide, and carboplatin are directly injected into the vitreous cavity to treat vitreous tumors [36].

18.5 Conclusion

Eye cancer has the least incidence rate among all other cancers and is most prominent in males than in females. Among eye cancers, retinoblastoma and uveal melanoma are the well-known and occur in the retina and uveal region of the eye, respectively. Mutation in the *RB1* gene is the major cause for the retinoblastoma and mutation in the *GNAQ* and *GNA11* genes is the major reason for the uveal melanoma. Size of the tumor can be detected by ultrasound; extrascleral extension is detected by magnetic resonance imaging and stage of the cancer can be detected by positron emission topography-CT scan. Various similar options are available for the treatment of both retinoblastoma and uveal melanoma. Chemotherapy with agents such as vincistrine, etoposide, and carboplatin are the best treatment options for the eye cancer; for large size tumors, focal therapy along with chemotherapy was recommended. In case of any fail in the chemotherapy, radiation therapy was recommended with dose of 40Gy to 45Gy in 180-cGy to 200-cGy fractions. Last option for the treatment of the eye tumor is surgery; unilateral intralocular retinoblastoma is treated by primary enucleation and large-sized uveal melanoma tumor can be treated by secondary enucleation. Exo-resection and endo-resection are suitable for tumors (uveal melanoma) that are larger than 8 mm in thickness.

References

1. Maheshwari A, Finger PT. Cancers of the eye. Cancer Metastasis Rev. 2018;37:677–90.
2. Lande K, Gupta J, Ranjan R, Kiran M, Torres Solis LF, Solís Herrera A, Aliev G, Karnati R. Exosomes: insights from retinoblastoma and other eye cancers. Int J Mol Sci. 2020;21(19):7055.
3. Sheehan AP. Retinoblastoma: early diagnosis is crucial. J Pediatr Health Care. 2020;34(6):601–5.
4. Ortiz MV, Dunkel IJ. Retinoblastoma. J Child Neurol. 2016;31(2):227–36.
5. Amaro A, Gangemi R, Piaggio F, Angelini G, Barisione G, Ferrini S, Pfeffer U. The biology of uveal melanoma. Cancer Metastasis Rev. 2017;36:109–40.
6. Kaliki S, Shields CL. Uveal melanoma: relatively rare but deadly cancer. Eye. 2017;31(2):241–57.
7. Wang H, Elsheikh M, Gilmour K, Cohen V, Sagoo MS, Damato B, Anguita R, Heimann H, Hussain R, Cauchi P, Chadha V. Impact of COVID-19 pandemic on eye cancer care in United Kingdom. Br J Cancer. 2021;124(8):1357–60.
8. Goldofsky E, Cohen BA, Greenstein AJ. Acute septic pancreatitis presenting as colonic necrosis. Am J Gastroenterol. 1984;79(7):548–52.
9. Chattopadhyay C, Kim DW, Gombos DS, Oba J, Qin Y, Williams MD, Esmaeli B, Grimm EA, Wargo JA, Woodman SE, Patel SP. Uveal melanoma: from diagnosis to treatment and the science in between. Cancer. 2016;122(15):2299–312.
10. Kivelä T, Kujala E. Prognostication in eye cancer: the latest tumor, node, metastasis classification and beyond. Eye (Lond). 2013;27(2):243–52. https://doi.org/10.1038/eye.2012.256. Epub 2012 Dec 21. PMID: 23258307; PMCID: PMC3574256
11. Kim JW, Abramson DH, Dunkel IJ. Current management strategies for intraocular retinoblastoma. Drugs. 2007;67(15):2173–85.
12. Dimaras H, Corson TW. Retinoblastoma, the visible CNS tumor: a review. J Neurosci Res. 2019;97(1):29–44.
13. Broggi G, Russo A, Reibaldi M, Russo D, Varricchio S, Bonfiglio V, Spatola C, Barbagallo C, Foti PV, Avitabile T, Longo A. Histopathology and genetic biomarkers of choroidal melanoma. Appl Sci. 2020;10(22):8081.
14. Kels BD, Grzybowski A, Grant-Kels JM. Human ocular anatomy. Clin Dermatol. 2015;33(2):140–6.
15. DelMonte DW, Kim T. Anatomy and physiology of the cornea. J. Cataract Refract Surg. 2011;37:588–98.
16. Willoughby CE, Ponzin D, Ferrari S, Lobo A, Landau K, Omidi Y. Anatomy and physiology of the human eye: effects of mucopolysaccharidoses disease on structure and function–a review. Clin Experiment Ophthalmol. 2010;38:2–11.
17. Dl N, Wallman J. The multifunctional choroid. Prog Retin Eye Res. 2010;29(2):144–68.
18. Eagle RC. The pathology of ocular cancer. Eye. 2013;27(2):128–36.
19. Dimas K, Ulukaya E, Sakellaridis N. Cancer of the eye (intraocular cancer). 2015.
20. Coupland SE, Lake SL, Zeschnigk M, Damato BE. Molecular pathology of uveal melanoma. Eye. 2012;1:13.
21. Griewank KG, Yu X, Khalili J, Sozen MM, Stempke-Hale K, Bernatchez C, Wardell S, Bastian BC, Woodman SE. Genetic and molecular characterization of uveal melanoma cell lines. Pigment Cell Melanoma Res. 2012;25(2):182–7.
22. AlAli A, Kletke S, Gallie B, Lam WC. Retinoblastoma for pediatric ophthalmologists. Asia-Pac J Ophthalmol. 2018;7(3):160–8.

23. Leclerc R, Olin J. An overview of retinoblastoma and enucleation in pediatric patients. AORN J. 2020;111(1):69–79.
24. Williams BK, Di Nicola M. Ocular oncology—primary and metastatic malignancies. Med Clin. 2021;105(3):531–50.
25. Singh M, Durairaj P, Yeung J. Uveal melanoma: a review of the literature. Oncol Ther. 2018;6:87–104.
26. Gündüz K, Bechrakis NE. Exoresection and endoresection for uveal melanoma. Middle East Afr J Ophthalmol. 2010;17(3):210.
27. Rodriguez-Galindo C, Orbach DB, VanderVeen D. Retinoblastoma. Pediatr Clin. 2015;62(1):201–23.
28. Stannard C, Sauerwein W, Maree G, Lecuona K. Radiotherapy for ocular tumours. Eye. 2013;27(2):119–27.
29. Chan HS, Gallie BL, Munier FL. Chemotherapy for retinoblastoma. Ophthalmol Clin N Am. 2005;18(1):55–63.
30. Suzuki S, Kaneko A. Management of intraocular retinoblastoma and ocular prognosis. Int J Clin Oncol. 2004;9:1–6.
31. Ray A, Gombos DS. Retinoblastoma: an overview. Indian J Pediatr. 2012;79:916–21.
32. Balmer A, Zografos L, Munier F. Diagnosis and current management of retinoblastoma. Oncogene. 2006;25(38):5341–9.
33. Rao R, Honavar SG. Retinoblastoma. Indian J Pediatr. 2017;84:937–44.
34. Shah CP, Shields CL, Shields JA. Chemotherapy for malignant intraocular tumors. Ret Pharmacotherap. 2016;55:337–43.
35. Wyse E, Handa JT, Friedman AD, Pearl MS. A review of the literature for intra-arterial chemotherapy used to treat retinoblastoma. Pediatr Radiol. 2016;46:1223–33.
36. Fabian ID, Onadim Z, Karaa E, Duncan C, Chowdhury T, Scheimberg I, Ohnuma SI, Reddy MA, Sagoo MS. The management of retinoblastoma. Oncogene. 2018;37(12):1551–60.

Adrenocortical Carcinoma 19

Manasa Desai, Prapthi Bathini, Hameeda Bee, and Rama Krishna Kancha

19.1 Introduction

Adrenocortical carcinoma (ACC) affects women more often than men, with five-year survival rate of about 50% [1]. It is the second most frequent endocrine cancer and the frequency of incidence is twice in females than in males [2, 3]. Approximately half of ACC patients have symptoms of hypersecretion of glucocorticoids and/or androgens while one-third of cases have symptoms related to the tumor mass [1, 4]. The majority of ACC instances are sporadic; however, germline alterations have been linked to 5–10% of ACCs. ACC was seen in several syndromes and develops in about 1% of Li-Fraumeni syndrome patients, usually before the age of 30 years [4–6]. The usage of oral contraceptives, alcohol consumption, and cigarette smoking were found to be linked to the development of ACC [7]. The diagnosis of cancer is based on a thorough evaluation of clinical history and examination for adrenal hormone excess, detailed hormonal workup, and imaging (CT or MRI) before surgery as well as a pathological examination after the tumor has been removed. In the majority of cases, traditional and functional imaging can correctly diagnose an adrenal tumor as ACC. The risk of ACC rises with tumor size, with a higher index of suspicion for larger tumors [8, 9].

M. Desai · R. K. Kancha (✉)
Molecular Medicine and Therapeutics Laboratory, CPMB, Osmania University, Hyderabad, India
e-mail: ramakancha@osmania.ac.in

P. Bathini
Apollo Institute of Medical Sciences and Research, Hyderabad, India

H. Bee
Deparment of Microbiology, Osmania University, Hyderabad, India

R. K. Kancha (ed.), *Biomedical Aspects of Solid Cancers*,
https://doi.org/10.1007/978-981-97-1802-3_19

19.2 Classification

According to WHO 2017 classification, cortical carcinoma, cortical adenoma, sex cord-stromal tumors, adenomatoid tumor, mesenchymal and stromal tumors, hematological tumors, and secondary tumors are the many types of adrenal cortex [10]. T stage: Stage I—tumor size <5 cm, localized to adrenals; Stage II—tumor >5 cm, localized to adrenals; Stage III—tumor of any size with positive regional lymph nodes, metastasis to the surrounding tissue; Stage IV—tumor of any size with metastasis to adjacent organs or venous tumor. N stage: N0: lymph nodes that are negative and N1 refers to lymph nodes that are positive. M stage: M0 denotes the absence of distant metastases and M1 denotes the presence of distant metastases [2]. According to TNM staging of ACC, stage 1 is T1 N0 M0, stage 2 is T2 N0 M0, stage 3 is T3 N0 M0, T1/2 N1 M0, T4 N0 M0, T3/4 N1 M0, and stage 4 is any T N M1 [2]. The survival rates for stages 1, 2, 3, and 4 are 66–82%, 58–64%, 24–55%, and 0–18%, respectively [3].

19.3 Pathophysiology

Anatomy and Cell of Origin: The adrenal glands are small paired organs located on the superior aspect of each kidney. They weigh about 5 grams each and account for less than 1% of the total body weight. Each gland is divided into two distinct regions: the cortex and the medulla. The cortex has distinct layers: zona glomerulosa, fasciculata, and reticularis (Fig. 19.1). In these zones, cholesterol is converted into aldosterone, cortisol, and androgen hormones. Zone glomerulosa cells are found in a series of irregular focal nests around the cortex's periphery. Zona glomerulosa produces mineralocorticoids such as the aldosterone. ACTH regulates the

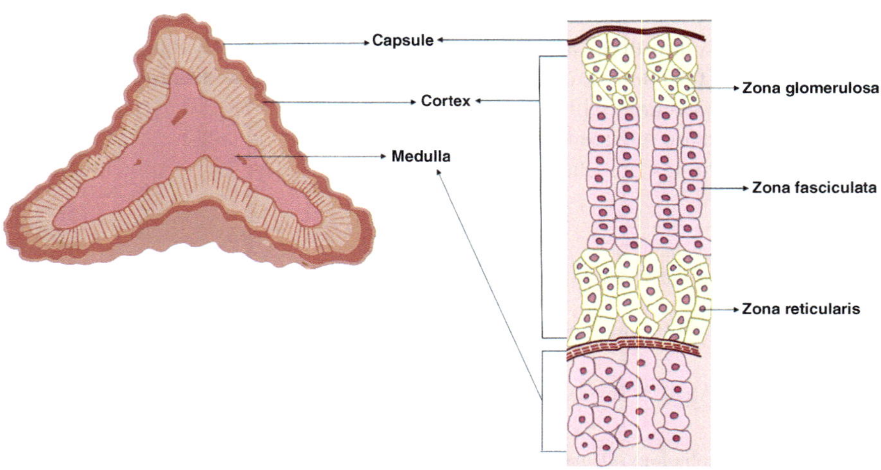

Fig. 19.1 Transverse section of adrenal gland and cells of adrenal cortex

zona fasciculata, which is the middle layer and is primarily responsible for glucocorticoid synthesis. Zona reticularis is the inner layer that secretes adrenal androgens such as DHEA and androstenedione as well as some glucocorticoids. Adrenal medulla, on the other hand, is a component of the sympathetic nervous system. It releases catecholamines on stimulation. Adrenocortical carcinoma is the cancer of adrenal cortex.

Genetics: Germline mutations in *TP53* gene were reported in about three-fourths of Li-Fraumeni syndrome families [9, 11]. Somatic mutations in *TP53* gene were found in only a quarter of sporadic ACC in adults [9, 12, 13]. Mutations of the *MEN1* gene are extremely uncommon in adrenocortical tumors; 25–40% of patients have mutations in *MEN1* [14]. Overexpression of IGF2, IGF1R, and IR are commonly observed in ACC [14], resulting in an auto-paracrine loop in which IGF2, via IGF1R and IR stimulation, activates IGF-downstream pathways that promote cancer [15]. In 3 out of the 28 cases, *FGFR1* amplification was reported. Genetic alterations of the FGFR pathway have been described in ACC cases ranging from 0% (for *FGFR1*) to 6% (for F*GFR4*) [16]. *CTNNB1* gene mutations are found in approximately 40% of ACC patients [17]. Several studies have found that copy number gains or amplifications in the CDK4 locus are common in ACC, with a prevalence ranging from 7% to 40%. Deletions in CDKN2A or CDKN2B were found in more than 10% of ACC patients [18].

19.4 Treatment

The best treatment option for ACC is a complete tumor resection. Surgery is the preferred treatment for nonmetastatic ACC and provides the best opportunity for long-term control of the cancer. The local control of ACC is critical for cure as well as improving symptomatic outcomes. Cytotoxic chemotherapy is now the standard treatment for advanced and metastatic ACC. When stable disease is counted as a response, approximately 30–50% of overall response was observed with chemotherapeutic regimens [19]. Radiotherapy was shown to be effective for ACC both in adjuvant and palliative settings, though such an improvement has not been demonstrated universally [20, 21]. The mTOR pathway was dysregulated in a fraction of ACC patients. Therefore, treatment with mTOR inhibitors as well as metformin was shown to be effective in vitro and in vivo [22, 23].

19.5 Conclusion

Adrenocortical carcinoma is a rare tumor with a good rate of survival. Women seem to be more affected than men. Risk factors mainly are genetic, and hormone excess is a common marker. Copy number alterations are significant contributing factors for this disease. Tumor resection seems to be the only solution; however, in cases of mTOR pathway dysregulation, temsirolimus and everolimus, either alone or in combination with other drugs were shown to be effective.

References

1. Altieri B, Ronchi CL, Kroiss M, Fassnacht M. Next-generation therapies for adrenocortical carcinoma. Best Pract Res Clin Endocrinol Metab. 2020;34(3):101434.
2. Lam AK. Adrenocortical carcinoma: updates of clinical and pathological features after renewed world health organisation classification and pathology staging. Biomedicines. 2021;9(2):175.
3. Wanis KN, Kanthan R. Diagnostic and prognostic features in adrenocortical carcinoma: a single institution case series and review of the literature. World J Surg Oncol. 2015;13(1):1–3.
4. Rodgers SE, Evans DB, Lee JE, Perrier ND. Adrenocortical carcinoma. Surg Oncol Clin. 2006;15(3):535–53.
5. Kamilaris CD, Hannah-Shmouni F, Stratakis CA. Adrenocortical tumorigenesis: lessons from genetics. Best Pract Res Clin Endocrinol Metab. 2020;34(3):101428.
6. Sameshima Y, Tsunematsu Y, Watanabe S, Tsukamoto T, Kawa-ha K, Hirata Y, Mizoguchi H, Sugimura T, Terada M, Yokota J. Detection of novel germ-line p53 mutations in diverse-cancer-prone families Identifiled by selecting patients with childhood Adrencortical carcinoma. JNCI J Natl Cancer Inst. 1992;84(9):703–7.
7. Hsing AW, Nam JM, Co Chien HT, McLaughlin JK, Fraumeni JF Jr. Risk factors for adrenal cancer: an exploratory study. Int J Cancer. 1996;65(4):432–6.
8. Sturgeon C, Shen WT, Clark OH, Duh QY, Kebebew E. Risk assessment in 457 adrenal cortical carcinomas: how much does tumor size predict the likelihood of malignancy? J Am Coll Surg. 2006;202(3):423–30.
9. Libe R, Fratticci A, Bertherat J. Adrenocortical cancer: pathophysiology and clinical management. Endocr Relat Cancer. 2007;14(1):13–28.
10. Lam AK. Update on adrenal tumours in 2017 World Health Organization (WHO) of endocrine tumours. Endocr Pathol. 2017;28:213–27.
11. Hisada M, Garber JE, Li FP, Fung CY, Fraumeni JF. Multiple primary cancers in families with Li-Fraumeni syndrome. JNCI J Natl Cancer Inst. 1998;90(8):606–11.
12. Ohgaki H, Kleihues P, Heitz PU. p53 mutations in sporadic adrenocortical tumors. Int J Cancer. 1993;54(3):408–10.
13. Reincke M, Karl MI, Travis WH, Mastorakos GE, Allolio BR, Linehan HM, Chrousos GP. p53 mutations in human adrenocortical neoplasms: immunohistochemical and molecular studies. J Clin Endocrinol Metabol. 1994;78(3):790–4.
14. De Martino MC, van Koetsveld PM, Feelders RA, de Herder WW, Dogan F, Janssen J, Hofste Op Bruinink D, Pivonello C, Waaijers AM, Colao A, et al. Igf and mtor pathway expression and in vitro effects of linsitinib and mtor inhibitors in adrenocortical cancer. Endocrine. 2019;64:673–84.
15. Altieri B, Tirabassi G, Casa SD, Ronchi CL, Balercia G, Orio F, Pontecorvi A, Colao A, Muscogiuri G. Adrenocortical tumors and insulin resistance: what is the first step? Int J Cancer. 2016;138(12):2785–94.
16. Zheng S, Cherniack AD, Dewal N, Moffitt RA, Danilova L, Murray BA, Lerario AM, Else T, Knijnenburg TA, Ciriello G, Kim S. Comprehensive pan-genomic characterization of adrenocortical carcinoma. Cancer Cell. 2016;29(5):723–36.
17. Lippert J, Appenzeller S, Liang R, Sbiera S, Kircher S, Altieri B, Nanda I, Weigand I, Gehrig A, Steinhauer S, Riemens RJ. Targeted molecular analysis in adrenocortical carcinomas: a strategy toward improved personalized prognostication. J Clin Endocrinol Metabol. 2018;103(12):4511–23.
18. Assié G, Jouinot A, Bertherat J. The 'omics' of adrenocortical tumours for personalized medicine. Nat Rev Endocrinol. 2014;10(4):215–28.
19. Else T, Kim AC, Sabolch A, Raymond VM, Kandathil A, Caoili EM, Jolly S, Miller BS, Giordano TJ, Hammer GD. Adrenocortical carcinoma. Endocr Rev. 2014;35(2):282–326.
20. Sabolch A, Feng M, Griffith K, Hammer G, Doherty G, Ben-Josef E. Adjuvant and definitive radiotherapy for adrenocortical carcinoma. Int J Radiat Oncol Biol Phys. 2011;80(5):1477–84.

21. Hermsen IG, Groenen YE, Dercksen MW, Theuws J, Haak HR. Response to radiation therapy in adrenocortical carcinoma. J Endocrinol Investig. 2010;33:712–4.
22. Non-Aldosterone-Producing UN. The role of insulin-like growth factor system in the adreno-cortical tumors. Minerva Endocrinol. 2019;44(1):43–57.
23. Poli G, Cantini G, Armignacco R, Fucci R, Santi R, Canu L, Nesi G, Mannelli M, Luconi M. Metformin as a new anti-cancer drug in adrenocortical carcinoma. Oncotarget. 2016;7(31):49636.

Thyroid Cancer

20

Manasa Desai, Mohammed Qudrathulla Khan Quadri,
Hameeda Bee, Prapthi Bathini, and Rama Krishna Kancha

20.1 Introduction

Thyroid cancer (TC) ranks ninth in incidence and is more common in young individuals [1, 2]. The disease's mortality rates are substantially lower, with women dying at a rate of 0.5 per 100,000 and males dying at a rate of 0.3 per 100,000 [1]. Incidence rates are higher in transitioned nations than in transitional countries [3]. Incidence is high in Eastern Asia with 260,692 new cases in 2020 and Cyprus has the highest global rates [1]. According to the National Cancer Registry Program (NCRP), there were 11,262 new cases of TC in India in 2020. Over screening and subsequent greater diagnosis rates were cited as a main reason for increasing incidence in high-income nations such as the United States and South Korea [4]. Women and ages between 20 and55 are at a higher risk for developing TCs. Childhood and adolescent exposure to ionizing radiation for diagnostic or therapeutic purposes such as the radiation therapy is a risk factor for papillary TC [5]. A dose-dependent relationship between exposure and the risk of TC was discovered in Chernobyl as well as Hiroshima and Nagasaki atomic bombings [6]. TC risk increases with an exposure at younger age and peaks at 15 to 19 years after exposure [7]. The risk of TC increases with a family history of TC or benign thyroid disease [4, 8]. Iodine deficiency is a risk factor for papillary TC, while excess iodine intake has been linked to follicular and anaplastic TC [9]. A thyroid nodule is a radiologically

M. Desai · M. Q. K. Quadri · R. K. Kancha (✉)
Molecular Medicine and Therapeutics Laboratory, CPMB, Osmania University, Hyderabad, India
e-mail: ramakancha@osmania.ac.in

H. Bee
Department of Microbiology, Osmania University, Hyderabad, India

P. Bathini (✉)
Apollo Institute of Medical Sciences and Research, Hyderabad, India

R. K. Kancha (ed.), *Biomedical Aspects of Solid Cancers*,
https://doi.org/10.1007/978-981-97-1802-3_20

distinguishable lesion within the thyroid gland [10]. Difficulty in swallowing, hoarseness or change in voice, and family history of TC, thyroid swellings require examination and investigation. Incidentally discovered nodules, which may be non-palpable when discovered on ultrasound or other anatomic imaging investigations and are just as likely to become cancerous as palpable nodules of the same size [10]. Higher TSH level in the serum is linked to increased risk of TC [11]. Fine needle aspiration biopsy is used to determine if it is cancerous or not.

20.2 Classification

There are two types of cells in thyroid tissue: follicular cells and parafollicular cells. Follicular cells are the source of differentiated thyroid carcinoma (DTC). Medullary thyroid cancer (MTC) is a type of TC that develops from parafollicular thyroid "C" cells [12]. TC can be broadly classified as (i) differentiated and (ii) undifferentiated. The most aggressive kind of TC is undifferentiated anaplastic thyroid cancer (ATC). According to the 2017 WHO histological categorization, there are three subclasses of differentiated thyroid cancer (DTC) that arise from epithelial thyroid cells: (a) papillary thyroid carcinoma (PTC), (b) follicular thyroid carcinoma (FTC), and (c) poorly differentiated thyroid carcinoma (PDTC) [13–16]. PTC accounts for more than 85% of cases. PTCs develop from follicular cells and are classified into three subtypes based on histotype: classical (most common) follicular, and tall cell variation (TCV) [17, 18]. The classical variant of PTC (50–60%) is a low-risk subtype while the tall-cell variant (5–11%) is more aggressive and the follicular variant of PTC (FV-PTC) can be either invasive encapsulated (24–33%) or noninvasive encapsulated FV-PTC [19, 20]. FTC accounts for 10–30% of all well-differentiated TCs [20, 21]. MTC arises from the C cells, accounts for about 3–5% of all cases, and is often associated with genetic mutations (e.g., *RET* gene). Anaplastic thyroid carcinoma (ATC) is a rare and aggressive form of TC that accounts for less than 2% of all cases. It usually affects older individuals and is associated with a poor prognosis. Poorly differentiated thyroid carcinoma (PDTC) is an aggressive type of TC that shares features with both DTC and ATC. It has a higher risk of distant metastasis and is associated with a poor prognosis [22].

The latest edition of WHO enlisted few changes classifying tumors of thyroid cancer based on their histopathology and their mutational profiles (Fig. 20.1) [23]. FTCs were categorized into benign, low risk, and malignant tumors [23]. Follicular variants of PTC with papillary structures were listed under benign neoplasm [23]. Multifocal benign nodules characterizing hyperplasia were newly introduced as follicular nodules [23]. In Malignant neoplasm, variants of PTC with BRAF-like mutations are differentiated from invasive encapsulated follicular variant papillary carcinomas that exhibit RAS-like mutational profiles into different subtypes [23]. Any differentiated TCs with high-grade features were listed under Follicular-derived carcinomas as differentiated high-grade TCs distinguishing it from poorly differentiated TCs [23]. Squamous cell carcinomas are now classified as undifferentiated ATCs [23]. Hurthle cell adenoma and Hurthle cell carcinoma are now renamed as oncocytic adenoma and oncocytic carcinoma (OCA), respectively [23].

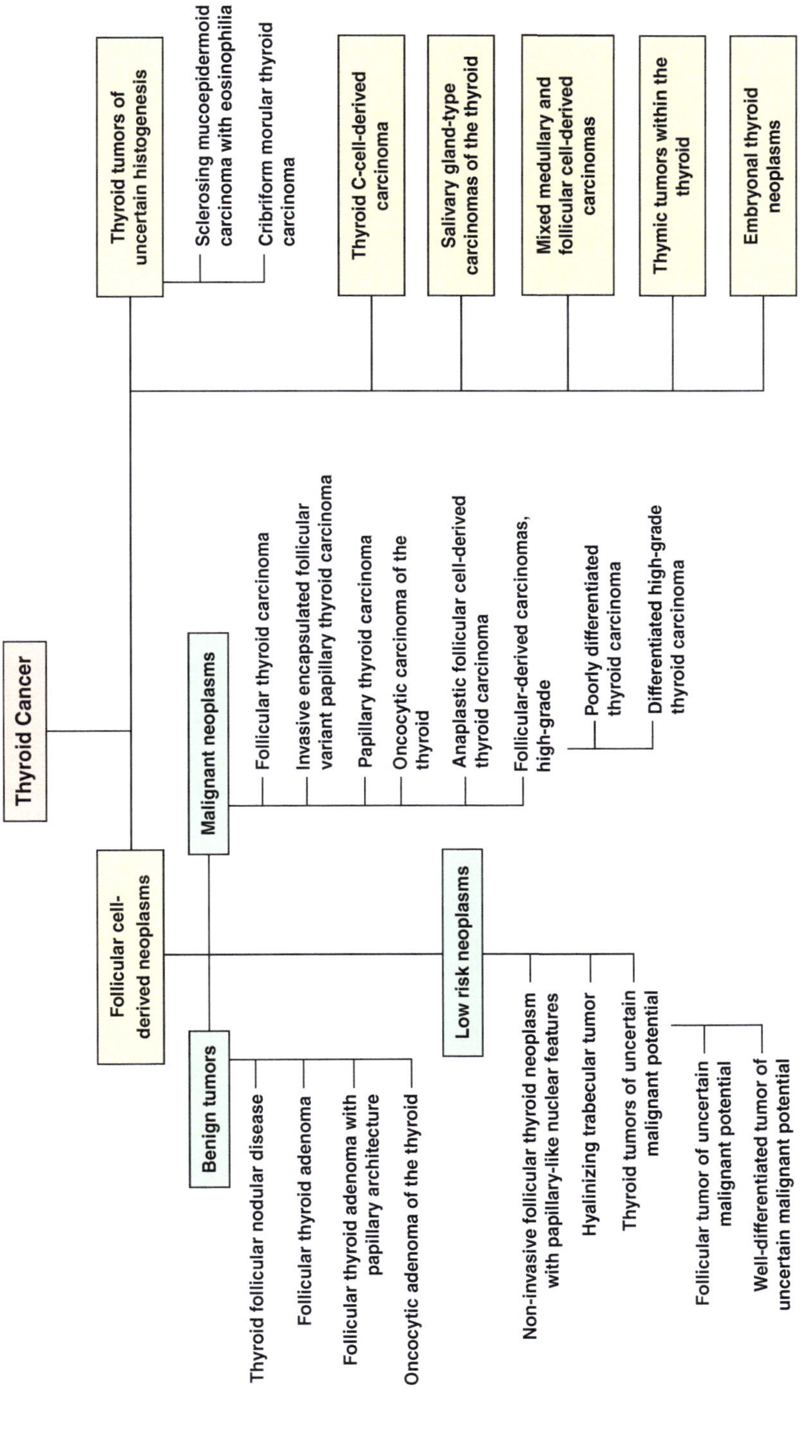

Fig. 20.1 WHO classification of thyroid cancer

Staging: Staging depends on size of the primary tumor, the extent of invasion into nearby tissues or organs, and the presence of lymph node or distant metastasis. For patients of <45 years of age with PTC or FTC, stage 1 refers to tumor that is localized to the thyroid gland, and stage 2 refers to the cancer that has spread to distant sites. For patients >45 years of age, stage 1 refers to tumor that is localized to the thyroid gland, stage 2 refers to the tumor size of 2–4 cm and localized to thyroid gland, stage 3 to a tumor size of <4 cm and still contained in the thyroid (T3) and no metastasis, and stage 4 when the tumor has spread locally, or to lymph nodes or if there is metastasis. For MTC, stage 0 is when the disease is detected by biochemical testing. Stage 1 refers to a tumor of <2 cm and stage 2 for 2–4 cm with no metastasis, or >4 cm with minimal extension. Stage 3 is when metastasis is till paratracheal or paralaryngeal lymph nodes. Stage 4A is moderately advanced with no distant metastasis. Stage 4B is when disease is advanced without any distant metastasis and Stage 4C is when there is a distant metastasis.

20.3 Pathophysiology

Anatomy and Cell of Origin: The thyroid gland regulates the basal metabolic rate (BMR), growth, and development, and is important for calcium metabolism [24]. Thyroid lobules are made up of several thyroid follicles (Fig. 20.2). Simple cuboidal epithelium is formed of thyroid follicular cells, which are organized in spherical thyroid follicles around the colloid, a fluid-filled cavity, lumen containing thyroglobulin. Thyroid hormone is secreted by these follicular cells. Thyroxine is a combination of predominant circulating version tetraiodothyronine (T4) and a little amount of triiodothyronine (T3). T3 is almost four times as effective as T4 and the

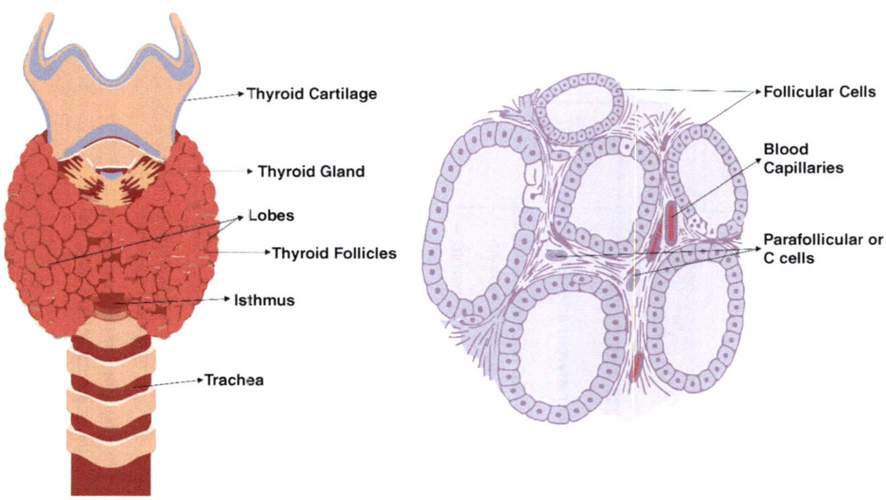

Fig. 20.2 Anatomy and physiology of TC

normal thyroid gland generates 80% of T4 and 20% of T3 [24, 25]. The small C cells are found in between these thyroid follicles or within the walls of the thyroid follicles. The lighter stained cytoplasm of parafollicular cells can be used to distinguish them from the follicular cells. The thyroid gland's normal follicular epithelium exhibits no detectable cytokeratin 19 (CK19) expression, whereas in PTC, it is overexpressed. Therefore, CK19 may serve as a reliable immunomarker for PTC diagnosis. Testing for thyroid tumors can be done by using cytochemical labeling to detect the up- or downregulation of E-cadherin, fibronectin, CD44, p27Kip, and BRAF [24, 26]. PTC, FTC, and ATC are generated by follicular epithelial thyroid cells that are involved in iodine metabolism [27, 28].

Genetics: As per molecular profiling, PTC is a less well-differentiated carcinoma than FTC [29]. WDTC is associated with 20–50% of undifferentiated tumors. Sometimes WDTC foci coexist with PDTC, indicating that the initial tumor was dedifferentiated [30]. The vast majority of TC instances are sporadic, with only 5% of DTC (mainly PTC) being familial and 25% of MTC being inherited as an autosomal trait [31]. According to the data from TCGA, approximately 70% of somatic driver mutations in PTC were identified as MAPK pathway activators such as *BRAF* and *RAS* as well as gene rearrangements in *RET* and *NTRK1* genes [17, 20, 32]. Mutations in *PTEN* and *PIK3CA* genes were observed at lesser frequencies at 2.32% and 3.48%, respectively [17, 33]. Up to 40% of all PTC have multifocality, which leads to aggressiveness and resistance to radioiodine treatment [17, 34–36]. In FTC, PI3K/Akt pathway has been found to have molecular changes, mutations, and/or gene copy number variations. FTC has a high prevalence in PIK3CA genetic copy gain (24%) [20, 37]. The BRAF-V600E mutation is quite uncommon in FTC [38]. Up to 40–50% of FTCs have *RAS* mutations; *PAX8-PPAR* gene fusions were reported in about one-third of FTC. When compared to WDTC, PDTC has a higher mutation rate. Mutations in *RAS* and *BRAF* are present in 20–50% and 35% of PDTC cases, respectively [30]. *TERT* promoter (20–50%) and *TP53* (10–35%) mutations that co-occur with *RAS* and *BRAF* mutations characterize PDTC [39]. Other genetic changes reported in PDTC are mutations in *CTNNB1* and *EIF1AX*, rearrangements in *ALK* gene, gain of chromosome 1q, and loss of 1p, 13q, 15q, and 22q chromosomes [40]. ATC has a substantially higher mutation burden than PTC and PDTC [17, 30]. ATC can develop on its own, but it frequently occurs in conjunction with well-differentiated tumors. The presence of *BRAF* and *RAS* mutations in ATC shows that it shares a genetic origin with the DTC [17, 41–43]. In ATC, *BRAF* (20–45%), *TP53* (70%), and *RAS* (20–40%) are the most common mutations. Many other changes implicated in ATC's aggressive behavior have been reported, which involve *EIF1AX*, *NF1*, *KMT*, and *PI3K/Akt* pathway genes [39]. Keratin, vimentin, and N-cadherin are found in ATC cells [20].

20.4 Treatment

The treatment of TC depends on several factors and may include surgery, radioactive iodine therapy, external beam radiation therapy, chemotherapy, and targeted therapy. Despite their numerous biological differences, PTC and FTC are quite often treated similarly [44]. Thyroidectomy is recommended for FTC with vascular infiltration and for FTC that has spread broadly. If lymph node metastases are found pre- or postoperatively, lymph node dissection is advised [45]. Thyroidectomy is advised for all PTCs that are larger than 1 cm in size as well as for all macroscopically invasive or metastasized PTCs, regardless of the size [45]. Total thyroidectomy is still advised in patients with metastatic DTC to facilitate radioiodine therapy [46]. Radioactive iodine therapy (RIT) refers to the systemic delivery of radioiodine in the form of sodium iodide or potassium iodide to irradiate and destroy thyroid remnants and DTC that are unresectable or have undergone incomplete resection. The benefit was demonstrated in DTC patients who were at a high risk of recurrence. Prospective studies have not shown that RIT has a positive effect on tumor-free and overall survival in patients with very low-risk DTC [45, 47]. Chemotherapy and radiotherapy have a limited role. Sorafenib, lenvatinib, and vandetanib were shown to be effective in papillary or follicular TC. Dabrafenib and trametinib are used to treat anaplastic TC in patients with mutation in the *BRAF* gene. Immunotherapy is also a treatment option for advanced or metastatic TC using immune checkpoint inhibitors [48]. Antitumor activity was demonstrated in vitro and in preclinical investigations with agents that target MAPK and PI3K/Akt pathways.

20.5 Conclusion

Incidence of TC has increased recently in both the sexes, of them mostly the middle-aged women. Mostly surgery is performed and complication rates also vary based on the type of surgery. With substantial information and advancement of studies on TC biology, contributions toward the development of novel diagnostic, prognostic, and prediction look practical. Efforts toward the molecular tests and gene expression markers can reduce the surgery for benign thyroid nodules. In addition, circulating miRNAs due to high stability and specificity can be considered as diagnostic and predictive biomarkers when compared to serum thyroglobulin assays. Successful drugs recommended include multikinase inhibitors such as sorafenib, lenvatinib, vancetabib, and cabozantinib, and few specific inhibitors such as larotrectinib, selpercatinib, and pralsetinib for the advanced MTC. Selpercatinib is recommended for those who require systemic therapy, with prior treatment of cabozantinib and/or vandetanib. In cases of ATC with BRAF V600E mutations, selective BRAF and MEK1/2 inhibitors appear to be the promising with manageable toxicity.

References

1. Sung H, Ferlay J, Siegel RL, Laversanne M, Soerjomataram I, Jemal A, Bray F. Global cancer statistics 2020: GLOBOCAN estimates of incidence and mortality worldwide for 36 cancers in 185 countries. CA Cancer J Clin. 2021;71(3):209–49.
2. Li M, Brito JP, Vaccarella S. Long-term declines of TC mortality: an international age–period–cohort analysis. Thyroid. 2020;30(6):838–46.
3. Ferlay J, Colombet M, Soerjomataram I, Mathers C, Parkin DM, Piñeros M, Znaor A, Bray F. Estimating the global cancer incidence and mortality in 2018: GLOBOCAN sources and methods. Int J Cancer. 2019;144(8):1941–53.
4. Kim J, Gosnell JE, Roman SA. Geographic influences in the global rise of TC. Nat Rev Endocrinol. 2020;16(1):17–29.
5. Cardis E, Kesminiene A, Ivanov V, Malakhova I, Shibata Y, Khrouch V, Drozdovitch V, Maceika E, Zvonova I, Vlassov O, Bouville A. Risk of TC after exposure to 131 I in childhood. J Natl Cancer Inst. 2005;97(10):724–32.
6. Seib CD, Sosa JA. Evolving understanding of the epidemiology of TC. Endocrinol Metab Clin. 2019;48(1):23–35.
7. Ron E, Lubin JH, Shore RE, Mabuchi K, Modan B, Pottern LM, Schneider AB, Tucker MA, Boice JD Jr. TC after exposure to external radiation: a pooled analysis of seven studies. Radiat Res. 1995;141(3):259–77.
8. Pal T, Vogl FD, Chappuis PO, Tsang R, Brierley J, Renard H, Sanders K, Kantemiroff T, Bagha S, Goldgar DE, Narod SA. Increased risk for nonmedullary TC in the first degree relatives of prevalent cases of nonmedullary TC: a hospital-based study. J Clin Endocrinol Metabol. 2001;86(11):5307–12.
9. Crnčić TB, Tomaš MI, Girotto N, Ivanković SG. Risk factors for TC: what do we know so far? Acta Clin Croat. 2020;59(Suppl 1):66.
10. Cooper DS, Doherty GM, Haugen BR, Kloos RT, Lee SL, Mandel SJ, Mazzaferri EL, McIver B, Pacini F, Schlumberger M, Sherman SI. Revised American Thyroid Association management guidelines for patients with thyroid nodules and differentiated TC: the American Thyroid Association (ATA) guidelines taskforce on thyroid nodules and differentiated TC. Thyroid. 2009;19(11):1167–214.
11. Boelaert K, Horacek J, Holder RL, Watkinson JC, Sheppard MC, Franklyn JA. Serum thyrotropin concentration as a novel predictor of malignancy in thyroid nodules investigated by fine-needle aspiration. J Clin Endocrinol Metabol. 2006;91(11):4295–301.
12. Carneiro RM, Carneiro BA, Agulnik M, Kopp PA, Giles FJ. Targeted therapies in advanced differentiated TC. Cancer Treat Rev. 2015;41(8):690–8.
13. Schlumberger M, Leboulleux S. Current practice in patients with differentiated TC. Nat Rev Endocrinol. 2021;17(3):176–88.
14. Hu MI, Vassilopoulou-Sellin R, Lustig R, Lamont JP. Thyroid and parathyroid cancers. Cancer management: a multidisciplinary approach. 2008;11.
15. Aboelnaga EM, Ahmed RA. Difference between papillary and follicular thyroid carcinoma outcomes: an experience from Egyptian institution. Cancer Biol Med. 2015;12(1):53.
16. Pacini F, Schlumberger M, Dralle H, Elisei R, Smit JW, Wiersinga W. European TC taskforce 2006 European consensus for the management of patients with differentiated thyroid carcinoma of the follicular epithelium. Eur J Endocrinol. 2006;154(6):787–803.
17. Pstrąg N, Ziemnicka K, Bluyssen H, Wesoły J. TCs of follicular origin in a genomic light: in-depth overview of common and unique molecular marker candidates. Mol Cancer. 2018;17:1–7.
18. Agrawal N, Akbani R, Aksoy BA, Ally A, Arachchi H, Asa SL, Auman JT, Balasundaram M, Balu S, Baylin SB, Behera M. Integrated genomic characterization of papillary thyroid carcinoma. Cell. 2014;159(3):676–90.
19. Greenebaum E, Koss LG, Elequin F, Silver CE. The diagnostic value of flow cytometric DNA measurements in follicular tumors of the thyroid gland. Cancer. 1985;56(8):2011–8.

20. Laha D, Nilubol N, Boufraqech M. New therapies for advanced TC. Front Endocrinol. 2020;11:82.
21. McHenry CR, Phitayakorn R. Follicular adenoma and carcinoma of the thyroid gland. Oncologist. 2011;16(5):585–93.
22. Lloyd RV, Osamura RY, Klöppel G, Rosai J. WHO classification of tumours of endocrine organs. 2017.
23. Jung CK, Bychkov A, Kakudo K. Update from the 2022 world health organization classification of thyroid tumors: a standardized diagnostic approach. Endocrinol Metab. 2022;37(5):703–18.
24. Khan YS, Farhana A. Histology, thyroid gland. 2019.
25. Levy O, Dai G, Riedel C, Ginter CS, Paul EM, Lebowitz AN, Carrasco N. Characterization of the thyroid Na+/I− symporter with an anti-COOH terminus antibody. Proc Natl Acad Sci. 1997;94(11):5568–73.
26. Naoum GE, Morkos M, Kim B, Arafat W. Novel targeted therapies and immunotherapy for advanced TCs. Mol Cancer. 2018;17(1):1–5.
27. Arribas J, Castellví J, Marcos R, Zafón C, Velázquez A. Expression of YY1 in differentiated TC. Endocr Pathol. 2015;26:111–8.
28. Nagy R, Ringel MD. Genetic predisposition for nonmedullary TC. Hormones Cancer. 2015;6:13–20.
29. Asa SL. The current histologic classification of TC. Endocrinol Metab Clin. 2019;48(1):1–22.
30. Jung CK, Little MP, Lubin JH, Brenner AV, Wells SA, Sigurdson AJ, Nikiforov YE. The increase in TC incidence during the last four decades is accompanied by a high frequency of BRAF mutations and a sharp increase in RAS mutations. J Clin Endocrinol Metabol. 2014;99(2):E276–85.
31. Lodish MB, Stratakis CA. RET oncogene in MEN2, MEN2B, MTC and other forms of TC. Expert Rev Anticancer Ther. 2008;8(4):625–32.
32. Society AC. Cancer facts & figures 2017. J Consum Health Internet. 2012;16:366–7.
33. Hou P, Liu D, Shan Y, Hu S, Studeman K, Condouris S, Wang Y, Trink A, El-Naggar AK, Tallini G, Vasko V. Genetic alterations and their relationship in the phosphatidylinositol 3-kinase/Akt pathway in TC. Clin Cancer Res. 2007;13(4):1161–70.
34. Kiriakopoulos A, Petralias A, Linos D. Multifocal versus solitary papillary thyroid carcinoma. World J Surg. 2016;40:2139–43.
35. Barczyński M, Konturek A, Stopa M, Nowak W. Prophylactic central neck dissection for papillary TC. J Br Surg. 2013;100(3):410–8.
36. Kim HJ, Sohn SY, Jang HW, Kim SW, Chung JH. Multifocality, but not bilaterality, is a predictor of disease recurrence/persistence of papillary thyroid carcinoma. World J Surg. 2013;37:376–84.
37. Poller DN, Nikiforov YE. Non-invasive follicular thyroid neoplasm with papillary-like nuclei: reducing overtreatment by reclassifying an indolent variant of papillary TC. J Clin Pathol. 2016;69(11):947–8.
38. Bae JS, Kim Y, Jeon S, Kim SH, Kim TJ, Lee S, Kim MH, Lim DJ, Lee YS, Jung CK. Clinical utility of TERT promoter mutations and ALK rearrangement in TC patients with a high prevalence of the BRAF V600E mutation. Diagn Pathol. 2016;11:21.
39. Landa I, Ibrahimpasic T, Boucai L, Sinha R, Knauf JA, Shah RH, Dogan S, Ricarte-Filho JC, Krishnamoorthy GP, Xu B, Schultz N. Genomic and transcriptomic hallmarks of poorly differentiated and anaplastic TCs. J Clin Invest. 2016;126(3):1052–66.
40. Garcia-Rostan G, Camp RL, Herrero A, Carcangiu ML, Rimm DL, Tallini G. β-catenin dysregulation in thyroid neoplasms: down-regulation, aberrant nuclear expression, and CTNNB1 exon 3 mutations are markers for aggressive tumor phenotypes and poor prognosis. Am J Pathol. 2001;158(3):987–96.
41. Ricarte-Filho JC, Ryder M, Chitale DA, Rivera M, Heguy A, Ladanyi M, Janakiraman M, Solit D, Knauf JA, Tuttle RM, Ghossein RA. Mutational profile of advanced primary and metastatic radioactive iodine-refractory TCs reveals distinct pathogenetic roles for BRAF, PIK3CA, and AKT1. Cancer Res. 2009;69(11):4885–93.

42. Santarpia L, El-Naggar AK, Cote GJ, Myers JN, Sherman SI. Phosphatidylinositol 3-kinase/akt and ras/raf-mitogen-activated protein kinase pathway mutations in anaplastic TC. J Clin Endocrinol Metabol. 2008;93(1):278–84.
43. Guerra A, Di Crescenzo V, Garzi A, Cinelli M, Carlomagno C, Tonacchera M, Zeppa P, Vitale M. Genetic mutations in the treatment of anaplastic TC: a systematic review. BMC Surg. 2013;13:1–6.
44. Hundahl SA, Fleming ID, Fremgen AM, Menck HR. A National Cancer Data Base report on 53,856 cases of thyroid carcinoma treated in the US, 1985-1995. Cancer. 1998;83(12):2638–48.
45. Schmidbauer B, Menhart K, Hellwig D, Grosse J. Differentiated TC—treatment: state of the art. Int J Mol Sci. 2017;18(6):1292.
46. Haugen BR, Sawka AM, Alexander EK, Bible KC, Caturegli P, Doherty GM, Mandel SJ, Morris JC, Nassar A, Pacini F, Schlumberger M. American Thyroid Association guidelines on the management of thyroid nodules and differentiated TC task force review and recommendation on the proposed renaming of encapsulated follicular variant papillary thyroid carcinoma without invasion to noninvasive follicular thyroid neoplasm with papillary-like nuclear features. Thyroid. 2017;27(4):481–3.
47. Perros P, Boelaert K, Colley S, Evans C, Evans RM, Gerrard Ba G, Gilbert J, Harrison B, Johnson SJ, Giles TE, Moss L. Guidelines for the management of TC. Clin Endocrinol. 2014;81:1–22.
48. Sherman SI. Evolution of targeted therapies for thyroid carcinoma. Trans Am Clin Climatol Assoc. 2019;130:255.

Skin Cancer

21

Anitha Kurva, Meghana Korikani, Vasavi Mohan, and Rama Krishna Kancha

21.1 Introduction

Epidemiology: The most prevalent types of cancer in white populations today are melanoma and nonmelanoma skin cancer (NMSC). While there is an increase in global incidence rates, their fatality rates are either steady or declining. The incidence of nonmelanoma (18–20%) is higher compared to that of the melanoma [1]. According to the worldwide cancer data, nonmelanoma skin cancer (NMSC) is ranked fifth among the world's most widespread cancers, followed by melanoma of skin at 17th place. All skin-related malignant neoplasms other than melanoma are referred to as NMSC. Basal cell carcinoma (BCC) and squamous cell carcinoma (SCC) are the major types of NMSC, which make up to nearly 99%, while sebaceous carcinoma, apocrine adenocarcinoma, and Merkel cell carcinoma are the examples of other NMSCs [2]. The incidence of skin cancer depends on ethnicity, increase in sun exposure, age, gender, clothing style, ozone depletion, immunosuppression, and genetics [3]. BCC accounts for 80% of nonmelanoma skin malignancies globally, making it the most frequent type of skin tumor followed by SCC, and is very common in ethnic groups such as Caucasians, Hispanics, and Asians [4]. There is a correlation between BCC and the range of pigmentation, as 35–45% of Caucasians are affected [5]. Individuals of 60 years of age and beyond account for nearly 80% of the NMSC cases. Patients with BCC varied in age from 18 to 101 years, and those with SCC ranged from 19 to 102 years. In the youngest group of NMSC patients, women made up most of the patients (18–44 years). There was

A. Kurva · M. Korikani · R. K. Kancha (✉)
Molecular Medicine and Therapeutics Laboratory, CPMB, Osmania University, Hyderabad, India
e-mail: ramakancha@osmania.ac.in

V. Mohan
Vasavi Medical and Research Centre, Hyderabad, India

R. K. Kancha (ed.), *Biomedical Aspects of Solid Cancers*,
https://doi.org/10.1007/978-981-97-1802-3_21

no discernible sex difference in patients aged 45–64 years. Men were found to predominate significantly in patients aged 65–79 years, whereas women were found to predominate significantly in patients aged 80–102 years [6].

The mortality rate of BCC is low; in the case of metastatic BCC, the death rate is 0.12 per 100,000 [7]. The case-fatality rate for SCC is in the range of 1–2%, while the mortality rates from NMSCs are extremely low [8]. Where it has been reported, the mortality rate for NMSC has been declining for most of this century, but in nations like Australia, it may be leveling out [9]. The cumulative risk varies by gender and geographic location; men have a greater cumulative risk than women. About 75% of skin cancer deaths are caused by cutaneous melanoma, although only accounting for 4% of diagnoses [10]. The cumulative risk for melanoma incidence is highest in Australia and New Zealand (3.29). The age-standardized rate of incidence per 100,000 is 3.8 for men (cumulative life-time risk: 0.42%) and 3.0 for women (cumulative life-time risk: 0.33%). White men (34.7/100,000) had a higher incidence than white women (22.1/100,000) [11].

Risk Factors: Exposure to UV radiation is the chief cause of NMSC; intermittent exposure to sun increases the risk of developing BCC [1] and cumulative exposure to the sun results in the progression to cutaneous SCC (cSCC) [4]. A 4:1 ratio of BCC to SCC is observed in patients who have a normal immune response; immunosuppression makes a person more liable to BCC [12]. The significant prognostic factors of BCC include initial truncal occurrence, age above 60 years, male gender, and renal transplant. The risk of SCC occurrence is directly proportional to the organ transplants (65–250%) [13]. A person who suffers from chronic lymphocytic leukemia has a risk of 8–10% of developing SC [14]. Infection with the HPV is associated with periungual and anogenital cSCC [15]. The exposure to environmental factors such as arsenic (well water and lead arsenate in pesticides), polycyclic hydrocarbons, and alkylating agents are also risk factors [16]. Any exposure to ionizing radiations makes the cSCC reoccur with a metastatic range of 10–30% [17]. Rare familial syndromes make the individuals prone to the multiple cSCC at a young age [18]. The risk factors of melanoma are multifactorial that include both genetic as well as environmental factors [19]. Most melanoma is caused by UV radiation of which UV-A and UV-B play an important role in melanoma pathogenesis [20]. Acquired melanocytic nevus is considered a risk factor [21]. UVA doses are 12 times greater in tanning beds compared to the sun exposure [22, 23]. The phenotypic characters such as blue eyes or green eyes as compared to that of black eyes showed greater risk [24]. Blonde hair and red hair individuals seem to have a higher risk than black hair persons [25]. Freckles are an important hallmark risk factor for melanoma. About 20% of individuals with Xeroderma pigmentosa will develop melanoma [19]. The chance of developing melanoma is 3–8% in those individuals having a family history of melanoma [24].

Diagnosis: Histological testing is used to provide a clinical diagnosis of skin cancer. BCC can be diagnosed by dermoscopy, direct inspection, and histopathological examinations. Nodular, superficial, infiltrative or morphoeic, and micronodular growth patterns are included in the histological reporting of basal cell carcinoma [26]. Other procedures for diagnosing BCC include optical coherence tomography (OCT) and confocal laser scanning microscopy. BCCs are positive for pan-cytokeratin markers like MNF116, cytokeratin 5/6, and 5/17. For diagnosing SCC, various noninvasive optical methods such as dermoscopy along with a complementary tool, Reflectance confocal microscopy (RCM), are used to improve clinical diagnostic accuracy and characterize the tumor in vivo [27]. The lesion thickens clinically as in situ SCC develops into microinvasive SCC, and hairpin and/or linear-irregular capillaries form on dermoscopic examination occasionally producing a picture like a red starburst. Diagnosis of SCC also includes RCM, High-Frequency Ultrasonography (HFUS), and OCT [28]. Melanoma diagnosis depends on ABCDEs: asymmetry, borders, change of color, diameter, and evolution of lesions. There is a consideration of a few criteria for diagnosing melanoma such as architectural features including asymmetry, growth confluence, conspicuous cellularity, and inadequate circumscription [29]. Melanoma can resemble a variety of cancers such as germ cell tumors, sarcomas, lymphomas, carcinomas, and neuroendocrine tumors. Therefore, the diagnosis of melanomas frequently uses immunohistochemical labeling for melanocytic markers of differentiation [30]. Also, Melan-A outperformed S-100 at differentiating between melanoma and nonmelanocytic neoplasms with a sensitivity and specificity of 93% and 98%, respectively [31]. Some serological markers such as serum lactate dehydrogenase (LDH) have 92% specificity but with only 79% sensitivity [32].

21.2 Classification

Classification of NMSC: According to the World Health Organization (WHO), the year 2020 saw 1.2 million cases of nonmelanoma skin cancer worldwide. Skin cancers are classified as nonkeratinocyte and keratinocyte skin tumors; both BCC and SCC are grouped together and are called keratinocyte tumors (Fig. 21.1). (1) BCC: a class of cancerous skin tumors distinguished by the presence of lobules, columns, bands or cords of basaloid cells. Superficial BCC accounts for 10–15% of BCC and appears as erythematous patches that are frequently numerous and range in size from a few millimeters to over 10 cm. Nodular BCC sometimes starts as raised pearly nodules connected to telangiectasia, which can develop into ulcerated or cystic lesions and accounts to 30–75% of all BCCs. Micronodular BCC has micronodules that typically appear as raised or flat infiltrative tumors; the back is the most typical location. Infiltrating BCC is made up of fine cords, strands, and columns of basaloid cells that invade the deeper tissues as well as the dermal collagen bundles and accounts for 10% of all BCC. Fibroepithelial BCC appears as elevated, flesh-colored or erythematous nodule. BCC with adnexal differentiation is distinguished by the presence of basaloid buds, ductal, sebaceous, and trichilemmal elements in the adnexa. Basosquamous carcinoma is characterized by squamous differentiation while keratotic BCC is distinguished by a pronounced keratin development in the tumor islands centers. Histologically, (1) BCC is of three major types: (i) Nodular BCC with three subtypes: adenoid BCC, basal cell epithelioma, and micronodular BCC, (ii) Superficial Basal Carcinoma, and (iii) Infiltrative BCC.

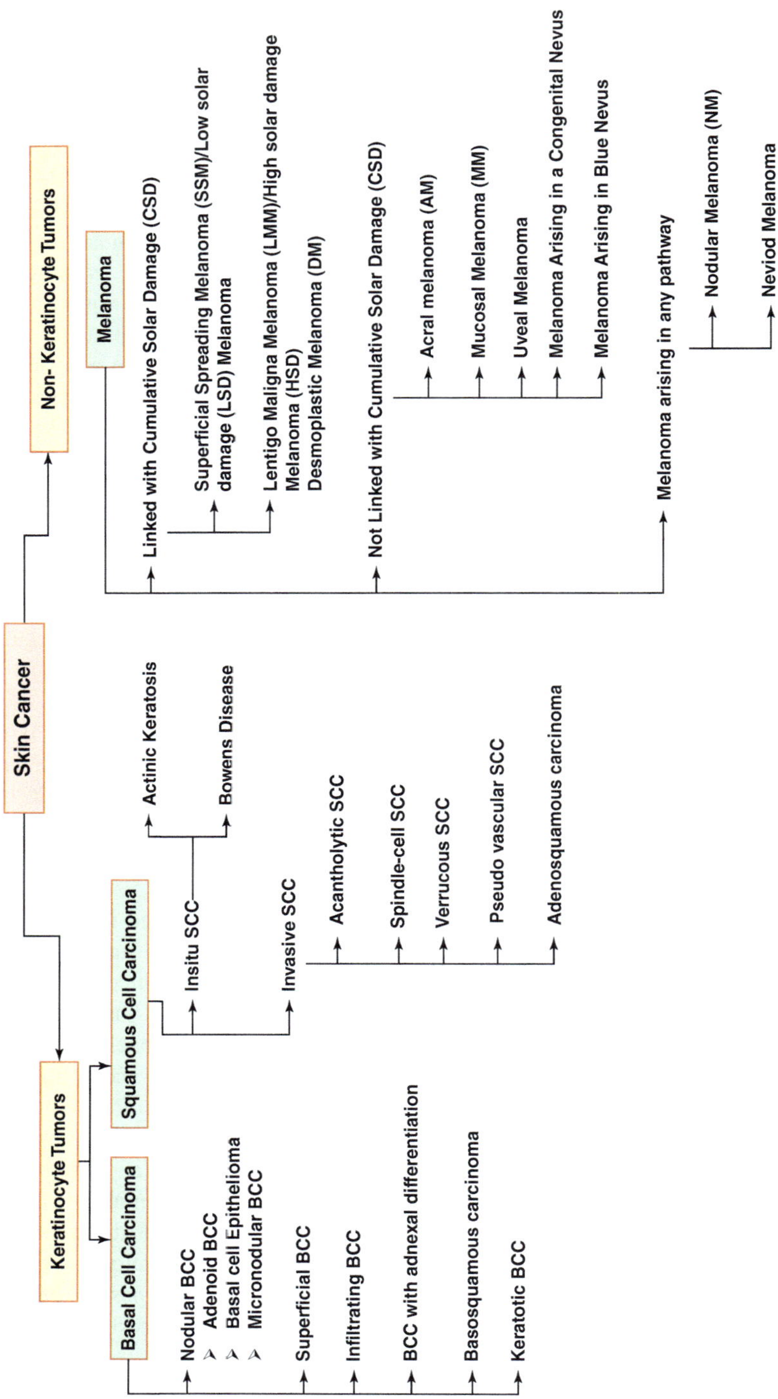

Fig. 21.1 WHO classification of skin cancer

(2) SCC: It is a malignant tumor of keratinocytes of the epidermis in which the component cells exhibit various squamous differentiating characteristics. According to the WHO, SCC is divided into major subtypes (Fig. 21.1). (2a) Acantholytic SCC (ASCC) is a histological type of cutaneous SCC that is characterized by acantholysis. (2b) Spindle cell SCC is a rare form of SCC with a noticeable spindle cell shape. (2c) Verrucous SCC is a rare type of SCC with a less malignant potential. (2d) Pseudo-vascular SCC is an aggressive form of SCC with pronounced acantholysis and regions that resemble angiosarcomas. (2e) Adenosquamous carcinoma is an uncommon subtype of SCC that develops from pluripotent acrosyringia-related cells and is defined by the development of mucin-secreting glands. Histologically, there are several subtypes of cSCC (i) Bowens Disease (BD) is an intraepidermal carcinoma with atypia of keratinocytes [33]. Five percent of in situ cases can develop into Invasive cSCC. (ii) Keratoacanthoma (KA) is a highly differentiated form of cSCC that has an extended layer of epidermis over the tumor and is symmetrical and restricted keratinocyte growth with a central horn plug. (iii) Invasive cSCC has dyskeratotic keratinocytes with pleomorphic nuclei, which also has atypical keratinocytes with local destructive proliferation and a high rate of metastasis. (iv) Desmoplastic, (v) Spindle cell, (vi) acantholytic, (vii) pseudo-vascular, (viii) verrucous, (ix) adeno squamous, and (x) neurotropic cSCC are other cSCC subtypes.

TNM staging (Tumor Diameter, Regional Lymph nodes, and Metastatic Sites): The pT categories are classified on the basis of diameter of tumor and depth of invasion. If the tumor diameter is 2 cm or less, it is classified under T1. If the tumor diameter is more than 2 cm, then it is staged as T2. In T3, there is an invasion of tumor into maxilla, mandible, orbit or temporal bone and if it is to the base or skull, it is T4. In the new edition, theT4 stage is further classified into T4a and T4b. T4a is defined by cortical or marrow invasion and T4b by invasion into the skull base. In nodal staging, the pN categories of skin cancer are based on ipsilateral nodes, while contralateral involvement nodes are considered distant metastases. In N1, the metastasis is in a single ipsilateral node measuring 3 cm or less than 3 cm. In N2a, the metastases in single ipsilateral node is more than 3 cm and less than 6 cm where as in N2b, the metastasis is in multiple ipsilateral lymph nodes of greater than 6 cm. N2c includes metastases of bilateral or contralateral lymph node but not more than 6 cm in size. If the nodal metastases are more than 6 cm, it classified as N3 [34].

Merkel Cell Carcinoma: A nonmelanoma skin cancer that develops typically in places that are exposed to the sun, with the tumor's maximum dimension of 2 cm or less is T1. In T2, the size is around 2–5 cm and if it is more than 5 cm, it is T3. T4 refers to the main tumor's extracutaneous invasion into bone, muscle, fascia, or cartilage. pN1 is divided into N1a and N1b; the tumor cells in the lymph node are categorized as micrometastases (N1a) and macrometastases (N1b). Transit metastases are pN2 while in distant metastasis, the stages are classified into M1 where it metastasizes beyond lymph nodes, which is further classified into M1a, M1b, and M1c. M1a is metastasis to skin or subcutaneous tissues, while M1b is to lung, and M1c to visceral sites [34].

Classification of Melanoma: According to the WHO classification, melanomas (nonkeratinocyte) are of three subtypes based on the solar damage (Fig. 21.1). (1)

Melanomas with Cumulative Solar Damage (CSD). (1a) Superficial Spreading Melanoma (SSM)/Low solar damage (LSD) melanoma is a common type and accounts for 60–70%; it normally occurs on the back in men and the calf region in women [35]. SSM at the early stage looks like asymmetrical and irregular scalloped papules of diameter less than 5 mm [36], the lesions of SSM can be de novo; the lesions arise rarely from individual nevi, but increase with nevi count [37]. (1b) Lentigo Maligna Melanoma (LMM)/High solar damage melanoma (HSD) is less common and comprises of 9% of cutaneous melanomas; affected individuals are mostly older and women [38]. It occurs in the cheek and neck region in women and in head and scalp regions in men. The precursor lesion is known as Lentigo malignant and the chance of progressing into LMM is 5% [39]. The lesions are indolent, asymmetric brown-to-black macules with irregular indentation [40]. (1c) Desmoplastic Melanoma (DM) comprises 4% of all cutaneous melanomas [41]. It is most common in older men. The lesions are developed in sun-exposed areas, they appear as plaque or skin-colored red or black nodules [42]. They are rarely metastatic and the survival rate is 67–89%.

(2) Melanomas are not always linked to cumulative sun damage; the other types include: (2a) Spitz melanoma (SM) commonly occurs in childhood. Spitz nevi (SN) are almost equivalent to Spitz melanoma. The characteristic features that differentiate between Spitz nevi and Spitz melanoma are distinctive large spindle/epithelioid melanocytes and different driver mutations responsible for their initiation [43]. The lesions of SM are large and ulcerated with growth and change whereas the SN are amelanotic papules with defined borders and symmetrical [44]. (2b) Acral melanoma (AM), an aggressive subtype follows the ABCDE characteristics, both radial and vertical growth phase occur in AM [45]. (2c) Mucosal Melanoma (MM) can only evolve through the RGP, which becomes difficult to identify as it occurs in visceral organs. They are bulky tumors and can be visible in the regions such as the vulva or conjunctivitis [46]. (2d) Melanoma arising from a congenital nevus where melanoma develops from the junctional or dermal point of the nevus [47]. The characteristics of both differ as the junctional point involves similar features of low CSD. They are masked by a background pigmented hairy nevus. (2e) Melanoma occurring in blue nevus is often composed of pigmented spindle cells with thin cytoplasm, which is often located in the thick reticular dermis of collagen bundle fibers [48].

(3) This third type comprises of melanoma arising in any pathway and has two subtypes. (3a) Nodular Melanoma (NM) comprises 15–20% of melanomas. It will mostly affect fair-skinned individuals. The incidence is greater in men on the head, trunk, and neck. At an early stage, the lesions are black or blue nodules with regular borders and with a small diameter. Around 2–80% of lesions are considered amelanotic. (3b) Nevoid Melanoma is heterogeneous group of lesions where benign nevus which is in dome shaped or verrucous has the apparent maturation in the dermis by descent and the nodule size is greater than 1 cm. Histologically, the NM comprises of subtypes which include SM, atypical fibroxanthoma-like melanoma, and collision tumors. AM consists of subungual melanoma as a major subtype. Uncommon

histological subtypes include spindle cell, neurotropic, and malignant blue nevus [36].

TNM staging: pT1 is when melanomas have thickness of 1.0 mm or less, melanomas of 1.01–2.0 mm are pT2. In pT3, the dimensions are 2.01–4.0 mm and more than 4.0 mm are pT4. The nodal category is divided on the basis of number of metastatic nodes and metastatic mass. The N1 is divided into N1a (micrometastasis) and N1b (macrometastasis) even though the number of nodes involved is 1. N2 is where the number of nodes are 2–3 which are further divided into N1a (micrometastases), N2b (macrometastases), and N2c (in transit metastasis), but in N2c, no metastatic nodes are involved. N3 has four or more metastatic nodes. The sites of the metastases and elevated serum LDH levels are utilized to divide the M1 into three categories [34].

21.3 Pathophysiology

The skin is considered the largest vital organ in the body and comprises of layers and cells and accounts for 15% of the total body weight. It carries out many functions such as protection against chemical, physical, and biological agents and plays a specific role in thermoregulation [49]. The skin comprises three layers: epidermis, dermis, and hypodermis (Subcutaneous tissue) and they differ in function and thickness. The epidermis, which is the skin's topmost layer, is made up of a particular kind of cells called keratinocytes that produce keratin. Keratinization process is controlled by several transcription factors, as well as the EGFR family of kinase signaling that is responsible for processes related to epidermal homeostasis. Collagen, a fibrillar structural protein, makes up the dermis. The subcutaneous tissue on which the dermis rests has tiny lobes of fat cells called lipocytes and depending on their location, their thickness varies greatly [50]. There are intercellular adhesion complexes with desmosomes and adherens junctions to hold keratinocytes together and provide mechanical strength to the epidermis. Abnormalities in tight junction proteins have been seen with several skin diseases, both common and rare ones.

The stratified squamous epithelium layer consists of keratinocytes and dendritic cells, which differ by the presence of intercellular bridges and cytoplasmic abundance (Fig. 21.2). Other cells of epidermis include melanocytes, Merkel cells, and Langerhans cells (Fig. 21.2). The keratinocytes make up to about 80% of the epidermis cells. They form a variety of compounds such as keratin and lamellar bodies which form epidermal water barriers and hold melanin that is derived from melanocytes, and protect from harmful UV radiation. Keratinocytes are formed in the stratum Basale and assembly of keratin fibers happens. When they reach the layer of stratum spinosum, keratinocytes get connected with the help of desmosomes with visible keratohyalin, lamellar bodies, and keratin molecules (Fig. 21.2). The organelles of keratinocytes are pushed into the stratum lucidum and further get degraded and the dead keratinocytes become corneocytes in the stratum corneum, which is filled with keratin and eventually shed off (Fig. 21.2) [51]. Keratinocytes express

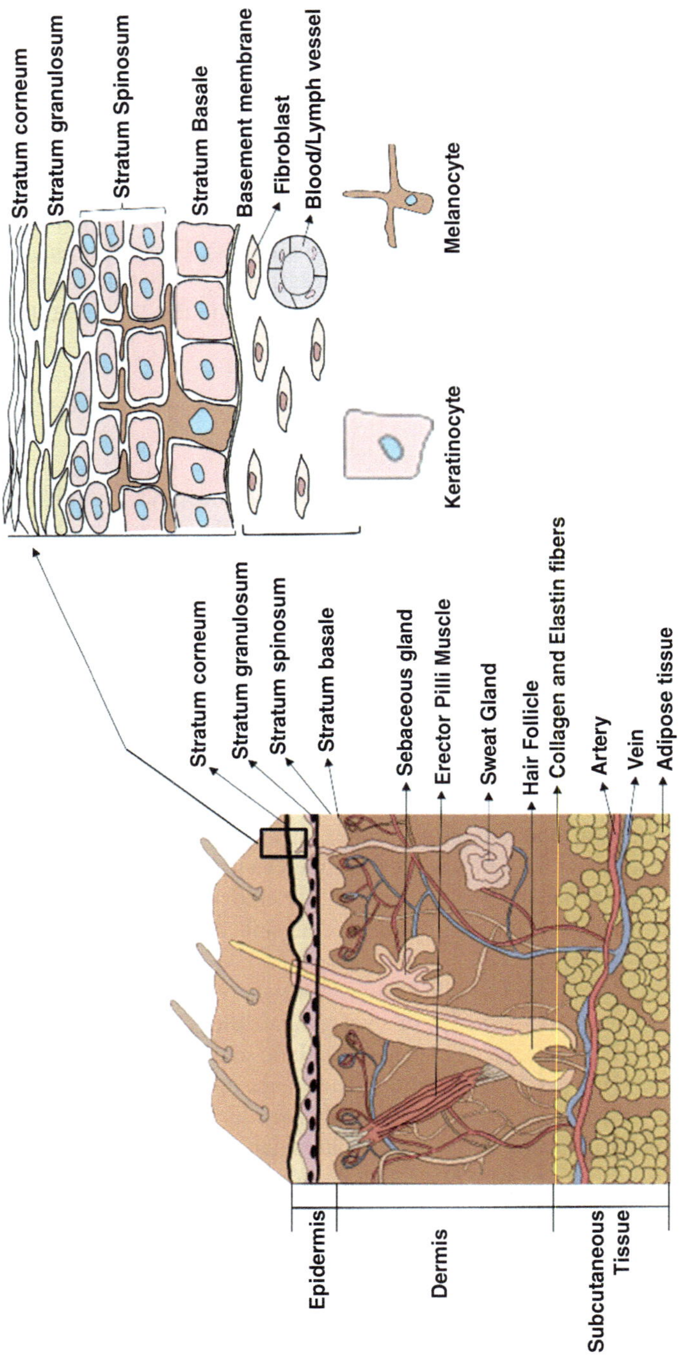

Fig. 21.2 Anatomy and pathophysiology of skin cancer

receptors that recognize microbial components and work to initiate host innate immune responses. However, commensal microflora activates a protective immune response suggesting their contribution to maintaining immune homeostasis [52].

The melanocyte is a pigment-producing cell that arises from the neural crest and is restricted to the basal layer of the skin. Even though melanocytes encounter keratinocytes they do not engage in any type of connection with them. Merkel cells can be found in the outer root sheath of hair follicles, lips, regions of the oral cavity, and digits. Langerhans cells recognize and process antigens within the epidermal tissue to participate in a variety of T-cell responses. Throughout life, Langerhans circulate and replenish the epidermis [51]. Nails, sweat glands, and pilosebaceous apparatuses are examples of derivative structures that are produced by the epidermis, which is a layer that is constantly renewing itself.

According to keratinocyte form and position, the epidermis is typically split into four layers: (a) Stratum germinativum also known as the basal cell layer, contains keratinocytes that adhere to the basement membrane zone [53]. The basal layer has most of the mitotically active cells that give rise to the cells of the outer epidermal layers [54]. (b) Stratum spinosum or squamous cell layer is thick with 5–10 cells that overlie on the basal layer, which has cells that differ in characteristics based on their location. (c) Stratum granulosum or granular cell layer is the superficial layer that contains live flattened cells that have a lot of keratohyalin granules. (d) Stratum corneum or cornified cell layer that has big, flat, polyhedral-shaped horny cells have lost their nuclei [53]. The cornified layer's horny cells (corneocytes) act as a barrier to stop water loss as well as mechanical protection for the underlying epidermis [55]. The dermal-epidermal junction is porous and binds the epidermis and the dermis together while allowing the flow of cells [56]. Arrector pili muscle emerges as down growths from the epidermis which contributes to wound healing and maintains homeostasis [50]. The dermis is an interconnected system of fibrous, filamentous, and amorphous connective tissue that contains mast cells, fibroblasts, macrophages, vascular networks, and appendages that are generated from the epidermis. The dermis, which makes up most of the skin, gives its elasticity and tensile strength. It also shields the body from mechanical harm, binds water, helps regulate body temperature, and has sensory receptors. About 70% of the dry weight of the skin is made up of collagen.

Cell of Origin: Interestingly, there is still a debate over BCC's anatomical origin. BCC is named after cells that histologically resemble basal keratinocytes seen in the Inter follicular epidermis (IFE) and Hair Follicles (HF). Utilizing mouse genetics, it was found that activating the Smoothened mutant (SmoM2) in the hair follicle bulge cells did not result in the formation of BCC [57]. Instead, it was discovered that the IFE and the higher follicular infundibulum's long-lived resident progenitor cells are where BCC is generated. When GLI2 activator (GLI2N) is induced, it encourages the growth of BCC-like tumors in mice. Superficial BCC-like cancers develop from the interfollicular epidermis, while nodular BCC-like tumors develop from the stem cells of hair follicles which follow high-level signaling [58]. The basal cell layer and pluripotent epithelial cells of the outer root sheath of hair follicles are the sources of BCC [59]. Activating mutation in *KRAS* and *TP53* deletion in IFE stem cells and HF stem cells leads to the development of well-differentiated cSCC and with characteristics of the epithelial to mesenchymal transition, respectively. TP63 and KLF5 influence IFE gene expression and the growth of well-differentiated cSCC, while SMAD2, NFATC1, and TCF7L1 influence HF gene expression and the growth of cSCC [60]. Melanocytes develop from neural crest cells and go to the basal layer of the skin's epidermis [61]. A tiny percentage also travels to the mucosal surfaces, uvea, and meninges. Malignant melanoma is produced by melanocytes that are atypical and genetically altered [62].

Genetics: The human genome has 54 functional keratin genes in two compact clusters. These genes are highly specific such that specific keratin expression profiles are present for different epithelial tissues. Epidermolysis bullosa simplex was the first known keratin-related genetic condition described, with mutations in keratins 5 and 14. There are eight different collagens present in the skin where the collagen fibrils exist as homo- or heterotrimers. Cancer cells are known to alter collagen biosynthesis through several gene mutations where collagen plays a role in fibrosis [63]. Current research has provided an understanding of Hedgehog (HH) signaling pathway in skin development and cancer. Activation of HH signaling is the hallmark of BCC pathogenesis [64]. In patients with Basal cell nevus syndrome (BCNS) or Gorlin syndrome, loss of one functional copy of *PTCH1* predisposes them to the BCC development. Loss-of-function mutations in *PTCH1* cause most of the sporadic BCC (85–90%) and impair the suppression of HH signaling.

Mutations in *SMO* gene, which make it resistant to *PTCH1* inhibition, may be responsible for 10–20% of the formation of sporadic BCC [65]. Mutations in the *PTCH2* gene were discovered in a small number of sporadic BCC [66]. The HH pathway interacts with several different oncogenic signaling networks, which together may help to promote the growth of BCC [67]. Mutations in *TP53,* CDKN2A locus, the *RAS* gene, and of the PI3K/AKT pathway were reported in a less percentage of sporadic BCCs [68]. Truncating mutations make up 61% of all genomic alterations [69]. WNTs are overexpressed in BCCs [70], and β-catenin with stabilizing mutations is localized in the nucleus in approximately 30% of BCC [71]. In 5% and 8% of BCC samples, respectively, detrimental mutations and Loss of Heterozygosity (LOH) events in the *FBXW7* gene have been discovered [69]. Many mutations are connected to functional loss indicating a tumor-suppressor function for *NOTCH* in the etiology of BCC [72]. TERT promoter mutations have been found to occur frequently in BCCs [73]. BCCs have been discovered to harbor noncoding mutations in the promoters of *DPH3* and *OXNAD1* genes [69]. Different miRNA profiles are associated with the BCC subtypes of nodular and infiltrative tumors [74].

In the SCC, despite the strong mutational background brought on by UV exposure, 23 putative driver genes for aggressive cSCC were reported [75]. It is generally known that a significant percentage of cSCC and precursor lesions have *TP53* mutations, which can account for up to 90% of all cSCC [76]. The elevated expression levels of mutant *p53* also indicate aggressive tumor behavior [77]. It is considered that the development from AK to cSCC is correlated with the deletion of *p16INK4a* [78]. Initial investigations have revealed *RAS* mutations in 12–20% of cSCC, implicating the dysregulation of the *RAS* gene in the development of cSCC [79]. Metastatic cSCC exhibits considerable overexpression as well as downregulation of several microRNAs [80]. The *HERC2/OCA2, DEF8,* and *RALY* genes have three additional previously unreported SCC-associated SNPs [81].

Most of the genetic changes that underlie this disease's genetic foundation arise as sporadically acquired mutations in melanocytes, and a buildup of genomic alterations aid in the development of melanoma [82]. About 20–40% of familial melanoma cases show the dominant inheritance of *CDKN2A* mutations. Due to a loss of binding to p16, R24C and R24H mutants of CDK4 behave as dominant oncoproteins [83]. Mutations in the *ACD* and *TERF2IP* genes were also found to predispose to melanoma [84]. The *BAP1* gene was reported as a rare high-risk germline melanoma susceptibility gene [85]. The risk of cutaneous melanoma was more than twice as high for carriers of two or more *MC1R* mutant alleles as it was for wild-type controls [86]. The gain-of-function mutation *MITF* gene was shown to predispose to familial melanoma [87]. Carriers of the p.E318K variant of *MITF* gene were identified to have a significantly greater risk of getting melanoma [88]. *BRAF* and *N-RAS* are the two genes in that melanoma that have been shown to have the greatest somatic mutations. The melanoma results were the most startling, with identical *BRAF* mutations present in 92% of all melanoma patients [89]. About 90% of *N-RAS* mutations occur at codon 61 [90]. Enhanced levels of activated *AKT* are caused by aberrant *PTEN* expression; enhanced *AKT3* activity has been noted in 40–60% of melanomas [91]. The *TRRAP* gene mutation S722F was the second most frequent recurring mutation after the *BRAF* V600E mutation [92]. Somatic mutations in MAP2K1 and MAP2K2 as well as in MAP3K5 and MAP3K9 were also reported in two recent melanoma exome sequencing investigations [93].

21.4 Treatment

Surgical or nonsurgical options are available for the treatment of BCC. Curettage and electrodessication, cryosurgery, surgical excision, and Mohs micrographic surgery are a few surgical techniques. For low-risk lesions tiny, well-defined primary lesions on the neck, torso, arms, and legs, with nonaggressive histologic characteristics, curettage and electrodesiccation or cryosurgery can achieve 5-year cure rates of 95% or more. Physicians may resort to chemical peels if actinic keratosis is seen, to remove the premalignant cells. Recurrent or morpheaform tumors should not be treated with curettage, electrodessication, or cryosurgery [4]. The best method for treating recurrent BCC is Mohs surgery, which has the lowest 5-year recurrence rate (1.0% for initial tumors and 5.6% for recurrent tumors). This is a time-consuming procedure where skin is removed layer by layer and checked for cancer cells and has better outcome than other surgical procedures. For BCC, two types of radiation therapy have been used: teletherapy (external beam RT) and brachytherapy [94]. Ionizing radiation therapy is not recommended for patients with certain genetic syndromes, such as BCNS or Gorlin-Goltz syndrome, due to the increased risk of inducing secondary cancers [95]. For superficial BCC, topical 5-fluorouracil and imiquimod have been approved; favorable results were seen with NBCCs also [96, 97]. Only superficial or small BCCs located in low-risk locations should be treated with topical treatment methods [98].

When surgery or radiotherapy is not acceptable, the FDA and the EMA have approved the targeted oral medicines vismodegib and sonidegib for the treatment of BCC [99]. Vismodegib is specifically indicated for both locally progressed and metastatic disease, whereas sonidegib is exclusively effective in the first setting. Vismodegib and sonidegib both work by inhibiting the hedgehog signaling [100]. In cSCC, one of the first systemic medicines tested to treat cSCC was EGFR inhibition [101]. Cetuximab is well tolerated, however, skin responses that typically can manifest as an acne-like rash or as a nail abnormality [102] that need to be treated, may occur as side effects in most patients. Patients with cSCC and AK have been treated with lapatinib [103]. Cemiplimab showed promise in treating immune competent patients with advanced cSCC and metastatic illness, with response rates of 50% and 47%, respectively [104]. Nonsurgical local treatments may be taken into consideration if surgical therapy is not possible or desired [105]. In situ or low-risk SCC may respond to imiquimod (3.75–5%) or 5-fluorouracil topical therapy or photodynamic therapy. Nonsurgical ablative techniques are used without surgery, including cryosurgery, electrocoagulation, and CO2 laser ablation. The recurrence rate of cSCC is higher with these methods due to the lack of histological margin control. Primary local radiation may also be employed when other treatments are either dangerous or not feasible [106].

Melanoma neoplasms have a high risk for aggressive metastasis, especially to the lymph nodes, brain, and lungs and the treatment varies with tumor stage or primary lesion. The best treatment for an early tumor is surgical removal, which is the main therapeutic strategy for melanoma. Additional therapies for cancers in advanced stages include adjuvant therapy, chemotherapy, and the use of many vaccinations [107]. Melanoma has previously been managed with interleukin 2 (IL-2). In a phase I/II trial, cutaneous malignant melanoma nodules were transfected with M11 cells using a retrovirus vector, making the transfected cells sensitive to ganciclovir. Both tumor necrosis and tumor size were observed to be moderately impacted [108].

21.5 Conclusion

Skin cancer is one of the most common cancers worldwide having rising incidences every year, as the risk factors mostly include UV exposure, life style habits, ethnicity, and age. Based on the cells, the skin cancer can be classified as nonmelanoma and melanoma; keratinocytes cause nonmelanoma and melanocytes cause melanoma. Nonmelanoma is majorly classified into Basal Cell Carcinoma and Squamous cell carcinoma, which accounts for 99% of all nonmelanoma skin cancer (NMSC). The histopathological examination is the golden standard for diagnosing skin cancers but there is a chance of misdiagnosing as the subtypes can have similar patterns. Surgery is the most effective treatment for skin cancer with low recurrence rates, in some conditions less invasive options are used; topical pharmacotherapy and photodynamic therapy were used for treating NMSC. As melanoma spreads quickly and aggressively, it becomes difficult to treat; new immunotherapy drugs have emerged for treating advanced stage of melanoma; drugs targeting tumors with specific *BRAF* mutations have improved the overall survival rate in melanoma. With all current therapies in place, it is important to educate individuals on identifying skin lesions that may require further medical investigation so that the chance for these individuals to receive early diagnosis and better management is high.

References

1. Armstrong BK, Kricker A. The epidemiology of UV induced skin cancer. J Photochem Photobiol B Biol. 2001;63(1–3):8–18.
2. Losquadro WD. Anatomy of the skin and the pathogenesis of nonmelanoma skin cancer. Facial Plast Surg Clin. 2017;25(3):283–9.
3. Leiter U, Keim U, Garbe C. Epidemiology of skin cancer: update 2019 sunlight, vitamin D and skin. Cancer. 2020;1268:123–39.
4. Rubin AI, Chen EH, Ratner D. Basal-cell carcinoma. N Engl J Med. 2005;353(21):2262–9.
5. Ridky TW. Nonmelanoma skin cancer. J Am Acad Dermatol. 2007;57(3):484–501.
6. Ciążyńska M, Kamińska-Winciorek G, Lange D, Lewandowski B, Reich A, Sławińska M, Pabianek M, Szczepaniak K, Hankiewicz A, Ułańska M, Morawiec J. The incidence and clinical analysis of non-melanoma skin cancer. Sci Rep. 2021;11(1):15705.
7. McDaniel B, Badri T, Steele RB. Basal cell carcinoma. In: StatPearls [Internet]. Treasure Island, FL: StatPearls Publishing; 2021.
8. Nixon RL, Marks R, Dorevitch AP. Squamous cell carcinoma of the skin: accuracy of clinical diagnosis and outcome of follow-up in Australia. Med J Aust. 1986;144(5):235–9.
9. Giles C. Trends in skin cancer in Australia: an overview of the available data. Trans Menzies Found. 1989;15:143–7.
10. American Cancer Society. Cancer facts & figures 2013. Atlanta, GA: American Cancer Society; 2013.
11. Sung H, Ferlay J, Siegel RL, Laversanne M, Soerjomataram I, Jemal A, Bray F. Global cancer statistics 2020: GLOBOCAN estimates of incidence and mortality worldwide for 36 cancers in 185 countries. CA Cancer J Clin. 2021;71(3):209–49.
12. Jemec GB, Holm EA. Nonmelanoma skin cancer in organ transplant patients. Transplantation. 2003;75(3):253–7.
13. Jensen P, Hansen S, Møller B, Leivestad T, Pfeffer P, Geiran O, Fauchald P, Simonsen S. Skin cancer in kidney and heart transplant recipients and different long-term immunosuppressive therapy regimens. J Am Acad Dermatol. 1999;40(2):177–86.
14. Velez NF, Karia PS, Vartanov AR, Davids MS, Brown JR, Schmults CD. Association of advanced leukemic stage and skin cancer tumor stage with poor skin cancer outcomes in patients with chronic lymphocytic leukemia. JAMA Dermatol. 2014;150(3):280–7.
15. zur Hausen H. Papillomaviruses in the causation of human cancers—a brief historical account. Virology. 2009;384(2):260–5.
16. Yuspa SH. Cutaneous chemical carcinogenesis. J Am Acad Dermatol. 1986;15(5):1031–44.
17. Edwards MJ, Hirsch RM, Broadwater JR, Netscher DT, Ames FC. Squamous cell carcinoma arising in previously burned or irradiated skin. Arch Surg. 1989;124(1):115–7.
18. Ransohoff KJ, Jaju PD, Tang JY, Carbone M, Leachman S, Sarin KY. Familial skin cancer syndromes: increased melanoma risk. J Am Acad Dermatol. 2016;74(3):423–34.
19. Dzwierzynski WW. Melanoma risk factors and prevention. Clin Plast Surg. 2021;48(4):543–50.

20. Volkovova K, Bilanicova D, Bartonova A, Letašiová S, Dusinska M. Associations between environmental factors and incidence of cutaneous melanoma. Rev Environ Health. 2012;11(1):1–3, S12
21. Syed DN, Mukhtar H. Botanicals for the prevention and treatment of cutaneous melanoma. Pigment Cell Melanoma Res. 2011;24(4):688–702.
22. Sample A, He YY. Autophagy in UV damage response. Photochem Photobiol. 2017;93(4):943–55.
23. Goldstein AM, Tucker MA. Etiology, epidemiology, risk factors, and public health issues of melanoma. Curr Opin Oncol. 1993;5(2):358–63.
24. O'Neill CH, Scoggins CR. Melanoma. J Surg Oncol. 2019;120(5):873–81.
25. Evans RD, Kopf AW, Lew RA, Rigel DS, Bart RS, Friedman RJ, Rivers JK. Risk factors for the development of malignant melanoma—I: review of case-control studies. J Dermatol Surg Oncol. 1988;14(4):393–408.
26. Sexton M, Jones DB, Maloney ME. Histologic pattern analysis of basal cell carcinoma: study of a series of 1039 consecutive neoplasms. J Am Acad Dermatol. 1990;23(6):1118–26.
27. Pan Y, Chamberlain AJ, Bailey M, Chong AH, Haskett M, Kelly JW. Dermatoscopy aids in the diagnosis of the solitary red scaly patch or plaque–features distinguishing superficial basal cell carcinoma, intraepidermal carcinoma, and psoriasis. J Am Acad Dermatol. 2008;59(2):268–74.
28. Warszawik-Hendzel O, Olszewska M, Maj M, Rakowska A, Czuwara J, Rudnicka L. Non-invasive diagnostic techniques in the diagnosis of squamous cell carcinoma. J Dermatol Case Rep. 2015;9(4):89.
29. McNutt NS, Urmacher C, Hakimian J, Hoss DM, Lugo J. Nevoid malignant melanoma: morphologic patterns and immunohistochemical reactivity. J Cutan Pathol. 1995;22(6):502–17.
30. Anstey A, Cerio R, Orchard G, Smith N, Jones EW. Desmoplastic malignant melanoma. An immunocytochemical study of 25 cases. Am J Dermatopathol. 1994;16(1):14–22.
31. Jing X, Michael CW, Theoharis CG. The use of immunocytochemical study in the cytologic diagnosis of melanoma: evaluation of three antibodies. Diagn Cytopathol. 2013;41(2):126–30.
32. Deichmann M, Benner A, Bock M, Jäckel A, Uhl K, Waldmann V, Näher H. S100-Beta, melanoma-inhibiting activity, and lactate dehydrogenase discriminate progressive from nonprogressive American joint committee on cancer stage IV melanoma. J Clin Oncol. 1999;17(6):1891.
33. Heidarpour M, Rajabi P, Sajadi F. CD10 expression helps to differentiate basal cell carcinoma from trichoepithelioma. J Res Med Sci. 2011;16(7):938.
34. Keohane SG, Proby CM, Newlands C, Motley RJ, Nasr I, Mohd Mustapa MF, British Association of Dermatologists (Squamous and Basal Cell Carcinoma Guideline Development Groups), Slater, D.N. and Royal College of Pathologists (Skin Cancer Lead). The new 8th edition of TNM staging and its implications for skin cancer: a review by the British Association of Dermatologists and the Royal College of pathologists, UK. Br J Dermatol. 2018;179(4):824–8.
35. Elder DE, Massi D, Scolyer RA, Willemze R. WHO classification of skin tumours. 2018.
36. Lipsker D, Engel F, Cribier B, Velten M, Hedelin G. Trends in melanoma epidemiology suggest three different types of melanoma. Br J Dermatol. 2007;157(2):338–43.
37. Swerdlow AJ, English J, MacKie RM, O'doherty CJ, Hunter JA, Clark J, Hole DJ. Benign melanocytic naevi as a risk factor for malignant melanoma. Br Med J (Clin Res Ed). 1986;292(6535):1555–9.
38. Weiss J, Bertz J, Jung EG. Malignant melanoma in southern Germany: different predictive value of risk factors for melanoma subtypes. Dermatology. 1991;183(2):109–13.
39. Weinstock MA, Sober AJ. The risk of progression of lentigo maligna to lentigo maligna melanoma. Br J Dermatol. 1987;116(3):303–10.
40. Argenziano G, Soyer HP, Chimenti S, Talamini R, Corona R, Sera F, et al. Dermoscopy of pigmented skin lesions: results of a consensus meeting via the internet. J Am Acad Dermatol. 2003;48(5):679–93.

41. Quinn MJ, Crotty KA, Thompson JF, Coates AS, O'Brien CJ, McCarthy WH. Desmoplastic and desmoplastic neurotropic melanoma: experience with 280 patients. Cancer. 1998;83(6):1128–35.
42. McCarthy SW, Scolyer RA, Palmer AA. Desmoplastic melanoma: a diagnostic trap for the unwary. Pathology. 2004;36(5):445–51.
43. Newman S, Fan L, Pribnow A, Silkov A, Rice SV, Lee S, Shao Y, Shaner B, Mulder H, Nakitandwe J, Shurtleff S. Clinical genome sequencing uncovers potentially targetable truncations and fusions of MAP3K8 in spitzoid and other melanomas. Nat Med. 2019;25(4):597–602.
44. Cerrato F, Wallins JS, Webb ML, McCarty ER, Schmidt BA, Labow BI. Outcomes in pediatric atypical spitz tumors treated without sentinel lymph node biopsy. Pediatr Dermatol. 2012;29(4):448–53.
45. Carrera C, Gual A, Díaz A, Puig-Butillé JA, Noguès S, Vilalta A, Conill C, Rull R, Vilana R, Arguis P, Vidal-Sicart S. Prognostic role of the histological subtype of melanoma on the hands and feet in Caucasians. Melanoma Res. 2017;27(4):315–20.
46. Saida T, Kawachi S, Takata M, Kurita H, Kurashina K, Kageshita T, Tonogi M, Okazaki Y, Yamane GY, Takubo K, Ueyama Y. Histopathological characteristics of malignant melanoma affecting mucous membranes: a unifying concept of histogenesis. Pathology. 2004;36(5):404–13.
47. Zaal LH, Mooi WJ, Smitt JS, Van der Horst CM. Classification of congenital melanocytic naevi and malignant transformation: a review of the literature. Br J Plast Surg. 2004;57(8):707–19.
48. Zembowicz A. Blue nevi and related tumors. Clin Lab Med. 2017;37(3):401–15.
49. Kanitakis J. Anatomy, histology and immunohistochemistry of normal human skin. Eur J Dermatol. 2002;12(4):390–401.
50. James WD, Berger TG, Elston DM. Viral diseases. Andrews' diseases of the skin. Clinical dermatology. 1st ed. Toronto, ON: Saunders Elsevier; 2006. p. 367–415.
51. Chu DH. Overview of biology, development, and structure of skin. Fitzpatrick's dermatology in general medicine. 2008;7:57–73.
52. Chieosilapatham P, Ogawa H, Niyonsaba F. Current insights into the role of human β-defensins in atopic dermatitis. Clin Exp Immunol. 2017;190(2):155–66.
53. Murphy G. Histology of the skin. In: Elenitsas R, Jaworsky C, Johnson B, editors. Lever's histopathology of the skin. Philadelphia, PA: Lippincott-Raven; 1997. p. 5–50.
54. Jones PH. Isolation and characterization of human epidermal stem cells. Clin Sci. 1996;91(2):141–6.
55. Haake AR. The structure and development of skin. Dermatology in general medicine. 1999:70–114.
56. Stepp MA, Spurr-Michaud S, Tisdale A, Elwell J, Gipson IK. Alpha 6 beta 4 integrin heterodimer is a component of hemidesmosomes. Proc Natl Acad Sci. 1990;87(22):8970–4.
57. Seykora JT, Cotsarelis G. Keratin 15-positive stem cells give rise to basal cell carcinomas in irradiated Ptch1+/− mice. Cancer Cell. 2011;19(1):5–6.
58. Grachtchouk M, Mo R, Yu S, Zhang X, Sasaki H, Hui CC, Dlugosz AA. Basal cell carcinomas in mice overexpressing Gli2 in skin. Nat Genet. 2000;24(3):216–7.
59. Paolino G, Donati M, Didona D, Mercuri SR, Cantisani C. Histology of non-melanoma skin cancers: an update. Biomedicines. 2017;5(4):71.
60. Sanchez-Danes A, Blanpain C. Deciphering the cells of origin of squamous cell carcinomas. Nat Rev Cancer. 2018;18(9):549–61.
61. Dupin E, Calloni GW, Coelho-Aguiar JM, Le Douarin NM. The issue of the multipotency of the neural crest cells. Dev Biol. 2018;444:S47–59.
62. Kozovska Z, Gabrisova V, Kucerova L. Malignant melanoma: diagnosis, treatment and cancer stem cells. Neoplasma. 2016;63(4):510–7.
63. Xu S, Xu H, Wang W, Li S, Li H, Li T, Zhang W, Yu X, Liu L. The role of collagen in cancer: from bench to bedside. J Transl Med. 2019;17(1):309.
64. Ingham PW, McMahon AP. Hedgehog signaling in animal development: paradigms and principles. Genes Dev. 2001;15(23):3059–87.

65. Aszterbaum M, Rothman A, Fisher M, Xie J, Bonifas JM, Zhang X, Epstein EH Jr, Johnson RL, Scott MP. Identification of mutations in the human PATCHED gene in sporadic basal cell carcinomas and in patients with the basal cell nevus syndrome. J Invest Dermatol. 1998;110(6):885–8.
66. Smyth I, Narang MA, Evans T, Heimann C, Nakamura Y, Chenevix-Trench G, Pietsch T, Wicking C, Wainwright BJ. Isolation and characterization of human patched 2 (PTCH2), a putative tumour suppressor gene in basal cell carcinoma and medulloblastoma on chromosome 1p32. Hum Mol Genet. 1999;8(2):291–7.
67. Epstein EH. Basal cell carcinomas: attack of the hedgehog. Nat Rev Cancer. 2008;8(10):743–54.
68. Marzuka AG, Book S. Basal cell carcinoma: pathogenesis, epidemiology, clinical features, diagnosis, histopathology, and management. Yale J Biol Med. 2015;88(2):167–79.
69. Bonilla X, Parmentier L, King B, Bezrukov F, Kaya G, Zoete V, Seplyarskiy VB, Sharpe HJ, McKee T, Letourneau A, Ribaux PG. Genomic analysis identifies new drivers and progression pathways in skin basal cell carcinoma. Nat Genet. 2016;48(4):398–406.
70. Doglioni C, Piccinin S, Demontis S, Cangi MG, Pecciarini L, Chiarelli C, Armellin M, Vukosavljevic T, Boiocchi M, Maestro R. Alterations of β-catenin pathway in non-melanoma skin tumors: loss of α-ABC nuclear reactivity correlates with the presence of β-catenin gene mutation. Am J Pathol. 2003;163(6):2277–87.
71. El-Bahrawy M, El-Masry N, Alison M, Poulsom R, Fallowfield M. Expression of β-catenin in basal cell carcinoma. Br J Dermatol. 2003;148(5):964–70.
72. Watt FM, Estrach S, Ambler CA. Epidermal Notch signalling: differentiation, cancer and adhesion. Curr Opin Cell Biol. 2008;20(2):171–9.
73. Griewank KG, Murali R, Schilling B, Schimming T, Möller I, Moll I, Schwamborn M, Sucker A, Zimmer L, Schadendorf D, Hillen U. TERT promoter mutations are frequent in cutaneous basal cell carcinoma and squamous cell carcinoma. PLoS One. 2013;8(11):e80354.
74. Heffelfinger C, Ouyang Z, Engberg A, Leffell DJ, Hanlon AM, Gordon PB, Zheng W, Zhao H, Snyder MP, Bale AE. Correlation of global microRNA expression with basal cell carcinoma subtype. G3. 2012;2(2):279–86.
75. Bukhari MH, Niazi S, Chaudhry NA. Relationship of immunohistochemistry scores of altered p53 protein expression in relation to patient's habits and histological grades and stages of squamous cell carcinoma. J Cutan Pathol. 2009;36(3):342–9.
76. Brown VL, Harwood CA, Crook T, Cronin JG, Kelsell DP, Proby CM. p16INK4a and p14ARF tumor suppressor genes are commonly inactivated in cutaneous squamous cell carcinoma. J Invest Dermatol. 2004;122(5):1284–92.
77. Chin SS, Romano RA, Nagarajan P, Sinha S, Garrett-Sinha LA. Aberrant epidermal differentiation and disrupted ΔNp63/Notch regulatory axis in Ets1 transgenic mice. Biol Open. 2013;2(12):1336–45.
78. Ota T, Takekoshi S, Takagi T, Kitatani K, Toriumi K, Kojima T, Kato M, Ikoma N, Mabuchi T, Ozawa A. Notch signaling may be involved in the abnormal differentiation of epidermal keratinocytes in psoriasis. Acta Histochem Cytochem. 2014;47(4):175–83.
79. Durinck S, Ho C, Wang NJ, Liao W, Jakkula LR, Collisson EA, Pons J, Chan SW, Lam ET, Chu C, Park K. Temporal dissection of tumorigenesis in primary cancers temporal dissection of tumorigenesis in primary cancers. Cancer Discov. 2011;1(2):137–43.
80. Gillespie J, Skeeles LE, Allain DC, Kent MN, Peters SB, Nagarajan P, Yu L, Teknos TN, Olencki T, Toland AE. Micro RNA expression profiling in metastatic cutaneous squamous cell carcinoma. J Eur Acad Dermatol Venereol. 2016;6(30):1043–5.
81. Leufke C, Leykauf J, Krunic D, Jauch A, Holtgreve-Grez H, Böhm-Steuer B, Bröcker EB, Mauch C, Utikal J, Hartschuh W, Purdie KJ. The telomere profile distinguishes two classes of genetically distinct cutaneous squamous cell carcinomas. Oncogene. 2014;33(27):3506–18.
82. Barrett JH, Taylor JC, Bright C, Harland M, Dunning AM, Akslen LA, Andresen PA, Avril MF, Azizi E, Bianchi Scarrà G, Brossard M. Fine mapping of genetic susceptibility loci for melanoma reveals a mixture of single variant and multiple variant regions. Int J Cancer. 2015;136(6):1351–60.

83. Puntervoll HE, Yang XR, Vetti HH, Bachmann IM, Avril MF, Benfodda M, Catricalà C, Dalle S, Duval-Modeste AB, Ghiorzo P, Grammatico P. Melanoma prone families with CDK4 germline mutation: phenotypic profile and associations with MC1R variants. J Med Genet. 2013;50(4):264–70.
84. Aoude LG, Pritchard AL, Robles-Espinoza CD, Wadt K, Harland M, Choi J, Gartside M, Quesada V, Johansson P, Palmer JM, Ramsay AJ. Nonsense mutations in the shelterin complex genes ACD and TERF2IP in familial melanoma. J Natl Cancer Inst. 2015;107(2):dju408.
85. Wiesner T, Obenauf AC, Murali R, Fried I, Griewank KG, Ulz P, Windpassinger C, Wackernagel W, Loy S, Wolf I, Viale A. Germline mutations in BAP1 predispose to melanocytic tumors. Nat Genet. 2011;43(10):1018–21.
86. Pasquali E, García-Borrón JC, Fargnoli MC, Gandini S, Maisonneuve P, Bagnardi V, Specchia C, Liu F, Kayser M, Nijsten T, Nagore E. MC1R variants increased the risk of sporadic cutaneous melanoma in darker-pigmented C aucasians: a pooled-analysis from the M-SKIP project. Int J Cancer. 2015;136(3):618–31.
87. Yokoyama S, Woods SL, Boyle GM, Aoude LG, MacGregor S, Zismann V, Gartside M, Cust AE, Haq R, Harland M, Taylor JC. A novel recurrent mutation in MITF predisposes to familial and sporadic melanoma. Nature. 2011;480(7375):99–103.
88. Ghiorzo P, Pastorino L, Queirolo P, Bruno W, Tibiletti MG, Nasti S, Andreotti V, Paillerets BB, Bianchi Scarrà G, Genoa Pancreatic Cancer Study Group. Prevalence of the E 318 K MITF germline mutation in Italian melanoma patients: associations with histological subtypes and family cancer history. Pigment Cell Melanoma Res. 2013;26(2):259–62.
89. Davies H, Bignell GR, Cox C, Stephens P, Edkins S, Clegg S, Teague J, Woffendin H, Garnett MJ, Bottomley W, Davis N. Mutations of the BRAF gene in human cancer. Nature. 2002;417(6892):949–54.
90. Omholt K, Platz A, Kanter L, Ringborg U, Hansson J. NRAS and BRAF mutations arise early during melanoma pathogenesis and are preserved throughout tumor progression. Clin Cancer Res. 2003;9(17):6483–8.
91. Stahl JM, Sharma A, Cheung M, Zimmerman M, Cheng JQ, Bosenberg MW, Kester M, Sandirasegarane L, Robertson GP. Deregulated Akt3 activity promotes development of malignant melanoma. Cancer Res. 2004;64(19):7002–10.
92. Wei X, Walia V, Lin JC, Teer JK, Prickett TD, Gartner J, Davis S, Stemke-Hale K, Davies MA, Gershenwald JE, NISC Comparative Sequencing Program. Exome sequencing identifies GRIN2A as frequently mutated in melanoma. Nat Genet. 2011;43(5):442–6.
93. Stark MS, Woods SL, Gartside MG, Bonazzi VF, Dutton-Regester K, Aoude LG, Chow D, Sereduk C, Niemi NM, Tang N, Ellis JJ. Frequent somatic mutations in MAP3K5 and MAP3K9 in metastatic melanoma identified by exome sequencing. Nat Genet. 2012;44(2):165–9.
94. Cameron MC, Lee E, Hibler BP, Giordano CN, Barker CA, Mori S, Cordova M, Nehal KS, Rossi AM. Basal cell carcinoma: contemporary approaches to diagnosis, treatment, and prevention. J Am Acad Dermatol. 2019;80(2):321–39.
95. Neville JA, Welch E, Leffell DJ. Management of nonmelanoma skin cancer in 2007. Nat Clin Pract Oncol. 2007;4(8):462–9.
96. Schulze HJ, Cribier B, Requena L, Reifenberger J, Ferrándiz C, Garcia Diez A, Tebbs V, McRae S. Imiquimod 5% cream for the treatment of superficial basal cell carcinoma: results from a randomized vehicle-controlled phase III study in Europe. Br J Dermatol. 2005;152(5):939–47.
97. Micali G, Pasquale RD, Caltabiano R, Impallomeni R, Lacarrubba F. Topical imiquimod treatment of superficial and nodular basal cell carcinomas in patients affected by basal cell nevus syndrome: a preliminary report. J Dermatol Treat. 2002;13(3):123–7.
98. Love WE, Bernhard JD, Bordeaux JS. Topical imiquimod or fluorouracil therapy for basal and squamous cell carcinoma: a systematic review. Arch Dermatol. 2009;145(12):1431–8.
99. Meiss F, Andrlová H, Zeiser R. Vismodegib. Small Mol Oncol. 2018:125–39.
100. Wahid M, Jawed A, Dar SA, Mandal RK, Haque S. Differential pharmacology and clinical utility of sonidegib in advanced basal cell carcinoma. Onco Targets Ther. 2017;10:515.

101. Wheeler DL, Dunn EF, Harari PM. Understanding resistance to EGFR inhibitors—impact on future treatment strategies. Nat Rev Clin Oncol. 2010;7(9):493–507.
102. Hu JC, Sadeghi P, Pinter-Brown LC, Yashar S, Chiu MW. Cutaneous side effects of epidermal growth factor receptor inhibitors: clinical presentation, pathogenesis, and management. J Am Acad Dermatol. 2007;56(2):317–26.
103. Jenni D, Karpova MB, Mühleisen B, Mangana J, Dreier J, Hafner J, Dummer R. A prospective clinical trial to assess lapatinib effects on cutaneous squamous cell carcinoma and actinic keratosis. ESMO Open. 2016;1(1):e000003.
104. Connolly SM, Baker DR, Coldiron BM, Fazio MJ, Storrs PA, Vidimos AT, et al. American Academy of Dermatology; American College of Mohs Surgery; American Society for Dermatologic Surgery Association; American Society for Mohs Surgery; Ad Hoc Task Force (Vol. 10, pp. 1582–1603). AAD/ACMS/ASDSA/ASMS 2012 appropriate use criteria for Mohs micrographic surgery: a report of the American Academy of Dermatology, American College of Mohs Surgery, American Society for Dermatologic Surgery Association, and the American Society for Mohs Surgery. Dermatol Surg. 2012:38.
105. Alam M, Armstrong A, Baum C, Bordeaux JS, Brown M, Busam KJ, Eisen DB, Iyengar V, Lober C, Margolis DJ, Messina J. Guidelines of care for the management of cutaneous squamous cell carcinoma. J Am Acad Dermatol. 2018;78(3):560–78.
106. Lansbury L, Bath-Hextall F, Perkins W, Stanton W, Leonardi-Bee J. Interventions for non-metastatic squamous cell carcinoma of the skin: systematic review and pooled analysis of observational studies. BMJ. 2013;347.
107. Rigel DS, Carucci JA. Malignant melanoma: prevention, early detection, and treatment in the 21st century. CA Cancer J Clin. 2000;50(4):215–36.
108. Bishop DT, Demenais F, Iles MM, Harland M, Taylor JC, Corda E, Randerson-Moor J, Aitken JF, Avril MF, Azizi E, Bakker B. Genome-wide association study identifies three loci associated with melanoma risk. Nat Genet. 2009;41(8):920–5.

Bone Cancer

22

Ayesha Rahmat Yadwad, Jahnavi Ramesh Iyer,
Meghana Korikani, Kishore Reddy Bhavanam,
and Rama Krishna Kancha

22.1 Introduction

Epidemiology: Primary malignant bone cancers have a global incidence of less than 1%; approximately one thousand new cases are diagnosed annually in the United States [1]. Chondrosarcoma is the most prevalent in adults whereas in children and teens, osteosarcoma and Ewing sarcoma are most prevalent. The occurrence of osteosarcoma mostly impacts the age group of 10–30 years with teens being the most affected. Only 10% of the osteosarcoma cases are identified in people of age > 60 years. The bimodal incidence of osteosarcoma can be observed at two peaks: a major peak at the age of 18 years (primary diagnosis) and a second peak with poor prognosis at 60 years of age [2, 3]. According to the SEER database, the 5-year survival rates of giant cell tumor of bone, chordoma, and chondrosarcoma were 76%, 79%, and 79%, respectively, for the period 2011–2017. Chondroma (66.8 months) has the highest mean survival rate followed by chondrosarcoma (63.5 months), Ewing sarcoma (58.0 months), and osteosarcoma (54.9 months) [1]. The incidence rates of osteosarcoma during 1992–2004 for American Indian/Alaska Native, Hispanic, non-Hispanic white, Black, and Asian/Pacific Islander were 2.4%, 3.3%, 3%, 4%, and 2.9%, respectively [3]. Males had a higher incidence of osteosarcoma than females [3]. In children to young adults, the median diagnostic age for Ewing sarcoma is 14–15 years [4]. The incidence of metastatic Ewing sarcoma in children (0–9 years old) and adolescents and young adults (15–19 years old) is 23.8% and 32.3%,respectively [4]. According to a retrospective study during

A. R. Yadwad · J. R. Iyer · M. Korikani · R. K. Kancha (✉)
Molecular Medicine and Therapeutics Laboratory, CPMB, Osmania University, Hyderabad, Telangana, India
e-mail: ramakancha@osmania.ac.in

K. R. Bhavanam (✉)
Amor Hospitals, Hyderabad, Telangana, India

R. K. Kancha (ed.), *Biomedical Aspects of Solid Cancers*,
https://doi.org/10.1007/978-981-97-1802-3_22

1973–2015, the 1-, 5-, and 10-year survival rates for Ewing sarcoma were 91.1%, 72.9%, and 68.2%, respectively [5]. Females had consistently better 1-, 5-, and 10-year survival rates for Ewing sarcoma, with rates 91.4%, 75.4%, and 71.1%, respectively, when compared to men with 90.8%, 70.3%, and 65.7%, respectively [5].

Risk factors: The major risk factors for osteosarcoma include age (highest risk observed in the 10–30 years age group), height (tall > short people), gender (males > females), race/ethnicity (African Americans and Hispanics/Latinos > whites in USA), and exposure to radiation. The risk of development of osteochondromas increases with the occurrence of Paget disease, fibrous dysplasia, hereditary syndromes such as the Li–Fraumeni syndrome, Rothmund–Thompson syndrome, Werner syndrome, Bloom syndrome, and retinoblastoma familial cancers [6–11]. Elevated levels of IL-6 are also linked to increased tumor growth [2, 12].

Diagnosis: Diagnosis of bone cancer (BC) is primarily based on histological analysis, biochemical tests, and imaging tests. Histological analysis is mainly done through biopsies. Scanning/Imaging tests for bone cancer include MRI scan and PET-CT scan. Biochemical tests include blood tests such as complete blood counts to check for anemia, clotting problems (low platelet count), elevated levels of alkaline phosphatase, and lactate dehydrogenase. Osteocalcin (bone sialoprotein) and alkaline phosphatase are the biochemical markers expressed by osteosarcoma cells [2].

22.2 Classification

According to the World Health Organization, bone cancer is categorized into various subtypes (Fig. 22.1). Based on their origin, bone cancers can be classified into primary bone cancers in which cancer originates in the bone and bone metastases in which cancer originates in a different organ but spreads/metastasizes to the bone. Depending on their rate of metastasis, primary bone cancers are: (A) chondrosarcomas are classified into 3 grades, namely low-grade or grade I, which includes atypical cartilaginous tumors, intermediate-grade or grade II, and high-grade or grade III. Moreover, there are some uncommon types of chondrosarcomas that show certain characteristic features different from other types which include mesenchymal chondrosarcomas and clear cell chondrosarcomas. Based on their cell morphology and rate of metastasis. (B) osteosarcomas are classified into 3 subtypes: High-grade osteosarcomas are the fastest growing subtype, Intermediate-grade osteosarcomas that consist of one subtype i.e. periosteal (juxtacortical intermediate grade), and Low-grade osteosarcomas consist of two subtypes that include Parosteal and Intramedullary/intraosseous well differentiated. Almost all types of cancer can metastasize to the bone, but the most commonly observed ones include the breast, lung, prostate, kidney, ovarian, and thyroid cancers, and melanoma. There are 2 main staging systems for bone cancer: (A) Musculoskeletal Tumor Society (MSTS) and (B) tumor, node, metastasis (TNM) staging systems.

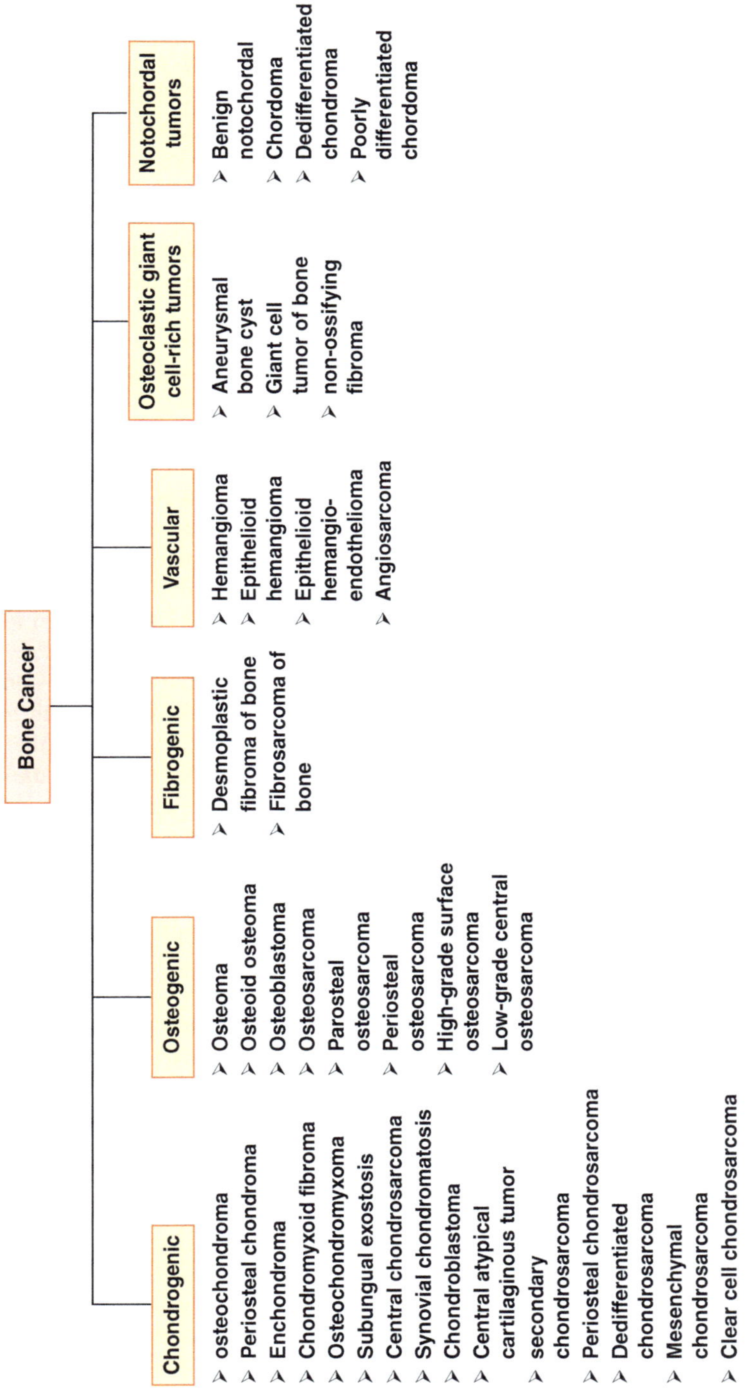

Fig. 22.1 World Health Organization classification of bone cancer

MSTS system: Depending on the tumor grade, size, and degree of metastasis, the MSTS system classifies bone cancers into the following stages: Stages IA and IB or low-grade, IIA and IIB or high-grade, and III or metastatic. *TNM system:* The AJCC proposed this system to categorize the cancer based on the size of the primary tumor (T), involvement of lymph nodes (N), extent of metastasis (M), and the cancer grade (abnormality of cells under a microscope) (G). There are 3 bone cancer grades: (a) Grade 1 (G1)—cancer tissue looks similar to the normal bone tissue; (b) Grade 2 (G2)—cancer tissue appears abnormal; (c) Grade 3 (G3)—cancer tissue has extremely abnormal appearance. The information about an individual's T, N, M, and G categories is then combined to assign an overall stage to the bone cancer, ranging from stages I–IV.

22.3 Pathophysiology

Bone serves as the supporting framework of the body. The compact (cortical) bone makes up the outermost hard-layer of the bone, which protects the inner lighter spongy (trabecular) bone. The fibrous tissue known as periosteum externally surrounds the bone. The medullary cavity is an internal space that is lined by tissue lining called endosteum and holds the spongy, soft tissue called the bone marrow. Majority of the bones start out as a more flexible and softer tissue known as the cartilage, which gets calcified to form the bone. A small amount of cartilage may remain after formation of the bone. Cartilage, ligaments, and other tissues connect bones to form joints. Adults often have cartilage at the terminals of certain bones that are part of a joint. The three types of bone cells are: (a) Osteoclasts are the cells that degrade and eliminate old components of the bone, (b) Osteoblasts are the cells that are involved in bone formation, and (c) Osteocytes that are nutrient-carrier cells of the bone. Any alterations in these bone cells may lead to bone cancer. Intramembranous ossification and endochondral ossification are the two bone formation processes [13]. Different subtypes of bone cancer show marked differences in their origin and the most commonly observed and widely studied subtypes are (a) Osteosarcomas, (b) Chondroblastomas, (c) Giant Cell Tumors, (d) Ewing Sarcoma, and (e) Chondrosarcoma (Fig. 22.2).

(a) Osteosarcomas (OS): Osteosarcomas are tumors which produce mechanically weaker, immature woven bone when compared to a normal lamellar bone [14]. The site of origin for primary OS are the long bones of the extremities such as the distal femur, proximal humerus, and proximal tibia with incidences accounting to 30%, 15%, and 15% [15]. In 90% of the cases, the origin of tumor is within the metaphysis of long bones [16]. In certain situations, fully differentiated osteocytes may act as OS-initiating cells [17]. *(b) Chondroblastomas:* They are uncommon, invasive bone cancers that originate from the immature chondrocytes, which are situated within the epiphyses of long bones [14]. *(c) Giant Cell Tumors of the Bone (GCTB):* GCTB are invasive, locally aggressive rare cancers which causes wearing down of the neighboring bones and joints [14]. They commonly originate within the appendicular skeleton, in the epiphysis of long bones [14]. They are diverse and

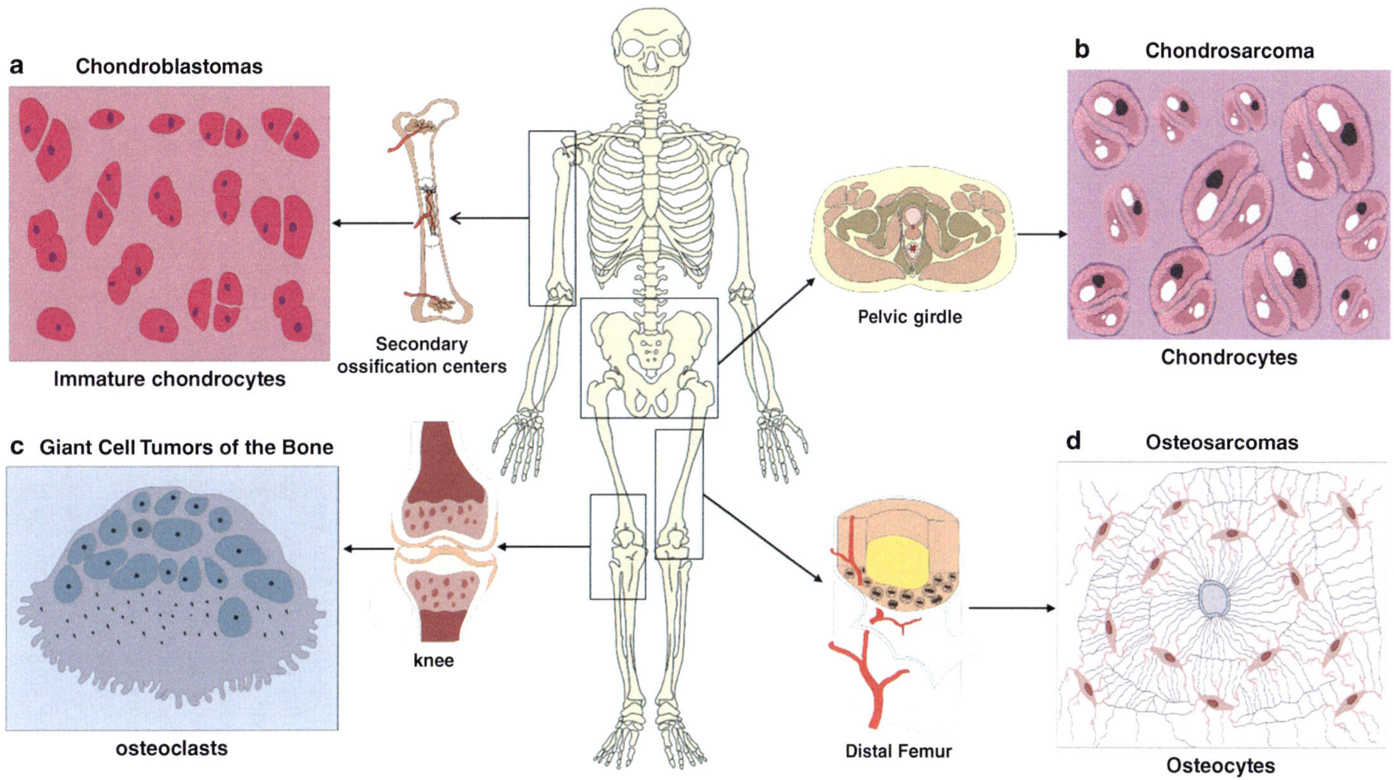

Fig. 22.2 Representation of bone cancer subtypes and their origin. (**a**) Chondroblastomas originate in the epiphysis of long bones from immature chondrocytes. (**b**) Chondrosarcoma develops in the pelvic girdle from chondrocytes. (**c**) Giant cell tumors of bone originate near the knee in multiple nucleated osteoclasts. (**d**) Osteosarcomas originate in the distal femur from osteocytes

comprises of three cell types: (i) Mesenchymal cells of the osteoblast lineage represent the neoplastic component of the tumors that express mutant H3.3 proteins and produces osteoblast products such as osteocalcin and alkaline phosphatase, (ii) Mononuclear histiocytic cells, and (iii) multi-nucleated giant cells that originate from the hematopoietic progenitors which express CD68 and also support the mutant osteoblastic cells [14]. *(d) Ewing Sarcoma:* Despite being classified in the group of small, round blue cell tumors based on its microscopic criteria, there still exists uncertainty in the cell of origin [18]. It is anticipated to arise from the primitive stem cells and the stage of differentiation arrest may have an impact on its degree of malignancy [18, 19]. *(e) Chondrosarcoma:* They are malignant bone cancers originating in the cartilage-producing cells [18] and occur commonly in the central skeleton and within the vertebrae, pelvic girdle, and proximal long bones [20].

Genetics: Ewing sarcomas are often characterized by somatic mutations in *TP53* [21], *STAG2* [22], and *CDKN2* [2, 23] genes. Mutations in *KDR*, *STK11*, *MLH1*, *KRAS*, and *PTPN11* genes are associated with increased proliferation and tumor heterogeneity in bone cancer [24]. Heat shock proteins also act as potential diagnostic markers and play a significant role in osteosarcoma development [25]. In addition to mutations in various oncogenes, *RB1* and *TP53* genes are also found to have a strong association with sporadic and hereditary osteosarcoma [26, 27]. In few cases, development of osteosarcoma is often initiated by the inactivation of *TP53* gene [28, 29]. About 10% of OS cases have a deletion in the *INK4A/ARF* locus [30]. Amplification of the 12q13 chromosome that contains *CDK4* and *MDM2* is often observed in approximately 10% of OS cases [27, 31]. Decreased survival in pediatric osteosarcoma is associated with a lack of expression of *P16INK4A* gene [27], whereas development of metastasis in OS is linked to amplification of *MDM2* [32].

Amplification or enhanced expression of cyclin D1 and E was observed in OS [33, 34]. The progression of OS is linked to expression and activation of *C-FOS* and *C-JUN* genes [35, 36]. Amplification of *C-MYC* is detected in sporadic OS [37]. High levels of *C-MYC* expression are associated with unfavorable outcomes in osteosarcoma patients [38]. Mutations in *MET*, *TWIST*, and *APC* genes which are prevalent in pediatric high-grade osteosarcoma are associated with worse prognosis [39]. Genes such as *LATS2, MCM4, BIRC2, BIRC3, COPS3, CCT3*, and *WWP1* are known to be potential drivers of osteosarcoma; Rothmund–Thomson syndrome, which occurs due OS-predisposition, is commonly associated with mutations in the *RECQL4* gene [26, 40–43]. Mutation and amplification of *RUNX2*, and loss of heterozygosity of *BUB3* and *FGFR2* were associated with the OS pathogenesis [43, 44]. Various bone tumors including OS were found to form due to the expression of intracellular domain of NOTCH1 (NICD) in osteoblast cells [45]. High-penetrance OS develop due to enhanced expression of Hedgehog (HH) signaling pathway in mature osteoblasts and in the presence of *TP53* heterozygous background [46]. Somatic mutations within *HIST1H3B* and *H3F3A* genes were frequently reported in osteosarcoma, *H3F3B* mutations in chondroblastoma, and *H3F3A* mutations in GCTB cases [47, 48]. *H3F3-AG34W/R* mutations in osteosarcoma are linked to dysregulation of epigenetic oncogenic pathways such as phosphatase and tensin homolog pathway [49]. Germline SNPs of the DNA excision repair pathway such as *ERCC1* and *ERCC2,* are associated to osteosarcoma survival [50, 51].

22.4 Treatment

The treatment options for bone cancer can vary depending on type (Primary/secondary) and subtype of cancer, size of tumor, location of cancer, stage/grade of the cancer, possible side effects, age, general health, and preference of the patient. The most common treatment methods include surgery (limb-salvage tumor resection or amputation), cryosurgery, chemotherapy, high-dose chemotherapy with stem cell rescue, radiation therapy, targeted therapy, and immunotherapy. Osteosarcoma and Ewing sarcoma are typically treated with a combination of surgery, chemotherapy, and long-term polychemotherapy (6–12 months) [12]. The standard treatment for osteosarcoma includes preoperative/neoadjuvant chemotherapy, surgical resection, and postoperative/adjuvant chemotherapy [18].

Conventionally used front-line treatment for children and young adult patients include high-dose methotrexate, ifosfamide, doxorubicin, etoposide, and cisplatin [52–54]. But high-dose methotrexate does not show high efficacy in adult patients with osteoblastoma [55, 56]. In Ewing sarcoma, liposome-encapsulated clodronate targets tumor-associated macrophages (TAMs) and simultaneously inhibits macrophage differentiation into M1 and M2 types, which further decreases the tumor growth [57]. Radiation therapy can be used to treat primary Ewing lesions that cannot be surgically resected due to the tumor location or size [18]. Malignant cartilage cells have poor vasculature and is therefore difficult for the delivery of chemotherapeutic agents to chondrosarcoma [58, 59]. Therefore, the primary choice of treatment for chondrosarcoma is surgical resection, while radiation therapy is employed for instances with poor surgical margins, much like it is for the treatment of Ewing sarcoma [18]. For patients affected with refractory sarcoma including osteosarcoma, a combination of gemcitabine (GEM) and docetaxel (DOC) is used, and the overall survival rate was better in patients who received GEM + DOC as adjuvant (postoperative) chemotherapy than those who received it as palliative therapy in a Korean patient cohort [60]. When compared to surgery alone, combinational management of chemotherapy and surgery for high-grade, localized osteosarcoma increased disease-free survival (DFS) probability from less than 20% to greater than 60% [61]. Although, there is lack of evidence indicating that preoperative chemotherapy increases survival, the histological responsiveness to preoperative chemotherapy can be evaluated, which further helps in predicting patient survival [62].

For patients with unresectable osteosarcoma, carbon ion radiotherapy [63], and proton-based radiotherapy [64] can be used to deliver high doses, especially in pediatric or young adult patients. The treatment strategies for recurrent osteosarcoma are based on the time period for recurrences and the frequency and locations of metastases [61]. First, all resectable metastases must be completely removed because more than one-third of patients with a complete second surgical remission survive for more than 5 years [65]. Radiofrequency ablation (RFA) and stereotactic radiotherapy can be used as alternative treatment options for bone metastases [66]. Multiagent regimens including vincristine, doxorubicin, cyclophosphamide/ifosfamide, and etoposide are used to treat primary Ewing sarcoma cases [67–69]. Administration of busulfan and melphalan (Bu-Mel) increases the survival in patients with Ewing sarcoma showing poor response to vincristine, ifosfamide, doxorubicin, and etoposide [70].

22.5 Conclusion

Bone cancer (BC) is heterogeneous by nature and the osteosarcoma subtype has the highest incidence. Minor differences in incidence between races and gender are also evident. Age, gender, height, race, and radiation exposure are a few of the variables that affect the incidence risk. Presence of hereditary syndromes also increases the incidence rate. According to the WHO, there are eight subtypes of BC including chondrogenic, vascular, osteogenic, osteoclastic, giant cell-rich, notochondral, other mesenchymal tumors, and hematological neoplasms. The present diagnosing process comprises preliminary biochemical tests, imaging, and histological analysis. Biochemical and cell-specific markers play a significant role in detection and diagnosis. Choosing a course of treatment frequently involves combining two or more modalities, such as chemotherapy, immunotherapy, radiation, and targeted therapy.

References

1. Xu G, Wu H, Xu Y, Zhang Y, Lin F, Baklaushev VP, Chekhonin VP, Peltzer K, Wang X, Mao M, Wang G. Homogenous and heterogenous prognostic factors for patients with bone sarcoma. Orthop Surg. 2021;13(1):134–44.
2. Brown HK, Schiavone K, Gouin F, Heymann MF, Heymann D. Biology of bone sarcomas and new therapeutic developments. Calcif Tissue Int. 2018;102:174–95.
3. Mirabello L, Troisi RJ, Savage SA. Osteosarcoma incidence and survival rates from 1973 to 2004: data from the surveillance, epidemiology, and end results program. Cancer: interdisciplinary international journal of the American cancer. Society. 2009;115(7):1531–43.
4. Worch J, Ranft A, DuBois SG, Paulussen M, Juergens H, Dirksen U. Age dependency of primary tumor sites and metastases in patients with Ewing sarcoma. Pediatr Blood Cancer. 2018;65(9):e27251.
5. Martin E, Radomski S, Harley EH. Pediatric Ewing sarcoma of the head and neck: a retrospective survival analysis. Int J Pediatr Otorhinolaryngol. 2019;117:138–42.
6. Correa H. Li–Fraumeni syndrome. J Pediatr Genet. 2016;5(02):084–8.
7. Simon T, Kohlhase J, Wilhelm C, Kochanek M, De Carolis B, Berthold F. Multiple malignant diseases in a patient with Rothmund–Thomson syndrome with RECQL4 mutations: Case report and literature review. Am J Med Genet A. 2010;152(6):1575–9.
8. Murata K, Hatamochi A, Shinkai H, Ishikawa Y, Kawaguchi N, Goto M. A case of Werner's syndrome associated with osteosarcoma. J Dermatol. 1999;26(10):682–6.
9. Lu L, Jin W, Wang LL. RECQ DNA helicases and osteosarcoma. In: Current advances in the science of osteosarcoma: research perspectives: tumor biology, organ microenvironment, potential new therapeutic targets, and canine models; 2020. p. 37–54.

10. Ng AJ, Walia MK, Smeets MF, Mutsaers AJ, Sims NA, Purton LE, Walsh NC, Martin TJ, Walkley CR. The DNA helicase recql4 is required for normal osteoblast expansion and osteosarcoma formation. PLoS Genet. 2015;11(4):e1005160.
11. Ren W, Gu G. Prognostic implications of RB 1 tumour suppressor gene alterations in the clinical outcome of human osteosarcoma: a meta-analysis. Eur J Cancer Care. 2017;26(1):e12401.
12. Heymann D, Ory B, Blanchard F, Heymann MF, Coipeau P, Charrier C, Couillaud S, Thiery JP, Gouin F, Redini F. Enhanced tumor regression and tissue repair when zoledronic acid is combined with ifosfamide in rat osteosarcoma. Bone. 2005;37(1):74–86.
13. Karsenty G. Regulation of bone formation. Annu Rev Cell Dev Biol. 2009;25:629.
14. Taylor EL, Westendorf JJ. Histone mutations and bone cancers. In: Histone Mutations and Cancer; 2021. p. 53–62.
15. Abarrategi A, Tornin J, Martinez-Cruzado L, Hamilton A, Martinez-Campos E, Rodrigo JP, González M, Baldini N, Garcia-Castro J, Rodriguez R. Osteosarcoma: cells-of-origin, cancer stem cells, and targeted therapies. Stem Cells Int. 2016;2016:3631764.
16. Alfranca A, Martinez-Cruzado L, Tornin J, Abarrategi A, Amaral T, de Alava E, Menendez P, Garcia-Castro J, Rodriguez R. Bone microenvironment signals in osteosarcoma development. Cell Mol Life Sci. 2015;72:3097–113.
17. Sottnik JL, Campbell B, Mehra R, Behbahani-Nejad O, Hall CL, Keller ET. Osteocytes serve as a progenitor cell of osteosarcoma. J Cell Biochem. 2014;115(8):1420–9.
18. Ferguson JL, Turner SP. Bone cancer: diagnosis and treatment principles. Am Fam Physician. 2018;98(4):205–13.
19. Rajwanshi A, Srinivas R, Upasana G. Malignant small round cell tumors. J Cytol. 2009;26(1):1.
20. Lanzkowsky P, Lipton J, Fish JD. Lanzkowsky's manual of pediatric hematology and oncology. Elsevier; 2010.
21. Huang HY, Illei PB, Zhao Z, Mazumdar M, Huvos AG, Healey JH, Wexler LH, Gorlick R, Meyers P, Ladanyi M. Ewing sarcomas with p53 mutation or p16/p14ARF homozygous deletion: a highly lethal subset associated with poor chemoresponse. J Clin Oncol. 2005;23(3):548–58.
22. Brohl AS, Solomon DA, Chang W, Wang J, Song Y, Sindiri S, Patidar R, Hurd L, Chen L, Shern JF, Liao H. The genomic landscape of the Ewing sarcoma family of tumors reveals recurrent STAG2 mutation. PLoS Genet. 2014;10(7):e1004475.
23. Bühnemann C, Li S, Yu H, Branford White H, Schäfer KL, Llombart-Bosch A, Machado I, Picci P, Hogendoorn PC, Athanasou NA, Noble JA. Quantification of the heterogeneity of prognostic cellular biomarkers in Ewing sarcoma using automated image and random survival forest analysis. PLoS One. 2014;9(9):e107105.
24. Zhang N, Liu H, Yue G, Zhang Y, You J, Wang H. Molecular heterogeneity of Ewing sarcoma as detected by ion torrent sequencing. PLoS One. 2016;11(4):e0153546.
25. Lallier M, Marchandet L, Moukengue B, Charrier C, Baud'huin M, Verrecchia F, Ory B, Lamoureux F. Molecular chaperones in osteosarcoma: diagnosis and therapeutic issues. Cells. 2021;10(4):754.
26. Ng AJ, Mutsaers AJ, Baker EK, Walkley CR. Genetically engineered mouse models and human osteosarcoma. Clinical sarcoma research. 2012;2(1):1–4.
27. Tang N, Song WX, Luo J, Haydon RC, He TC. Osteosarcoma development and stem cell differentiation. Clin Orthop Relat Res. 2008;466(9):2114–30.
28. Berman SD, Calo E, Landman AS, Danielian PS, Miller ES, West JC, Fonhoue BD, Caron A, Bronson R, Bouxsein ML, Mukherjee S. Metastatic osteosarcoma induced by inactivation of Rb and p53 in the osteoblast lineage. Proc Natl Acad Sci. 2008;105(33):11851–6.
29. Walkley CR, Qudsi R, Sankaran VG, Perry JA, Gostissa M, Roth SI, Rodda SJ, Snay E, Dunning P, Fahey FH, Alt FW. Conditional mouse osteosarcoma, dependent on p53 loss and potentiated by loss of Rb, mimics the human disease. Genes Dev. 2008;22(12):1662–76.
30. López-Guerrero JA, López-Ginés C, Pellín A, Carda C, Llombart-Bosch A. Deregulation of the G1 to S-phase cell cycle checkpoint is involved in the pathogenesis of human osteosarcoma. Diagn Mol Pathol. 2004;13(2):81–91.

31. Lonardo F, Ueda T, Huvos AG, Healey J, Ladanyi M. p53 and MDM2 alterations in osteosarcomas: correlation with clinicopathologic features and proliferative rate. Cancer. 1997;79(8):1541–7.
32. Ladanyi M, Cha C, Lewis R, Jhanwar SC, Huvos AG, Healey JH. MDM2 gene amplification in metastatic osteosarcoma. Cancer Res. 1993;53(1):16–8.
33. Benassi MS, Molendini L, Gamberi G, Ragazzini P, Sollazzo MR, Merli M, Asp J, Magagnoli G, Balladelli A, Bertoni F, Picci P. Alteration of pRb/p16/cdk4 regulation in human osteosarcoma. Int J Cancer. 1999;84(5):489–93.
34. Lockwood WW, Stack D, Morris T, Grehan D, O'Keane C, Stewart GL, Cumiskey J, Lam WL, Squire JA, Thomas DM, O'Sullivan MJ. Cyclin E1 is amplified and overexpressed in osteosarcoma. J Mol Diagn. 2011;13(3):289–96.
35. Gamberi G, Benassi MS, Bohling T, Ragazzini P, Molendini L, Sollazzo MR, Pompetti F, Merli M, Magagnoli G, Balladelli A, Picci P. C-myc and c-fos in human osteosarcoma: prognostic value of mRNA and protein expression. Oncology. 1998;55(6):556–63.
36. Wu JX, Carpenter PM, Gresens C, Keh R, Niman H, Morris JW, Mercola D. The protooncogene c-fos is over-expressed in the majority of human osteosarcomas. Oncogene. 1990;5(7):989–1000.
37. Smida J, Baumhoer D, Rosemann M, Walch A, Bielack S, Poremba C, Remberger K, Korsching E, Scheurlen W, Dierkes C, Burdach S. Genomic alterations and allelic imbalances are strong prognostic predictors in OsteosarcomaGenomic alterations and prognosis in osteosarcoma. Clin Cancer Res. 2010;16(16):4256–67.
38. Scionti I, Michelacci F, Pasello M, Hattinger CM, Alberghini M, Manara MC, Bacci G, Ferrari S, Scotlandi K, Picci P, Serra M. Clinical impact of the methotrexate resistance-associated genes C-MYC and dihydrofolate reductase (DHFR) in high-grade osteosarcoma. Ann Oncol. 2008;19(8):1500–8.
39. Entz-Werle N, Lavaux T, Metzger N, Stoetzel C, Lasthaus C, Marec P, Kalita C, Brugieres L, Pacquement H, Schmitt C, Tabone MD. Involvement of MET/TWIST/APC combination or the potential role of ossification factors in pediatric high-grade osteosarcoma oncogenesis. Neoplasia. 2007;9(8):678–88.
40. Kuijjer ML, Rydbeck H, Kresse SH, Buddingh EP, Lid AB, Roelofs H, Bürger H, Myklebost O, Hogendoorn PC, Meza-Zepeda LA, Cleton-Jansen AM. Identification of osteosarcoma driver genes by integrative analysis of copy number and gene expression data. Genes Chromosom Cancer. 2012;51(7):696–706.
41. Xiong Y, Wu S, Du Q, Wang A, Wang Z. Integrated analysis of gene expression and genomic aberration data in osteosarcoma (OS). Cancer Gene Ther. 2015;22(11):524–9.
42. Wang LL, Gannavarapu A, Kozinetz CA, Levy ML, Lewis RA, Chintagumpala MM, Ruiz-Maldanado R, Contreras-Ruiz J, Cunniff C, Erickson RP, Lev D. Association between osteosarcoma and deleterious mutations in the RECQL4 gene in Rothmund–Thomson syndrome. J Natl Cancer Inst. 2003;95(9):669–74.
43. Jones KB. Osteosarcomagenesis: modeling cancer initiation in the mouse. Sarcoma. 2011;2011:1.
44. Mendoza S, David H, Gaylord GM, Miller CW. Allelic loss at 10q26 in osteosarcoma in the region of the BUB3 and FGFR2 genes. Cancer Genet Cytogenet. 2005;158(2):142–7.
45. Tao J, Jiang MM, Jiang L, Salvo JS, Zeng HC, Dawson B, Bertin TK, Rao PH, Chen R, Donehower LA, Gannon F. Notch activation as a driver of osteogenic sarcoma. Cancer Cell. 2014;26(3):390–401.
46. Chan LH, Wang W, Yeung W, Deng Y, Yuan P, Mak KK. Hedgehog signaling induces osteosarcoma development through Yap1 and H19 overexpression. Oncogene. 2014;33(40):4857–66.
47. Castel D, Philippe C, Calmon R, Le Dret L, Truffaux N, Boddaert N, Pagès M, Taylor KR, Saulnier P, Lacroix L, Mackay A. Histone H3F3A and HIST1H3B K27M mutations define two subgroups of diffuse intrinsic pontine gliomas with different prognosis and phenotypes. Acta Neuropathol. 2015;130:815–27.

48. Behjati S, Tarpey PS, Presneau N, Scheipl S, Pillay N, Van Loo P, Wedge DC, Cooke SL, Gundem G, Davies H, Nik-Zainal S. Distinct H3F3A and H3F3B driver mutations define chondroblastoma and giant cell tumor of bone. Nat Genet. 2013;45(12):1479–82.
49. Koelsche C, Schrimpf D, Tharun L, Roth E, Sturm D, Jones DT, Renker EK, Sill M, Baude A, Sahm F, Capper D. Histone 3.3 hotspot mutations in conventional osteosarcomas: a comprehensive clinical and molecular characterization of six H3F3A mutated cases. Clin Sarcoma Res. 2017;7(1):1–1.
50. Serra M, Hattinger CM. The pharmacogenomics of osteosarcoma. Pharmacogenomics J. 2017;17(1):11–20.
51. Vos HI, Coenen MJ, Guchelaar HJ, Te Loo DM. The role of pharmacogenetics in the treatment of osteosarcoma. Drug Discov Today. 2016;21(11):1775–86.
52. Marina NM, Smeland S, Bielack SS, Bernstein M, Jovic G, Krailo MD, Hook JM, Arndt C, van den Berg H, Brennan B, Brichard B. Comparison of MAPIE versus MAP in patients with a poor response to preoperative chemotherapy for newly diagnosed high-grade osteosarcoma (EURAMOS-1): an open-label, international, randomised controlled trial. Lancet Oncol. 2016;17(10):1396–408.
53. Whelan JS, Bielack SS, Marina N, Smeland S, Jovic G, Hook JM, Krailo M, Anninga J, Butterfass-Bahloul T, Böhling T, Calaminus G. EURAMOS-1, an international randomised study for osteosarcoma: results from pre-randomisation treatment. Ann Oncol. 2015;26(2):407–14.
54. Ferrari S, Smeland S, Mercuri M, Bertoni F, Longhi A, Ruggieri P, Alvegard TA, Picci P, Capanna R, Bernini G, Müller C. Neoadjuvant chemotherapy with high-dose Ifosfamide, high-dose methotrexate, cisplatin, and doxorubicin for patients with localized osteosarcoma of the extremity: a joint study by the Italian and Scandinavian sarcoma groups. J Clin Oncol. 2005;23(34):8845–52.
55. Bajpai J, Chandrasekharan A, Talreja V, Simha V, Chandrakanth MV, Rekhi B, Khurana S, Khan A, Vora T, Ghosh J, Banavali SD. Outcomes in non-metastatic treatment naive extremity osteosarcoma patients treated with a novel non-high dosemethotrexate-based, dose-dense combination chemotherapy regimen 'OGS-12'. Eur J Cancer. 2017;85:49–58.
56. Piperno-Neumann S, Ray-Coquard I, Occean BV, Laurence V, Cupissol D, Perrin C, Penel N, Bompas E, Rios M, Le Cesne A, Italiano A. Results of API–AI based regimen in osteosarcoma adult patients included in the French OS2006/Sarcome-09 study. Int J Cancer. 2020;146(2):413–23.
57. Fujiwara T, Fukushi JI, Yamamoto S, Matsumoto Y, Setsu N, Oda Y, Yamada H, Okada S, Watari K, Ono M, Kuwano M. Macrophage infiltration predicts a poor prognosis for human Ewing sarcoma. Am J Pathol. 2011;179(3):1157–70.
58. Lieberman JR. AAOS comprehensive orthopaedic review. Rosemont, IL: American Academy of Orthopaedic Surgeons; 2009.
59. Giuffrida AY, Burgueno JE, Koniaris LG, Gutierrez JC, Duncan R, Scully SP. Chondrosarcoma in the United States (1973 to 2003): an analysis of 2890 cases from the SEER database. JBJS. 2009;91(5):1063–72.
60. Song BS, Seo J, Kim DH, Lim JS, Yoo JY, Lee JA. Gemcitabine and docetaxel for the treatment of children and adolescents with recurrent or refractory osteosarcoma: Korea cancer center hospital experience. Pediatr Blood Cancer. 2014;61(8):1376–81.
61. Strauss SJ, Frezza AM, Abecassis N, Bajpai J, Bauer S, Biagini R, Bielack S, Blay JY, Bolle S, Bonvalot S, Boukovinas I. Bone sarcomas: ESMO–EURACAN–GENTURIS–ERN PaedCan clinical practice guideline for diagnosis, treatment and follow-up. Ann Oncol. 2021;32(12):1520–36.
62. Smeland S, Bielack SS, Whelan J, Bernstein M, Hogendoorn P, Krailo MD, Gorlick R, Janeway KA, Ingleby FC, Anninga J, Antal I. Survival and prognosis with osteosarcoma: outcomes in more than 2000 patients in the EURAMOS-1 (European and American osteosarcoma study) cohort. Eur J Cancer. 2019;109:36–50.

63. Ciernik IF, Niemierko A, Harmon DC, Kobayashi W, Chen YL, Yock TI, Ebb DH, Choy E, Raskin KA, Liebsch N, Hornicek FJ. Proton-based radiotherapy for unresectable or incompletely resected osteosarcoma. Cancer. 2011;117(19):4522–30.
64. Matsunobu A, Imai R, Kamada T, Imaizumi T, Tsuji H, Tsujii H, Shioyama Y, Honda H, Tatezaki SI. Working Group for Bone and Soft Tissue Sarcomas. Impact of carbon ion radiotherapy for unresectable osteosarcoma of the trunk. Cancer. 2012;118(18):4555–63.
65. Kempf-Bielack B, Bielack SS, Jürgens H, Branscheid D, Berdel WE, Exner GU, Göbel U, Helmke K, Jundt G, Kabisch H, Kevric M. Osteosarcoma relapse after combined modality therapy: an analysis of unselected patients in the cooperative osteosarcoma study group (COSS). J Clin Oncol. 2005;23(3):559–68.
66. de Baere T, Tselikas L, Gravel G, Hakime A, Deschamps F, Honoré C, Mir O, Lecesne A. Interventional radiology: role in the treatment of sarcomas. Eur J Cancer. 2018;94:148–55.
67. Schuck A, Ahrens S, Paulussen M, Kuhlen M, Könemann S, Rübe C, Winkelmann W, Kotz R, Dunst J, Willich N, Jürgens H. Local therapy in localized Ewing tumors: results of 1058 patients treated in the CESS 81, CESS 86, and EICESS 92 trials. International journal of radiation oncology* biology*. Physics. 2003;55(1):168–77.
68. Womer RB, West DC, Krailo MD, Dickman PS, Pawel BR, Grier HE, Marcus K, Sailer S, Healey JH, Dormans JP, Weiss AR. Randomized controlled trial of interval-compressed chemotherapy for the treatment of localized Ewing sarcoma: a report from the Children's oncology group. J Clin Oncol. 2012;30(33):4148.
69. Le Deley MC, Paulussen M, Lewis I, Brennan B, Ranft A, Whelan J, Le Teuff G, Michon J, Ladenstein R, Marec-Bérard P, van den Berg H. Cyclophosphamide compared with ifosfamide in consolidation treatment of standard-risk Ewing sarcoma: results of the randomized noninferiority euro-EWING99-R1 trial. J Clin Oncol. 2014;32(23):2440–8.
70. Whelan J, Le Deley MC, Dirksen U, Le Teuff G, Brennan B, Gaspar N, Hawkins DS, Amler S, Bauer S, Bielack S, Blay JY. High-dose chemotherapy and blood autologous stem-cell rescue compared with standard chemotherapy in localized high-risk Ewing sarcoma: results of euro-EWING 99 and Ewing-2008. J Clin Oncol. 2018;36(31):3110.

23 Thymic Cancer

Mohammed Qudrathulla Khan Quadri,
Sai Sandeep Annamaraju, and Rama Krishna Kancha

23.1 Introduction

Epidemiology: Thymus cancers are rare heterogeneous group of malignancies that account for an incidence of 1.5 cases/100,000 each year in the US. In accordance with the SEER database, 13,586 new cases were reported with thymus cancer in the US, for the years 2001–2015 [1]. The number of new cases for different subtypes of thymic cancer in the US, for the years 2001–2015, include thymoma (9041 cases, 66.3% of total thymic cancers), thymic carcinoma (2772 cases, 20.4% of total thymic cancers), thymic neuroendocrine tumors (TNET) (481 cases, 3.5% of total thymic cancers), and other types of tumors (1319 cases, 9.7% of total thymic cancers) [1]. The cumulative SEER 5-year survival rates of thymoma, thymic carcinoma, and thymic NET were 90%, 55%, and 28–75%, respectively [2]. The peak incidence for thymus cancers was observed in the age group of 70–74 years (1.06 cases/100,000) [1]. The peak incidence was reported at a slightly younger age group in thymic NET (60–74-year-old age group) when compared to thymic carcinoma (70–74 years of age) and thymoma (70–79 years of age) [1]. The median age of diagnosis was 65.5 years during 2009–2015 (range include 16–96 years of age) [3]. In the US, thymic cancers occur more often in males (66%) compared to females (34%) [3].

Risk factors: Information on risk factors for thymus cancers are limited due to less available data for epidemiology and etiology [4]. A European case-control study revealed that smoking and high intake of alcohol significantly increases the risk of thymoma [5]. The MEN1 syndrome is associated with increased risk of developing thymoma and thymic carcinoma [6]. Epstein–Barr virus (EBV) infection may partially impact in the pathogenesis of thymic epithelial tumors (TETs) [7]. Myasthenia

M. Q. K. Quadri · S. S. Annamaraju · R. K. Kancha (✉)
Molecular Medicine and Therapeutics Laboratory, CPMB, Osmania University, Hyderabad, Telangana, India
e-mail: ramakancha@osmania.ac.in

R. K. Kancha (ed.), *Biomedical Aspects of Solid Cancers*,
https://doi.org/10.1007/978-981-97-1802-3_23

gravis is the most frequent autoimmune disease associated with the thymoma [4]. Nearly one-half to one-third of thymoma patients were affected with myasthenia gravis and less than 20% of myasthenia gravis patients develop thymoma [4, 8]. A very high risk of developing secondary malignancies such as the non-Hodgkin lymphoma within thymoma patients was observed [4, 9]. The other diseases that are associated with thymus cancer are pure red cell aplasia (PRCA), systemic lupus erythematosus, rheumatoid arthritis, and few other non-thymic cancers [8].

Diagnosis and screening: TETs account for 35% of anterior mediastinal tumors [10]. Chest radiographs are the most common imaging tests which are used for the initial detection of thymic mass [11]. CT scan helps to differentiate thymic tumors from benign thymic lesions and other malignancies of anterior mediastinum [6, 12]. PET scan is optional for tumors with advanced-stage cancer [11]. When CT scan is inconclusive, MRI with chemical shift imaging is useful in distinguishing thymic neoplasms from benign thymic hyperplasia [6, 11]. Though the usage of PET/CT is uncertain, aggressive tumors can be differentiated from less aggressive tumors [11]. For detection of thymic cancers from other anterior mediastinal tumors, various tests such as AFP (α-fetoprotein), βHCG (β-human chorionic gonadotropin), and LDH (lactate dehydrogenase) are taken into consideration [6, 10]. The pre-treatment biopsy is determined by whether or not the tumor can be surgically removed [6]. Pathologically, thymic carcinomas should be differentiated from its rare variants such as the lung squamous carcinomas [12]. Nearly 40% of thymoma patients report autoimmune diseases [13]. Thymic lesions should be considered for diagnosis, when autoimmune diseases such as myasthenia gravis were detected [6]. Type AB, B1, and B2 thymomas with myasthenia gravis usually exhibit AChR (acetylcholine receptor) antibodies in their serum [6]. PRCA and hypogammaglobulinemia are associated with thymoma and can be used as a diagnostic feature [6]. To detect the thymic tumors of mediastinal carcinomas, immunohistochemistry analysis has to be performed with anti-CD117/KIT antibodies [6]. The proliferation marker Ki67 can be used for differentiating large cell neuroendocrine carcinoma and small cell carcinoma, although it is not accurate for typical and atypical carcinoids of thymic NET [14].

23.2 Classification

Thymic epithelial tumors are the most prevalent cancers of the anterior mediastinum [13] and can be classified based on (I) WHO criteria, (II) histology (Suster and Moran classification), (III) molecular features, and (IV) staging.

(I) In accordance with the latest version of WHO classification of thymic neoplasm, TETs were classified into (a) thymoma, (b) thymic carcinoma, and (c) thymic NET; additionally, few rarer types which occur in combinations were also included [14]. (a) Based on the histology of the cancer cell and immunohistochemistry, thymomas were classified into type A (spindle/oval), type B (round/epithelioid), type AB (mixed thymoma), micronodular thymoma with lymphoid stroma, metaplastic thymoma, and lipofibroadenoma (Fig. 23.1) [14, 15]. Type A and AB

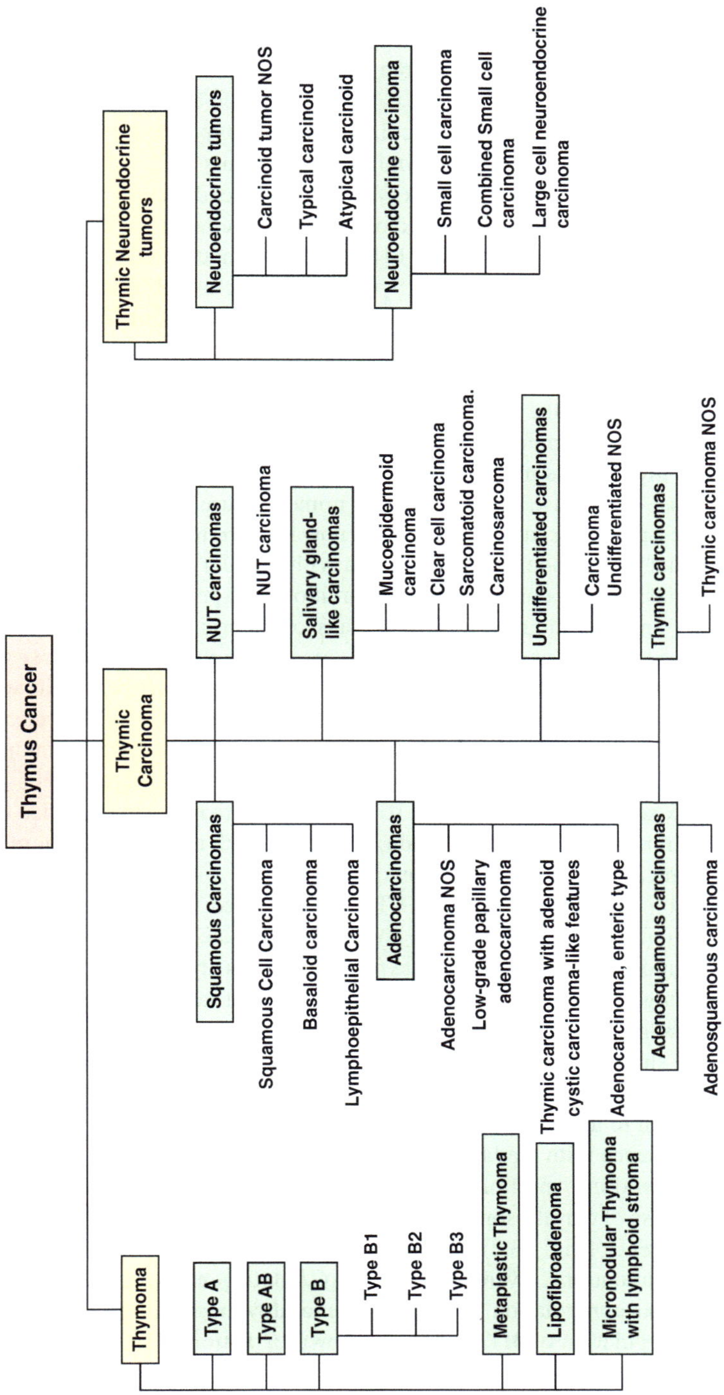

Fig. 23.1 **Histological classification of thymus cancer.** NOS: Not otherwise specified

thymomas are generally benign; however, type B thymomas are malignant and more aggressive. B3 thymomas exhibit a higher tendency of intrathoracic spread [16]. Type A thymoma was distinguished by the presence of spindle- or oval-shaped epithelial cells with obscure nucleoli, type B by the presence of round epithelial cells with excessive cytoplasm and large vesicular nuclei, and type AB by the presence of a combination of type A and type B thymoma constituents [15]. (b) Thymic carcinomas constitute extreme malignancies with a higher tendency of lymphatic and hematogenous metastasis [16, 17]. Based on morphologic features, WHO classified thymic carcinoma into seven subtypes [14]. (c) Thymic neuroendocrine tumors are very rare and highly aggressive type of thymic malignancies [2]. Based on the morphological characteristics, presence of necrosis and mitoses count, WHO classified thymic NETs as neuroendocrine tumors and neuroendocrine carcinomas [14, 18, 19].

The latest version of the WHO classification (2021) for TETs enlisted a few changes: microscopic thymoma is now considered as nodular epithelial hyperplasia and sclerosing thymoma is now classified within the typical thymoma with regressive nature [14]. WHO also introduced new nomenclature for the existing pathological subtypes: papillary adenocarcinoma is now referred to as low-grade papillary adenocarcinoma; high-grade adenocarcinoma with papillary features is referred as adenocarcinomas; lymphoepithelioma-like carcinoma is specified as lymphoepithelial carcinoma and mucinous adenocarcinomas or enteric type adenocarcinomas [14]. WHO also included new subtypes in thymic carcinoma such as micronodular thymic carcinoma with lymphoid hyperplasia (a squamous cell carcinoid variant with less aggressive and non-organotypic lymphoid stroma), hyalinizing clear cell carcinoma, and thymic sebaceous carcinoma [14]. Further, few thymic tumors that exhibit carcinoid-like morphological characteristics along with high mitotic count and ki67, index similar to that of grade III NET of pancreas, were classified under LCNEC of thymic carcinoma (high grade); however, such tumors were more similar to typical and atypical carcinoids (low grade) [14].

(II) Based on histologic grading, TETs are classified into well-differentiated tumors as thymoma (typical thymoma), poorly differentiated tumors as thymic carcinoma, and tumors that exhibit moderate proliferation as atypical thymoma [15]. A cytologic grading system was proposed where cells that lack cytologic atypia are classified as low-grade tumors, irrespective of the structure or count of lymphocytes [15]. Cells that show enlarged nucleus with moderate cytologic atypia are classified as intermediate-grade lesions [15]. Cells that show immense malignant cytological atypia are referred to as high-grade lesions (thymic carcinoma) [15].

(III) In accordance with the latest version of WHO classification, thymus cancer can be characterized into multiple clusters of same clinical subtypes based on various mutations, loss of chromosomal segments, and overexpression and downregulation of specific genes (Fig. 23.2) [14]. A-like cluster include type A thymoma that exhibits *GTF2I* mutations, overexpression of *C19MC* gene, upregulation of P53 tetramer complex, upregulation of *XBP1–2* gene, downregulation of MYC/MAX complex, downregulation of *MYB* gene, and downregulation of *FOXM1* gene [14]. B-like cluster include all the subtypes of type B thymoma which exhibits mutation

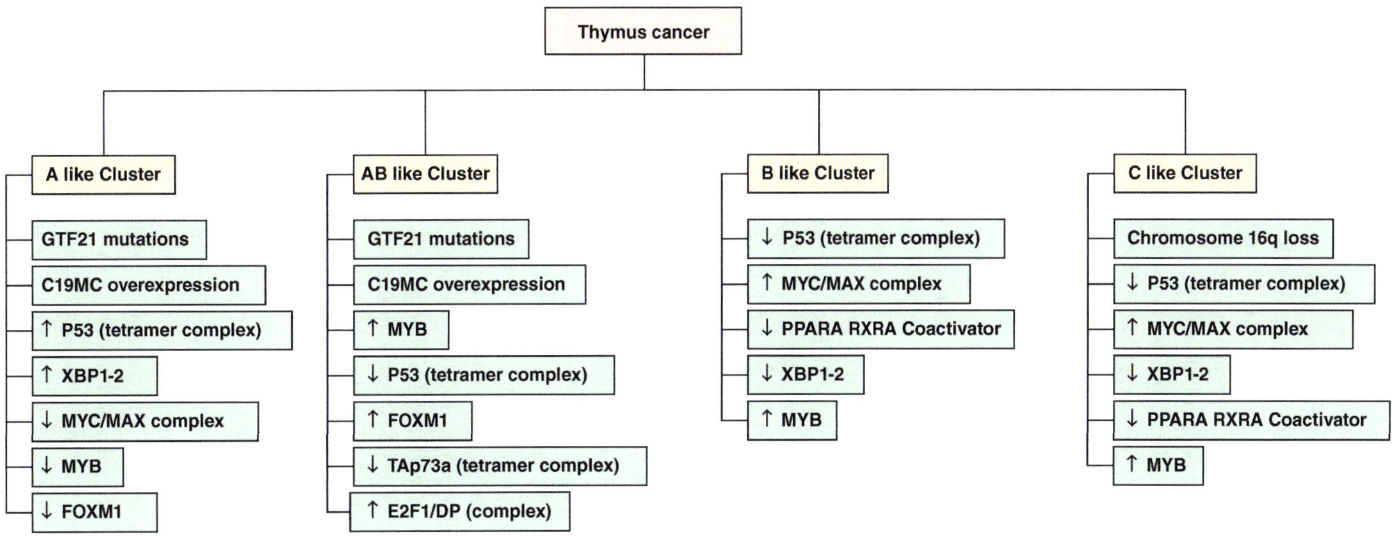

Fig. 23.2 **Molecular classification of thymus cancer based on the fifth edition of WHO**. A-like cluster denotes type A thymoma, B-like cluster denotes type B thymoma, AB-like cluster denotes type AB thymoma, and C-like cluster denotes thymic carcinoma. ↑: upregulation, ↓: downregulation of various protein coding genes

in the *GTF2I* gene, overexpression of *C19MC* gene, upregulation of *MYB* gene, downregulation of P53 tetramer complex, upregulation of *FOXM1* gene, downregulation of Tap 73a tetramer complex, and upregulation of E2F1/DP complex [14]. AB-like cluster include type AB thymoma, which is characterized by the downregulated P53 tetramer complex, upregulated MYC/MAX complex, downregulated PPARA RXRA coactivator, downregulated *XBP1–2* gene, and upregulated *MYB* gene [14]. C-like cluster include all the subtypes of thymic carcinoma which is distinguished by the deletion of Chr-16q, downregulated P53 tetramer complex, upregulated MYC/MAX complex, downregulated *XBP1–2* gene, downregulated PPARA/RXRA coactivator, and upregulated *MYB* gene.

(IV) Staging: IASLC and ITMIG proposed a TNM staging classification [20]. Tumor (T): T1 is classified into T1a that refers to encapsulated or unencapsulated, with or without invasion into adipose tissue of the mediastinum and T1b refers to invasion of tumor into the pleura [20]. T2 specifies infiltration of pericardium while T3 refers to infiltration into the lung, chest wall, and phrenic nerves [12, 21]. T4 refers to the infiltration into the aorta, myocardium, trachea, and esophagus [21]. Regional lymph node (N): N0 indicates the absence of lymph node involvement [10]. N1 and N2 refer to involvement of lymph nodes present in the peri-thymic and intra-thymic regions, respectively [10]. Metastasis (M): M0 specifies no evidence of metastasis [10]. M1a indicates metastasis to pleura or pericardial nodules and M1b specifies distant metastasis [10]. Stage I refers to T1, N0, and M0, stage II to T2, N0, and M0, stage IIIa to T3, N0, and M0, stage IIIb to T4, N0, and M0, stage IVa to any T, N0–1, and M0–1a, and stage IVb to any T, N0–2, M0–1b [12]. In addition to TNM staging, Masaoka-Koga staging that is associated with surgical pathology is also widely used [11]. According to the Masaoka-Koga staging system, stage I refers to an encapsulated tumor, stage II-A to microscopic level of trans-capsular tumor spread, stage II-B to tumor grossly adhered to, but does not extend into pleura or invasion of neighboring fatty tissue, stage III to infiltration into the surrounding tissues including lungs, pericardium, and great vessel, stage IV-A to metastasis to pleura or pericardium, and stage IV-B to distant metastasis through blood or lymph [22]. Due to their similar prognosis, the Masaoka Koga stages I, II and a few stage III tumors can be merged with the TNM stage I, stage III can be merged with TNM stage II, IIIa, and IIIb, stage IV-A can be equated with TNM stage IVa and IVb, and IV-B can be merged with TNM stage IVb [12].

23.3 Pathophysiology

Thymus is a pyramidal-shaped bilobed gland of ecto-endodermal origin that is located in the midline anterosuperior mediastinum [23, 24]. A sheath of connective fibrous tissue layer encapsulates thymus and divides each lobe into several lobules (Fig. 23.3) [23]. The right lobe is little larger in size compared to the left lobe and each thymic lobe consists of an outer cortex and an inner medulla [23, 25]. The cortex and medulla contain cells of hematopoietic origin [25]. Thymus gland weighs around 10–15 g at birth and gradually increases to its maximum weight of nearly

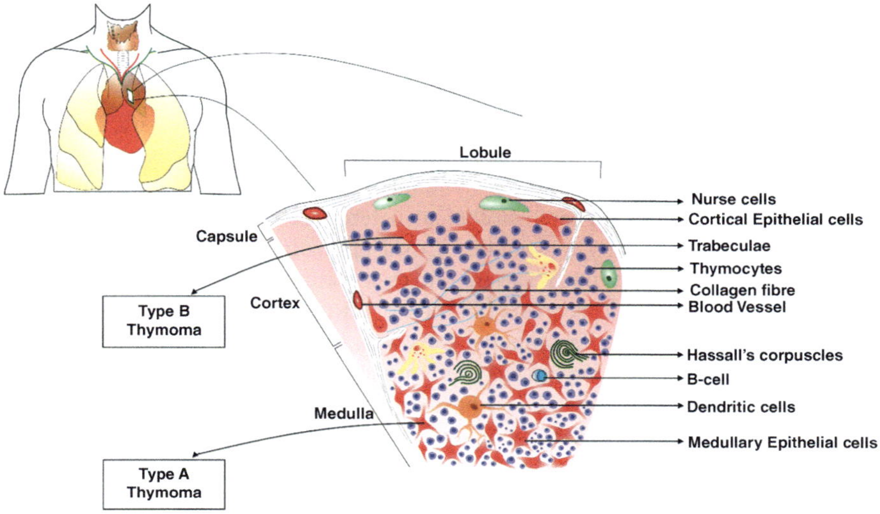

Fig. 23.3 Cross-sectional view of thymus gland indicating different types of cells and cell of origin of thymoma variants

40 g, but subsequently diminishes after adolescence and converts to a retrosternal adipose tissue by physiological involution [26]. Due to involution after puberty, thymus gland produces fewer T cells [27]. Epithelial cells and T lymphocytes are the major cell types of thymus gland [28]. In addition, thymus gland includes cells such as B lymphocytes, several white blood cells, neuroendocrine cells, myoid cells, germ cells, interdigitating reticulum cells (interacts lymphocytes and epithelial cells), and keratinized epithelial cells (Hassall's corpuscles) (Fig. 23.3) [28]. Thymic epithelial cells exhibit dual germ layer origins; cortical epithelial cells and medullary epithelial cells arise from ectoderm and endoderm, respectively [29].

Histologically, six distinct types of thymic epitheliocytes, which are a network of finely branched epithelial reticular cells, are present in the thymus [26]. Type-1 epitheliocytes are flat with distinct basal lamina, present in the subcapsular and perivascular locations [26]. Epitheliocytes of cortex include type-2 cells that are larger in size with long cytoplasmic processes, type-3 cells that are enlarged with pale appearance, and type-4 cells that are denser and very small in size [26]. Epitheliocytes of medulla comprises of type-5 cells that are very small in size and type-6 cells that are spindle-shaped cells, which produce thymic hormones, whereas flat cells that develop into Hassall's corpuscles [26]. Epitheliocytes of medulla features solid cord-like, keratinized, and stratified-like appearances while forming Hassall's corpuscles [26]. Thymic lymphocytes show extrathymic origin in the bone marrow [30]. Cells of origin for the thymoma and thymic carcinoma are thymic epithelial cells with non-cancerous lymphocytes that are present in variable amounts within the tumor [31, 32]. Type A thymoma originates from epithelial cells of medullary region, whereas type B thymoma arises from the cortical region of thymus.

Cell of origin for thymic NET is neuroendocrine cells, which are present in very low number and produce peptides and amines [28, 33].

Thymoma: TETs show more than one histological subtype of thymoma [14]. Malignant potential of thymoma is comparatively lower than thymic carcinoma [34]. Various morphological shapes of epithelial cells are mixed with T lymphocytes in thymoma [9]. Thymocytes are absent in type A and B3 thymomas, while they are present focally in type AB thymoma, and extensively in type B1 and B2 [35]. Thymoma shows higher histological heterogeneity [14]. Type A thymoma shows low mitotic activity of spindle or oval epithelial cells with inconspicuous nucleoli [24]. Atypical type A variant shows hypercellularity, cytological atypia, and increased mitoses and necrosis [24]. Type AB is distinguished by the presence of a mixture of small spindle epithelial cells with lymphocytes i.e., type A and type B thymoma [15]. Type B1 thymoma are lymphocyte-rich in cortical areas and few medullary islands (clear Hassall's corpuscles-like structure with scattered epithelial components) [24]. Type B2 thymoma comprises of poorly developed lymphoepithelial irregular lobules with or without medullary islands [24]. Type B3 thymoma exhibit predominant large epithelial component of cells with rare lymphocytes component [15]. Rare types of thymoma includes micronodular thymoma with lymphoid stroma, lipofibroadenoma, and metaplastic thymoma [24, 36].

Thymic carcinoma: Thymic carcinoma of any type can develop within thymoma of all types [34]. Thymic carcinoma exhibits cytological atypia and shows smaller mass spread than that of thymoma [34]. Squamous cell carcinoma exhibits large infiltrative keratinizing or non-keratinizing squamous cells [24]. Basaloid carcinoma cells exhibit peripheral palisades and comprise cystic-papillary, and nesting growth pattern [24]. Mucoepidermoid thymic carcinoma comprises of a mixture of squamous and mucinous cells that exhibit nests or lining cystic spaces [24]. Lymphoepithelial carcinoma comprises of a mixture of poorly dividing cancer cells with numerous lymphocytes and plasma cells [24]. Sarcomatoid carcinoma consists of a combination of spindle cells of type A thymoma and cytologically malignant spindle cells similar to that of sarcoma [24]. Clear cell thymic carcinoma comprises of predominantly polygonal cells with clear cytoplasm showing lobulated infiltrative growth pattern [24]. Adenocarcinoma is further subdivided based on histological growth patterns (papillary, adenoid cystic-like carcinoma, mucinous, and NOS) [24]. Undifferentiated thymic carcinoma comprises of polygonal cells that exhibit pleomorphic features with infiltrative islands and a coagulative necrosis pattern [24].

Thymic neuroendocrine tumors: Considering morphological characteristics, necrosis and mitoses counts, thymic NETs are classified into 3 grades which include (a) low-grade typical carcinoid (TC) with <2 mitoses/2 mm^2 with no necrosis, (b) intermediate-grade atypical carcinoid (AC) with <2 mitoses/2 mm^2 with necrosis or 2–10 mitoses/2 mm^2 with or without necrosis, and (c) high-grade malignancies with >10 mitoses/2 mm^2 which include LCNEC and SCC [18, 19]. TNETs exhibit polygonal cells with a round nucleus, monotonous cellular proliferation presenting numerous unusual spindle cell features, abundant oncocytic cytoplasm and microfilament attachments or mucin-rich stroma [37]. Typical carcinoid tumor is more benign with no necrosis, showing fine granular chromatin in round or oval cells with pale eosinophilic cytoplasm [38]. Foci of necrosis, hemorrhage, and calcification may also be observed [37]. The lesions are soft, little brown in color, and ranges from 3 to 20 cm in diameter [39]. Tumor cells usually show trabeculae, festoons, solid nests, rosette, glandular, and ribbon-like growth patterns [38].

Genetics and genomics: Mutational load in TETs is generally low in thymic cancers except in a few cases of thymic carcinoma [13]. The progression of TETs is significantly influenced by the stimulation of PI3K/AKT pathway [40]. Dysregulation of *RAD51L1* and/or *BMP2* as well as t(14;20) (q24.1; p12.3) chromosomal translocation were observed in familial thymomas [9, 41]. Loss of 6p chromosomal segment that consists of *FOXC1* gene, and gain in 1q chromosome were most common structural aberrations in all histotypes of thymoma [42]. A high frequency of mutations in the *GTF2I* was observed in low-grade tumors (thymoma type A and type AB) while it was very rarely observed in high-grade tumors (thymoma type B and thymic carcinoma) [14, 16, 42]. Overexpression of *HRAS* and *NRAS* genes is a significant feature of a typical thymoma. Mutations in the *TP53* gene is a characteristic feature of type B thymoma and thymic carcinoma [13, 14]. In thymic carcinoma, deletion of chr-16q was commonly observed [40]. PD-1 and PD-L1 are overexpressed in thymoma and thymic carcinoma [43]. The p63 immunoreactivity differentiates SCC from the B3 thymoma [34]. *YAP1-MAML2* translocation was unique for metaplastic thymoma [14]. Recurrent translocation of *KMT2A-MAML2* was observed in nearly 6% of type B2 and B3 thymomas patients [42]. A higher frequency of cytosine compared to thymine mutations within CpG dinucleotides related to aging was observed in thymoma [13, 14]. *CHRNA1* and *RYR3* were overexpressed in myasthenia gravis positive thymomas [13]. In carcinoids, *MEN1* mutations and *CDKN2A* alterations were usually seen [44]. Mutations in *RB1, TP53, PTEN,* and amplification of *MYC* gene was commonly observed in high-grade carcinomas [44].

23.4 Treatment

Complete surgical excision of the tumor was the most recommended option for treating early thymic tumors (stages I and II) [45]. Thymectomy may range from complete thymectomy to extended thymectomy [6]. Complete thymectomy involves the removal of entire thymus gland along with the surrounding mediastinal fat and was suggested in patients without myasthenia gravis [6]. Extended thymectomy that involves the excision of pleura, adipose tissue in the mediastinum and pericardiophrenic areas, was preferred in myasthenia gravis patients [6]. Thymectomy of invasive tumors include complete removal of infiltrated lung parenchymal tissues, pleural implants, great vessels, and nerves [12]. Excision of anterior mediastinal nodes was the most preferred option for stage III/IV tumors [12]. Radical resection was usually preferred in advanced stages due to which the prognosis was improved and the tumor burden was reduced from advanced stage tumor to stage I tumor along with improvement of long-term survival [6]. Five-year survival rates following radical surgery was 90% for stages I and II, 60% for stage III, and less than 25%

for the stage IV TETs [46]. To allow postoperative radiotherapy, the areas of the unresectable margins were precisely marked with clips [12]. Administration of corticosteroids preoperatively in advanced-stage thymomas facilitates surgical resection by inducing degenerative changes in epithelial cells and lymphocytes of TETs, thus reducing the tumor size [24].

Chemotherapy: Depending on the stage, margin of infiltration, and histological subtype, the postoperative treatment can be considered with either chemotherapy, radiotherapy, or concomitant chemoradiotherapy [46]. Systemic polychemotherapy was specified for unresectable TETs [46]. Different platinum-based combinations represent the standard first-line chemotherapy in thymomas, with overall response rate of 50% with PE (cisplatin and etoposide), 75% with PAC or CAP (cisplatin, doxorubicin, and cyclophosphamide), and 92% with ADOC (cisplatin, doxorubicin, cyclophosphamide, and vincristine) [47]. Other combinations for the first-line chemotherapy in thymoma were VIP (combined ifosfamide, cisplatin, and etoposide), CODE (cisplatin, vincristine, doxorubicin, etoposide), and CAMP (cisplatin, doxorubicin, methylprednisolone) [48, 49]. Regimen of carboplatin combined with paclitaxel was preferred for treating the thymic carcinoma [46]. Thymic carcinoma, upon treatment with a combination of carboplatin and amrubicin, showed a response rate of 42% for no previous chemotherapy and 30% with previous chemotherapy [40]. For the treatment of relapsed thymoma and thymic carcinoma, national comprehensive cancer network (NCCN) recommended single-agent, non-platinum-based chemotherapy along with a combination of octreotide plus prednisolone [40, 48]. Everolimus, a potent oral mTOR inhibitor, was clinically active in the treatment of advanced/recurrent thymoma and thymic carcinoma, in patients who were previously treated with cisplatin chemotherapy [50].

TETs show a higher expression of receptor PD-1 and PD-L1 [9]. Pembrolizumab is used in treating advanced thymic epithelial tumors [9]. KIT expression is a possible diagnostic marker of thymic carcinoma and KIT inhibitors, notably imatinib and sunitinib (potent angiogenic inhibitors) or sorafenib can be beneficial in thymic carcinomas [12]. In accordance with the outcomes of phase-II clinical trials, sunitinib was considered as an option for refractory TETs that show low relapse rates (greater than 80%) [12]. For recurrence in the non-resectable tumors, numerous consecutive lines of systemic treatment were administered that include PAC chemotherapy, carboplatin plus paclitaxel, and platin plus etoposide regimen as second-line treatment [12]. Sunitinib and imatinib are TKI receptor inhibitors used to treat thymic NETs [44]. Cisplatin-based regimens in combination with anthracyclines and/or etoposide were considered for thymic NETs [51]. Carboplatin plus nab-paclitaxel proved to be effective for treating thymic LCNEC [52].

Radiotherapy: Since TETs tend to relapse both locally and regionally, radiotherapy has been an important postoperative treatment strategy [12]. Multi-field three-dimensional conformal radiation therapy (3D-CRT) was used to target tumor and its extensions in the mediastinum with a total radiation dose of 45–50 Gy after primary resection and 50–54 Gy following R1 resection [12]. For treating advanced TETs, a combination of therapeutic drugs (cisplatin, etoposide) with a radiation exposure of 60 Gy may be considered [12]. Standard-fraction scheme that consists of daily dose from 1.8 to 2 Gy for an extended duration of 4–6 weeks and proton-beam radiotherapy were the current modalities of postoperative radiotherapy [12]. Postoperative radiation therapy for the stage I thymic tumors was very rare since the recurrence rates were very low [45]. Stage II tumors with gross adhesion to microscopic pleural invasion show a recurrence rate of 36.4% after surgery and 0% in the patients with no adhesion [45]. Relapse rates for the surgically excised tumors of stage II and stage III thymoma was 23% and 30%, respectively, with postoperative radiotherapy, and 25% each without postoperative radiotherapy [45]. The 5-year and 10-year survival rates were 95% and 86% for the patients who have undergone postoperative radiotherapy after surgical excision when compared to 90% and 79% for the patients who received resection alone [12].

23.5 Conclusion

Thymus is a primary lymphoid organ; hence, when a cancer develops in the thymus, it is highly associated with the immune despair and development of other secondary malignancies. Thymic cancers are very uncommon and are typically diagnosed in the patients within the age group of 70–74 years. Thymic cancers exhibit a wide range of pathological subtypes among which thymoma is usually benign and thymic carcinoma is highly malignant with prominent metastasis. Myasthenia gravis is the most well-known paraneoplastic disorder that affects up to 45 percent of thymoma patients. Thymic cancers exhibit low mutational burden and have a very limited information on risk factors. A higher frequency of mutation in genes such as *GTF2I*, *HRAS*, *NRAS*, and *TP53* was observed in patients of thymoma. TETs exhibit higher expression of PD-1 and PD-L1 and can be used as potent targets for immunotherapy. Complete surgical resection is highly preferred for early thymic tumors; however, for high-grade tumors when invasion to the surrounding pleura and metastasized to distant regions are observed, surgical resection is followed by chemotherapy and radiotherapy. Radiotherapy is crucial as postoperative or preoperative treatment strategy for targeting tumors in different angles, thus eventually eliminating the tumor on site and thus reducing the higher chances of relapse. Identification of potential biomarkers will aid in characterization and development of new thymic cancer treatment strategies.

References

1. Hsu CH, Chan JK, Yin CH, Lee CC, Chern CU, Liao CI. Trends in the incidence of thymoma, thymic carcinoma, and thymic neuroendocrine tumor in the United States. PLoS One. 2019;14(12):e0227197.
2. Bakhos CT, Salami AC, Kaiser LR, Petrov RV, Abbas AE. Thymic neuroendocrine tumors and thymic carcinoma: demographics, treatment, and survival. Innovations. 2020;15(5):468–74.
3. Koizumi T, Otsuki K, Tanaka Y, Noguchi T, Fukushuima T, Kobayashi T, Ozawa T, Sekiguchi N, Hamanaka K. National incidence and initial therapy for thymic carcinoma in Japan:

based on analysis of hospital-based cancer registry data, 2009–2015. Jpn J Clin Oncol. 2020;50(4):434–9.
4. Engels EA. Epidemiology of thymoma and associated malignancies. J Thorac Oncol. 2010;5(10):S260–5.
5. Eriksson M, Kaerlev L, Johansen P, Afonso N, Ahrens W, Costa-Pereira A, Guénel P, Jöckel KH, Gonzalez AL, Merletti F, Suárez-Varela MM. Tobacco smoking and alcohol consumption as risk factors for thymoma–a European case-control study. Cancer Epidemiol. 2019;61:133–8.
6. Girard N, Ruffini E, Marx A, Faivre-Finn C, Peters S. Thymic epithelial tumours: ESMO clinical practice guidelines for diagnosis, treatment and follow-up. Ann Oncol. 2015;26:v40–55.
7. Zhang G, Yu Z, Shen G, Chai Y, Liang C. Association between Epstein-Barr virus and Thymic epithelial tumors: a systematic review. Infect Agent Cancer. 2019;14:1–8.
8. Nishino M, Ashiku SK, Kocher ON, Thurer RL, Boiselle PM, Hatabu H. The thymus: a comprehensive review. Radiographics. 2006;26(2):335–48.
9. Soomro IN. Pathology of thymoma—where are we today? J Thorac Dis. 2020;12(12):7545.
10. Carter BW, Benveniste MF, Madan R, Godoy MC, Groot PM, Truong MT, Rosado-de-Christenson ML, Marom EM. IASLC/ITMIG staging system and lymph node map for thymic epithelial neoplasms. Radiographics. 2017;37(3):758–76.
11. Strange CD, Ahuja J, Shroff GS, Truong MT, Marom EM. Imaging evaluation of thymoma and thymic carcinoma. Front Oncol. 2022;11:810419.
12. Basse C, Girard N. Thymic tumours and their special features. Eur Respir Rev. 2021;30(162):200394.
13. Radovich M, Pickering CR, Felau I, Ha G, Zhang H, Jo H, Hoadley KA, Anur P, Zhang J, McLellan M, Bowlby R. The integrated genomic landscape of thymic epithelial tumors. Cancer Cell. 2018;33(2):244–58.
14. Marx A, Chan JK, Chalabreysse L, Dacic S, Detterbeck F, French CA, Hornick JL, Inagaki H, Jain D, Lazar AJ, Marino M. The 2021 WHO classification of tumors of the thymus and mediastinum: what is new in thymic epithelial, germ cell, and mesenchymal tumors? J Thorac Oncol. 2022;17(2):200–13.
15. Suster S, Moran CA. Histologic classification of thymoma: the World Health Organization and beyond. Hematol Oncol Clin North Am. 2008;22(3):381–92.
16. Enkner F, Pichlhöfer B, Zaharie AT, Krunic M, Holper TM, Janik S, Moser B, Schlangen K, Neudert B, Walter K, Migschitz B. Molecular profiling of thymoma and thymic carcinoma: genetic differences and potential novel therapeutic targets. Pathol Oncol Res. 2017;23:551–64.
17. Tseng YL. Thymic carcinoma: a rare cancer requiring special attention. Formos J Surg. 2011;44:136–40.
18. Marx A, Chan JK, Coindre JM, Detterbeck F, Girard N, Harris NL, Jaffe ES, Kurrer MO, Marom EM, Moreira AL, Mukai K. The 2015 World Health Organization classification of tumors of the thymus: continuity and changes. J Thorac Oncol. 2015;10(10):1383–95.
19. Dinter H, Bohnenberger H, Beck J, Bornemann-Kolatzki K, Schütz E, Küffer S, Klein L, Franks TJ, Roden A, Emmert A, Hinterthaner M. Molecular classification of neuroendocrine tumors of the thymus. J Thorac Oncol. 2019;14(8):1472–83.
20. Smith A, Cavalli C, Harling L, Harrison-Phipps K, Routledge T, Pilling J, King J, Bille A, Nonaka D. Impact of the TNM staging system for thymoma. Mediastinum. 2021;5:32.
21. Ried M, Eicher MM, Neu R, Sziklavari Z, Hofmann HS. Evaluation of the new TNM-staging system for thymic malignancies: impact on indication and survival. World J Surg Oncol. 2017;15:1–8.
22. Venuta F, Rendina EA, Anile M, de Giacomo T, Vitolo D, Coloni GF. Thymoma and thymic carcinoma. Gen Thorac Cardiovasc Surg. 2012;60:1–2.
23. Safieddine N, Keshavjee S. Anatomy of the thymus gland. Thorac Surg Clin. 2011;21(2):191–5.
24. Valavanis C, Stanc GM, Baltayiannis N. Classification, histopathology and molecular pathology of thymic epithelial tumors: a review. J BUON. 2021;26:1198–207.
25. Liu D, Ellis H. The mystery of the thymus gland. Clin Anat. 2016;29(6):679–84.
26. Palumbo C. Embryology and anatomy of the thymus gland. In: Thymus gland pathology: clinical, diagnostic, and therapeutic features; 2008. p. 13–8.

27. Rezzani R, Franco C, Hardeland R, Rodella LF. Thymus-pineal gland axis: revisiting its role in human life and ageing. Int J Mol Sci. 2020;21(22):8806.
28. Suster S, Rosai J. Histology of the normal thymus. Am J Surg Pathol. 1990;14(3):284–303.
29. Wang HX, Pan W, Zheng L, Zhong XP, Tan L, Liang Z, He J, Feng P, Zhao Y, Qiu YR. Thymic epithelial cells contribute to thymopoiesis and T cell development. Front Immunol. 2020;10:3099.
30. Marino M, Marx A, Anemona L, Lauriola L, Ströbel P, Müller-Hermelink HK. Juan Rosai as master of our comprehensive understanding of thymus and thymoma. Pathologica. 2021;113(5):360.
31. Alexiev BA, Drachenberg CB, Burke AP. Thymomas: a cytological and immunohistochemical study, with emphasis on lymphoid and neuroendocrine markers. Diagn Pathol. 2007;2(1):3.
32. Sun L, Li H, Luo H, Zhao Y. Thymic epithelial cell development and its dysfunction in human diseases. Biomed Res Int. 2014;2014:206929.
33. Ströbel P, Zettl A, Shilo K, Chuang WY, Nicholson AG, Matsuno Y, Gal A, Laeng RH, Engel P, Capella C, Marino M. Tumor genetics and survival of thymic neuroendocrine neoplasms: a multi-institutional clinicopathologic study. Genes Chromosom Cancer. 2014;53(9):738–49.
34. Kim SH, Minn YK. Pathologic finding of thymic carcinoma accompanied by myasthenia gravis. J Clin Neurol. 2015;11(4):372–5.
35. Den Bakker MA, Roden AC, Marx A, Marino M. Histologic classification of thymoma: a practical guide for routine cases. J Thorac Oncol. 2014;9(9):S125–30.
36. Qu G, Yu G, Zhang Q, Ma J, Wang X. Lipofibroadenoma of the thymus: a case report. Diagn Pathol. 2013;8:1–3.
37. Berman K, Kirsch J, Bejarano P, Drexler I, Martinez F. Primary neuroendocrine tumor of the thymus: radiological and pathological correlation. J Radiology Case Rep. 2020;14(1):1.
38. Bohnenberger H, Dinter H, König A, Ströbel P. Neuroendocrine tumors of the thymus and mediastinum. J Thorac Dis. 2017;9(Suppl 15):S1448.
39. Moran CA, Suster S. Primary neuroendocrine carcinoma (thymic carcinoid) of the thymus with prominent oncocytic features: a clinicopathologic study of 22 cases. Mod Pathol. 2000;13(5):489–94.
40. Kitadai R, Okuma Y. Future perspective of chemotherapy and pharmacotherapy in thymic carcinoma. Cancers. 2021;13(20):5239.
41. Nicodème F, Geffroy S, Conti M, Delobel B, Soenen V, Grardel N, Porte H, Copin MC, Laï JL, Andrieux J. Familial occurrence of thymoma and autoimmune diseases with the constitutional translocation t (14; 20)(q24. 1; p12. 3). Genes Chromosom Cancer. 2005;44(2):154–60.
42. Marx A, Belharazem D, Lee DH, Popovic ZV, Reißfelder C, Schalke B, Schölch S, Ströbel P, Weis CA, Yamada Y. Molecular pathology of thymomas: implications for diagnosis and therapy. Virchows Arch. 2021;478:101–10.
43. Suster D, Pihan G, Mackinnon AC, Suster S. Expression of PD-L1/PD-1 in lymphoepithelioma-like carcinoma of the thymus. Mod Pathol. 2018;31(12):1801–6.
44. Bertero L, Metovic J, Vittone F, Cassoni P, Papotti M. Overview of the pathology of thymic neuroendocrine tumors. Mediastinum. 2017;1:10.
45. Rajan A, Giaccone G. Treatment of advanced thymoma and thymic carcinoma. Curr Treat Options in Oncol. 2008;9:277–87.
46. Tateo V, Manuzzi L, De Giglio A, Parisi C, Lamberti G, Campana D, Pantaleo MA. Immunobiology of thymic epithelial tumors: implications for immunotherapy with immune checkpoint inhibitors. Int J Mol Sci. 2020;21(23):9056.
47. Conforti F, Pala L, Giaccone G, De Pas T. Thymic epithelial tumors: from biology to treatment. Cancer Treat Rev. 2020;86:102014.
48. Wei ML, Kang D, Gu L, Qiu M, Zhengyin L, Mu Y. Chemotherapy for thymic carcinoma and advanced thymoma in adults. Cochrane Database Syst Rev. 2013;8:CD008588.
49. Zucali PA, De Vincenzo F, Perrino M, Digiacomo N, Cordua N, D'Antonio F, Borea F, Santoro A. Systemic treatments for thymic tumors: a narrative review. Mediastinum. 2021;5:24.
50. Zucali PA, De Pas T, Palmieri G, Favaretto A, Chella A, Tiseo M, Caruso M, Simonelli M, Perrino M, De Vincenzo F, Toffalorio F. Phase II study of everolimus in patients with thymoma

and thymic carcinoma previously treated with cisplatin-based chemotherapy. J Clin Oncol. 2018;36(4):342–9.
51. Girard N. Neuroendocrine tumors of the thymus: the oncologist point of view. J Thorac Dis. 2017;9(Suppl 15):S1491.
52. Igawa S, Yanagisawa N, Niwa H, Ishihara M, Hiyoshi Y, Otani S, Katono K, Sasaki J, Satoh Y, Masuda N. Successful chemotherapy with carboplatin and nab-paclitaxel for thymic large cell neuroendocrine carcinoma: a case report. Oncol Lett. 2015;10(6):3519–22.

Soft Tissue Sarcoma

24

Mounika Sabhavath, Sai Sandeep Annamaraju, Nageswara Rao Amanchi, Kishore Reddy Bhavanam, and Rama Krishna Kancha

24.1 Introduction

Epidemiology: Soft tissue sarcomas (STS) account for about 1% of all cancers with an estimated overall incidence of 1.8–5.0 cases/100,000 per year [1, 2]. As per the United States SEER data, the mortality rate was 1.3 deaths/100,000 during 2015–2019 with a median age of diagnosis of 60 years [3]. STS was one of the top 5 cancers among children in terms of incidence and death. According to the SEER 2017 data, the 5-year and 10-year survival rates for soft tissue sarcoma were 65% and 50%, respectively [3]. Soft tissue cancer incidence was more predominant in black people (0.5 cases/APT; APT: average calculation over a period of time) compared to white people (0.1 cases/APT). The frequency of soft tissue sarcoma occurrence is higher in males compared to females with an incidence ratio of 1.9:1.0 [4]. The annual incidence rates reached 230 cases/100,000 in the age group of 85 years [4]. For the year 2022, the estimated number of new cases in the US were 13,460 cases (males-7720 cases; females-5740 cases) and the estimated mortality was 5350 deaths (males-2840 deaths; females-2510 deaths). Overall, STS incidence in China for the year 2014 was 2.91 cases/100,000 (males-2.21 cases/100,000; females-2.13 cases/100,000) [5]. In China, 3.1% of STS occur between the age of 0–19 years [5]. During the years 2014–2019, the incidence rate in India was 1% in adults and 15% in children [6]. Based on the histology, STS were classified into different types

M. Sabhavath · S. S. Annamaraju · R. K. Kancha (✉)
Molecular Medicine and Therapeutics Laboratory, CPMB, Osmania University, Hyderabad, India
e-mail: ramakancha@osmania.ac.in

N. R. Amanchi
Departmernt of Zoology, Osmania University, Hyderabad, India

K. R. Bhavanam
Amor Hospitals, Hyderabad, India

R. K. Kancha (ed.), *Biomedical Aspects of Solid Cancers*,
https://doi.org/10.1007/978-981-97-1802-3_24

which include leiomyosarcoma (12% of incidence), liposarcoma (12%), undifferentiated pleomorphic sarcoma (11%), myxofibrosarcoma (3%) and angiosarcoma (3%) [1]. STS may originate from different anatomic sites with nearly 20% such as lower extremity, 15% in the trunk region, 12% in the head and neck and about 8% in the upper extremity [7].

Risk factors: The major risk factors for the soft tissue sarcoma include various chemicals, genetic syndromes, oncogenic viruses, radiation and immunodeficiency [8]. Exposure to chemicals such as chlorophenols and phenoxy herbicides may increase the rate of the soft tissue sarcoma [9]. Exposure to vinyl chloride causes the angiosarcoma [9]. The common genetic disorders include Li–Fraumeni syndrome (causes liposarcoma and rhabdomyosarcoma), retinoblastoma (causes fibrosarcoma) and neurofibromatosis type 1 (causes rhabdomyosarcoma and gastrointestinal stroma tumors) [10]. Viral infections such as HHV8 (human herpesvirus 8) infection is associated with kaposi sarcoma [11]. Immunodeficiency due to EBV (Epstein–Barr Virus) infection leads to the formation of smooth muscle tumors [11]. STS may arise due to radiation therapy of breast cancer and non-Hodgkins's lymphoma [10]. Angiosarcoma was associated with radiation therapy for the breast cancer [10].

Diagnosis: Soft tissue sarcomas are rare carcinomas [3]. Due to its heterogeneity, soft tissue cancers are explored at three different levels for diagnosis, which include local exploration, histological exploration and staging [3]. All deep masses or superficial tumors with diameter of >5 cm can be diagnosed by MRI and CT scan [8]. MRI scanning is being used for detection of primary site in the extremities, trunk, head and neck lesions [8]. The main aim of the MRI was to evaluate concerning features like size, location (subcutaneous or below the fascia), relation to the adjacent structures and homogeneity [12]. For retroperitoneal and thoracic primary tumors, CT scan is preferred. CT scan is used for metastatic disease in patients with high-grade lesions in lungs [8]. Histological diagnosis defines the histological subtype [8]. The deep tumors with infiltrations greater than 5 cm need to be examined by the biopsy [8]. All soft tissue sarcomas in extremities and trunk regions that undergo surgical excision should have biopsies performed before excision [12]. Biopsy can be performed by core needle, incisional technique, fine needle aspiration and by the excision of small lesions [8]. Diagnosis based on staging include exploration of metastatic risk [3]. Soft tissue metastasis in lung can be explored by the CT scan [3].

24.2 Classification

Different classifications were made based on (i) tumor grading, (ii) histology and (iii) staging. (i) The French Federation of Cancer Centers Sarcoma Group (FNCLCC) defined grading based on the histological features such as tumor differentiation, mitotic rate and necrosis. The 2002 AJCC staging system classified tumors into four grades: G1 for well differentiated (low-grade), G2 for moderately differentiated (high-grade), G3 for poorly differentiated (high-grade) and G4 for undifferentiated [13].

(ii) The fourth edition of WHO classification was based on histology, immunohistochemical markers and molecular as well as genetic alterations [14]. The fifth edition of the WHO classification followed the same criteria as that of the fourth edition; however, additional criteria such as cytology, diagnostic molecular pathology and staging were included [14]. Some salient features of the different classes in fifth edition of WHO include (a) atypical spindle cell lipomatous tumor (ASCLT), myxoid pleomorphic tumors and atypical pleomorphic lipomatous tumors that were the three newly added entities in the adipocytic tumors [14]. ASCLT is a rename of spindle cell liposarcoma, which was represented as variant of the well-differentiated liposarcoma in the previous edition [11]. Myxoid pleomorphic sarcoma shows the morphological characters of both myxoid and pleomorphic sarcoma and it was introduced as a new entity [15]. Atypical pleomorphic sarcoma was newly added as an example of pleomorphic lipoma [15]. (b) Fibroblastic and myofibroblastic tumor was one of the largest categories with many types of entities [15]. In the new classification, three benign types were added to this category: angiofibroma of soft tissue, EWSRI-SMAD3 positive fibroblastic tumors and superficial CD34-positive fibroblastic tumors [15]. Calcifying fibrous tumors were removed from this category in the fifth edition [14]. Mammary-type myofibroblastoma was renamed as myofibroblastoma [14]. (c) Anstomosing hemangioma and epithelioid hemangioma were newly added to the vascular tumors in the fifth edition [15]. More information about pseudo myogenic hemangioendothelioma was characterized in the latest edition [15]. Tufted angioma and kaposiform hemangio endothelioma are now grouped together based on their morphological features [14]. Due to insufficient data, polymorphous hemangioendothelioma and giant cell angiobalstoma were phased out from the vascular tumors [14. (d) Cellular myofibroma/myopericytoma, which is characterized as increased cellularity, is added into perivascular (pericytoma) tumors [15]. (e) In the 2013 edition, EBV associated muscle tumors (EBV-SMTS) were classified as a subtype in the leiomyosarcoma; in the latest 2020 edition, it was considered as a different entity [15]. Inflammatory leiomyosarcoma was added as a new entity in the smooth muscle tumor [14]. (f) According to the fifth edition, rhabdosarcoma was subclassified into 4 types, namely embryonal, alveola, pleomorphic and spindle cell rhabdomyosarcoma [14]. Three subtypes were added into the spindle cell/sclerosing rhabdomyosarcoma based on the molecular and clinicopathological features [14]. Ectomesenchymoma (previously classified as nerve sheath tumors) shows genetic overlap with the embryonal rhabdosarcoma; hence, it was reclassified into skeletal muscle tumors. (g) No significant changes were observed in the fifth edition in the chondroosseus tumors subtype [15]. (h) Melanotic schwannoma consists of Schwann cells, which shows melanocytic differentiation, was classified as benign in the 2013 classification [14]. Now, it is reclassified as malignant based on the aggressive behavior and renamed as malignant melanotic nerve sheath tumor [14]. (i) NTRK-rearranged soft tissue sarcoma is an emerging entity, was included in the tumors of uncertain differentiation [14]. This tumor occurs in children and adolescents [15]. Angiomyolipoma was now recategorized into the class of tumors of uncertain differentiation which was previously grouped in the class of adipocytic tumors [14].

(iii) According to AJCC, soft tissue sarcomas were classified based on TNMG system. Size of the tumor was specified as Tx if assessment of tumor is not possible, T0 if there is no evidence of tumor, T1 if the size of the tumor is less than 5 cm, T2 if the size is between 5 cm and 10 cm, T3 if the size of tumor is between 10 cm and 15 cm and T4 if the tumor size is greater than 15 cm [1]. N0 refers to the absence of regional lymph node metastasis and N1 specifies regional lymph node metastasis. M0 indicates no distant metastasis and M1 refers to distant metastasis [1]. Six stages of the soft tissue are: stage IA (T1, N0, M0, G1), IB (T2/T3/T4, N0, M0, G1/GX), II (T1, N0, M0, G1/GX), IIIA (T2, N0, M0, G1/GX), IIIB (T3, N0, M0, G2/G3) and IV (any T, N1, M1, any G) [1]. SEER 5-year survival rates for the stage I, II and III were 71.2%, 53.4% and 5.2%, respectively [16].

24.3 Pathophysiology

Soft tissue is an extra-skeletal tissue that include muscle, fat and supporting fibrous structure that arise from embryonal mesoderm along with neuroectoderm [17]. Soft tissue cancers can arise from various anatomical sites [4].

Adipose tissue tumors: The white adipose tissue is made up of large adipocytes that contain a lipid droplet and consists of fewer mitochondria than that of brown adipose tissue [18]. The tumors which arise from the adipose tissue include ASCLT, well-differentiated liposarcoma, myxoid liposarcoma and myxoid pleomorphic liposarcoma (malignant) [4, 14]. ASCLT is a benign tumor characterized by prominent spindle cell component in a collagenous stroma [15, 19].

Skeletal muscle tumors: Skeletal muscle contains several bundles of muscle fiber (myofibers; also referred to as muscle cells), each myofiber is made up of many myofibrils and each myofibril is made up of a small repeating unit called sarcomere [20]. The tumors, which are arising from the skeletal muscle tissue include rhabdomyoma (benign), alveolar rhabdomyosarcoma, embryonal rhabdomyosarcoma and spindle cell/sclerosing rhabdomyosarcoma (malignant) [1]. Embryonal rhabdomyosarcoma is characterized by neoplastic spindle cell population and alveolar rhabdomyosarcoma by undifferentiated round cells [19].

Vascular tissue tumors: The blood vessels are made up of three layers that include tunica interna, tunica media and tunica externa [21]. The tunica interna was made up of a single layer of squamous epithelial cells called endothelium, the tunica media contains smooth muscle and elastin and the tunica externa has connective tissue fibers [21]. The malignant tumors arising from vascular tissue include hemangioendothelioma, angiosarcoma and hemanigopericytoma [4]. Angiosarcoma is the most common type that arises from the vascular tissue, which was characterized by the presence of abnormal, pleomorphic endothelial cells and the cell can be rounded, polygonal, pleomorphic, or fusiform and exhibit epitheliod appearance [22].

Peripheral nerve sheath tumors: The three layers of protective connective sheath of peripheral nerves are epineurium, perineurium and endoneurium [23]. The epineurium is the outer most layer of the peripheral nerve [23]. Perineurium is the middle layer that surrounds nerve fascicles [23]. Endoneurium is the inner most layer that surrounds small unmyelinated nerve fiber or myelin sheath [23]. The tumors that arise from peripheral nerve sheath are schwannoma, neurofibroma (benign), malignant peripheral nerve sheath, and malignant granular (malignant) [1]. Malignant nerve sheath tumors have fusiform appearance [24]. These lesions are white, solid and fleshy and the cells can be spindle, epithelioid, pleomorphic and elongated, with tapered and scanty amphophilic cytoplasm [24].

Gastrointestinal stromal tumors (GISTs): GISTs arise from the cajal cells or their stem cell like subset [25]. GISTs occur throughout the gastrointestinal tract from the esophagus to the anorectal part [25]. Esophageal GISTs arise from epithelioid cells [19]. Epithelioid gastrointestinal stromal cell borders are more distinct, the cells aggregate in sheets and the nuclei are round [15].

Fibrohistiocytic tumors: Characteristics of fibrous histiocytomas include polymorphous dermal infiltration of multinucleated giant cell, foamy histiocytes, hemosiderin, laden macrophages and bland spindle cells [26]. The lesion cell may extend into the superficial layers of subcutaneous fat [26]. The most common type of the fibrohistiocytic tumors include deep fibromastosis, fibrosarcoma, inflammatory fibrosarcoma and post-radiation fibrosarcoma [4].

Smooth muscle tumors: Smooth muscle cell contains a network of actin and myosin filaments which was surrounded by myosin-free cytoplasm [27]. Smooth muscle originates from the mesenchymal tissue that surrounds the epithelia of the gut, blood vessels, lungs, bladder, ureter and oviducts [27]. The tumors that arise from the smooth muscle tumors include leiomyoma (benign), leiomyosarcoma and epithelioid leiomyosarcoma (malignant) [4]. Smooth muscle tumors are well confined, unencapsulated, occasionally multi-nodular and peucicellular spindle cell lesions [28]. The tumor cells are bland and cigar shaped [28].

Pericytic (perivascular) tumors: Pericytes are the mesenchymal derived cells that surround small blood vessel walls that are closely connected with the endothelial cell layer [29]. Pericytes are further differentiated into multiple cell types that include myofibroblasts, osteoblasts and smooth muscle cells [30]. The tumors which arise from the pericytes include malignant glomus tumor and angioleiomyoma [1].

Fibroblastic and myofibroblastic soft tissue tumors: Fibroblasts are part of connective tissue that produce extracellular proteins (fibrous collagen and elastin), adhesive protein (lamina and fibronectin) and ground substance (glycosaminoglycans) [29]. Myofibroblasts originate from many precursor cells such as epithelial cells, pericytes, endothelial cells, fibrocytes and multipotent monocytes [29]. The tumors that arise from the fibroblastic and myofibroblastic tissue include dermatofibrosarcoma protuberans, solitary fibrous tumors, inflammatory myofibroblastic tumors, fibrosarcoma, EWSRI-SMAD3 fibroblastic tumors and superficial CD43 positive fibroblastic tumors [1, 4]. The fibromyxiod sarcoma was the most common type that arise from the fibroblastic cells [19]. Superficial CD43-positive fibroblastic tumors are characterized by spindle and epithelioid cells with numerous amounts of glossy cytoplasm while EWSRI-SMAD3 fibroblastic tumors were composed of fascicles of spindle cells [15].

Malignant chondro-ossesus tumors: Osteoblasts consist of abundant endoplasmic reticulum and golgi apparatus [30]. The tumor cells are small, round and are arranged in small clusters [19]. Malignant chondro-ossesus tumors include soft tissue chondroma and extra-skeletal osteosarcoma [1]. The common type of the chondro-ossesus tumor is soft tissue chondroma, which shows the morphological and molecular overlap with phosphaturic mesenchymal tumor [15].

Tumors of uncertain differentiation: The tumors which do not have the proper cell lineage of differentiation were included in the tumors of uncertain differentiation [15]. Myoepithelial carcinoma, synovial sarcoma, epithelioid sarcoma, alveolar soft part sarcoma and extra-skeletal Ewings sarcoma were included in the tumors of uncertain differentiation [1]. Synovial sarcoma is the most common type and the cells are uniformly spindled or epithelioid [19].

Cell of origin: Soft tissue sarcomas originate due to malignant transformation of the primitive, bone marrow-derived multipotent mesenchymal stem cells that differentiate into multiple cell lineages [31, 32]. Different subtypes of the soft tissue sarcoma can be evolved from multipotent mesenchymal stem cells [31]. Liposarcoma (adipose tissue tumors) originate from the adipose derived stem cells (ASC) [31]. Rhabdomyosarcoma (skeletal muscle tumor) arise from the myogenic precursors and malignant peripheral nerve sheath tumors from the precursors of post-natal Schwann-derived cells [31].

Genetics: Point mutations in *c-KIT* and *PDGFRA* genes were common in the GISTs [33]. These gene mutations were present in 85% of the gastrointestinal soft tissue tumors [34]. Point mutation in *MED12*, copy number gain/amplification of *MYOCD*, deletion of *TP53* and mutation in *PTEN* were altered in the leiomyosarcoma [33, 34]. Point mutations in *NF1*, *SUZ12*, *EED* genes and deletion of *CDKN2A* were observed in malignant peripheral nerve sheath tumors [33, 34]. A t(2;13) (q35;q14) translocation was observed in 25% of alveolar rhabdomyosarcoma cases [33, 34]. Embryonal rhabdomyosarcoma includes alterations in the *TP53*, *RAS* and *FGFR4* genes [33, 34]. Point mutation on the angiopoeitin and *KDR* genes were commonly mutated in angiosarcoma [33, 34]. The *YAP1-TFE3* gene fusion was found in young patients with epithelioid hemangioendothelioma [34]. Infantile fibrosarcoma include translocations such as t(12;15) (p13;q26) and the low-grade fibromyxoid sarcomas include the t(7;16)(q33;p11) translocation [34]. Myxoid liposarcoma has either a t (12;16) (q13; p11) reciprocal translocation between the *DDIT3* (*CHOP*) and *FUS* gene or *DDIT3* and *EWS* gene [34]. Point mutation on the *PIK3CA* is also common in the myxoid liposarcoma [33].

24.4 Treatment

Surgery: The standard treatment for all the localized soft tissue sarcomas was surgery, which was performed after considering the tumor stage and co-morbidity in patients [35]. The surgery involves the *en bloc* removal of the primary tumor and normal tissue around the tumor [36]. There are four types of surgical margins: radical, marginal, wide and intralesional [37]. Radical resection is the removal of full compartment, whereas wide resection is the removal of the tumor with an edge of the normal tissue [38]. In marginal resection, the resection margin goes through the reactive zone (pseudo-capsule) and in intralesional resection, pseudo-capsule of the tumor will be opened during the surgery [37]. The sarcomas of the extremities can be cured by the limb-sparing amputation alone or with the radiotherapy [36]. Treatment with chemotherapy or radiotherapy after the surgery depends on the patient symptoms, co-morbidity, histological subtype and the extent of metastasis [35]. Isolated limb perfusion, a preoperative chemotherapy technique that employs melphalan and TNFα helps in reducing the size of the tumors that are difficult yet potentially resectable [35].

Radiotherapy: For the high-grade tumors that are larger than 5 cm, radiation therapy is the standard treatment; tumors less than 5 cm should be treated with the surgery followed by radiotherapy, either pre-operatively or post-operatively [12, 36, 39]. Post-operative radiotherapy was the standard treatment strategy for the intermediate or high-grade soft tissue sarcomas [35]. The post-operative recommended radiation dose is 66 Gy in 1.8-2Gy fraction [40]. Myxiod liposarcoma, a radiosensitive subtype, can be treated by the pre-operative radiotherapy and a significant tumor shrinkage can be achieved [35]. The standard pre-operative radiotherapy regimen is 50 Gy, followed by surgery upon 6 weeks of completion of the radiotherapy [35, 40]. The major types of radiation therapy are external beam radiation therapy (EBRT), intra operative radiation therapy (IORT), brachytherapy and hardon therapy [38]. Intra operative radiation therapy was an advanced treatment strategy in which a large dose of the radiation was administered during surgery [41]. Brachytherapy was also called as internal radiation therapy as it involves the direct placing of radioactive source (Iridium-192, Iodine-125) in the tumor bed with catheters during the surgery [38, 42]. In hardon therapy, tumors are irradiated by the charged particles [38]. Proton particles irradiate the tumors of the soft tissue sarcoma, this radiation therapy is called as the proton beam radiation therapy [38]. In heavy ion therapy, the particles higher than the proton or neutron were used; usually carbon particles were used [38].

Chemotherapy: Pre-operative chemotherapy was considered for the high-grade tumors, considering the age, co-morbidity and histological type of the patient [35]. The post-operative chemotherapy is not routinely recommended [35]. Factors such as response of the tumor, histology, patient's age and co-morbidities should be considered before selecting the first-line chemotherapy [43]. First-line chemotherapy includes doxorubicin either alone or in combination with ifosfamide [44]. A study by Tap et al. confirmed that the combination of doxorubicin and olaratumab can also be used as first-line therapy [45]. Ifosfamide, in combination of the anthracyclines, can be considered as the second-line treatment [35]. The other second-line treatments include dacarbazine, trabectedin and gemcitabine plus docetaxel combination [46]. High dosage of gemcitabine with docetaxel is used in the treatment of aggressive uterine leiomyosarcoma [17]. While facial and scalp angiosarcoma show favorable response to paclitaxel, angiosarcomas of the other sites respond to the taxen [17]. Cyclophosphamide and ifosfamide, etoposide, doxorubicin, vincristine and dactinomycin are used as second-line in the treatment of small round cell sarcomas and Ewing's sarcoma [17].

24.5 Conclusion

Soft tissue sarcoma are rare malignancies and are more prevalent in males than females. They originate from different anatomic sites within the body and are classified into many subtypes based on the histology. The major risk factors include mutations in various genes such as *KIT*, *PDGFRA*, *MED12*, *MYCOD*, *TP53*, *PTEN* and t (7;16) (q34;11), exposure to chemicals, genetic syndromes, oncogenic viruses and immune deficiency. Soft tissue sarcoma can be diagnosed by MRI (size, location), CT scan (primary tumor and metastasis) and biopsy. Treatment for soft tissue include surgery, radiotherapy and chemotherapy. Pre-operative chemotherapy was recommended for the high-grade tumors based on the age, comorbidity and the histological type of patient. Doxorubicin in combination with olaratumab can be used as the first-line therapy and dacarbazine, trabectedin are used as second-line therapy. Immunotherapeutic approaches are currently being tested for soft tissue sarcomas, albeit with limited success. Further investigations are going on to personalize the immunotherapy of soft tissue cancers based on the molecular subtypes.

References

1. Gamboa AC, Gronchi A, Cardona K. Soft-tissue sarcoma in adults: an update on the current state of histiotype-specific management in an era of personalized medicine. CA Cancer J Clin. 2020;70(3):200–29.
2. García-Ortega DY, Clara-Altamirano MA, Martín-Tellez KS, Caro-Sánchez CHS, Álvarez-Cano A, Lino-Silva LS, Salcedo-Hernández RA, Ruvalcaba-González CC, Martínez-Said H, Luna-Ortiz K, Villavicencio-Valencia SV, Cuellar-Hubbe M. Epidemiological profile of soft tissue sarcomas of the extremities: incidence, histological subtypes, and primary sites. J Orthop. 2021;25:70–4.
3. Bourcier K, Le Cesne A, Tselikas L, Adam J, Mir O, Honore C, de Baere T. Basic knowledge in soft tissue sarcoma. Cardiovasc Intervent Radiol. 2019;42(9):1255–61.
4. Vodanovich DA, Choong PF. Soft-tissue sarcomas. Indian J Orthop. 2018;52:35–44.
5. Yang Z, Zheng R, Zhang S, Zeng H, Li H, Chen W. Incidence, distribution of histological subtypes and primary sites of soft tissue sarcoma in China. Cancer Biol Med. 2019;16(3):565.
6. Patel D, Saldanha E, Mehta N, Dhakad V, Desai S. A study and evaluation of soft tissue sarcoma cases in Central India. National J Med Res. 2019;9(03):113–6.
7. Saltus CW, Calingaert B, Candrilli S, Lorenzo M, D'yachkova Y, Otto T, Wagner U, Kaye JA. Epidemiology of adult soft-tissue sarcomas in Germany. Sarcoma. 2018;2018:5671926.
8. Brownstein JM, DeLaney TF. Malignant soft-tissue sarcomas. Hematol Oncol Clin North Am. 2020;34(1):161–75.
9. Banerjee RA, Bandopadhyay DE, Abilash VG. Epidemiology, pathology, types and diagnosis of soft tissue sarcoma: a research review. Asian J Pharm Clin Res. 2013;6(suppl 3):18–25.
10. Hui JY. Epidemiology and etiology of sarcomas. Surg Clin North Am. 2016;96(5):901–14.
11. Sbaraglia M, Dei Tos AP. The pathology of soft tissue sarcomas. Radiol Med. 2019;124(4):266–81.
12. Roland CL. Soft tissue tumors of the extremity. Surg Clin. 2020;100(3):669–80.
13. Cormier JN, Pollock RE. Soft tissue sarcomas. CA Cancer J Clin. 2004;54(2):94–109.
14. Choi JH, Ro JY. The 2020 WHO classification of tumors of soft tissue: selected changes and new entities. Adv Anat Pathol. 2021;28(1):44–58.
15. Anderson WJ, Doyle LA. Updates from the 2020 World Health Organization classification of soft tissue and bone tumours. Histopathology. 2021;78(5):644–57.

16. Lee NC, Eskander A, Miccio JA, Park HS, Shah C, Rutenberg M, Hosni A, Husain ZA. Evaluation of head and neck soft tissue sarcoma 8th edition pathologic staging system and proposal of a novel stage grouping system. Oral Oncol. 2021;114:105137.
17. Clark MA, Fisher C, Judson I, Thomas JM. Soft-tissue sarcomas in adults. N Engl J Med. 2005;353(7):701–11.
18. Zwick RK, Guerrero-Juarez CF, Horsley V, Plikus MV. Anatomical, physiological, and functional diversity of adipose tissue. Cell Metab. 2018;27(1):68–83.
19. Cloutier JM, Charville GW. Diagnostic classification of soft tissue malignancies: a review and update from a surgical pathology perspective. Curr Probl Cancer. 2019;43(4):250–72.
20. Mukund K, Subramaniam S. Skeletal muscle: a review of molecular structure and function, in health and disease. Wiley Interdiscip Rev Syst Biol Med. 2020;12(1):e1462.
21. Jarvis S, Saman S. Cardiac system 1: anatomy and physiology. Nurs Times. 2018;114(2):34–7.
22. Robin JY, Nicola JB, Malcolm W, Reed DH, Woll PJ. Angiosarcomas. Lancet Oncol. 2010;11:983–1.
23. Liu Q, Wang X, Yi S. Pathophysiological changes of physical barriers of peripheral nerves after injury. Front Neurosci. 2018;12:597.
24. Thway K, Fisher C. Malignant peripheral nerve sheath tumor: pathology and genetics. Ann Diagn Pathol. 2014;18(2):109–16.
25. Miettinen M, Lasota J. Gastrointestinal stromal tumors: review on morphology, molecular pathology, prognosis, and differential diagnosis. Arch Pathol Lab Med. 2006;130(10):1466–78.
26. Romano RC, Fritchie KJ. Fibrohistiocytic tumors. Clin Lab Med. 2017;37(3):603–31. https://doi.org/10.1016/j.cll.2017.05.007.
27. Jaslove JM, Nelson CM. Smooth muscle: a stiff sculptor of epithelial shapes. Philos Trans R Soc Lond B Biol Sci. 2018;373(1759):20170318.
28. McCarthy AJ, Chetty R. Benign smooth muscle tumors (leiomyomas) of deep somatic soft tissue. Sarcoma. 2018;2018:2071394.
29. Kendall RT, Feghali-Bostwick CA. Fibroblasts in fibrosis: novel roles and mediators. Front Pharmacol. 2014;5:123. The authors illustrate a central role for fibroblasts in the pathology of fibrosis, including ECM production in relation to fibrosis, and provide some examples of critical chemical signaling and myofibroblast differentiation
30. Florencio-Silva R, Sasso GR, Sasso-Cerri E, Simões MJ, Cerri PS. Biology of bone tissue: structure, function, and factors that influence bone cells. Biomed Res Int. 2015;2015:421746.
31. Genadry KC, Pietrobono S, Rota R, Linardic CM. Soft tissue sarcoma cancer stem cells: an overview. Front Oncol. 2018;8:475.
32. Iwasaki H, Nabeshima K, Nishio J, Jimi S, Aoki M, Koga K, Hamasaki M, Hayashi H, Mogi A. Pathology of soft-tissue tumors: daily diagnosis, molecular cytogenetics and experimental approach. Pathol Int. 2009;59(8):501–21.
33. Mariño-Enríquez A, Bovée JV. Molecular pathogenesis and diagnostic, prognostic and predictive molecular markers in sarcoma. Surg Pathol Clin. 2016;9(3):457–73.
34. Smith SM, Coleman J, Bridge JA, Iwenofu OH. Molecular diagnostics in soft tissue sarcomas and gastrointestinal stromal tumors. J Surg Oncol. 2015;111(5):520–31.
35. Grimer R, Judson I, Peake D, Seddon B. Guidelines for the management of soft tissue sarcomas. Sarcoma. 2010;2010:1.
36. Arifi S, Belbaraka R, Rahhali R, Ismaili N. Treatment of adult soft tissue sarcomas: an overview. Rare Cancers Ther. 2015;3(1–2):69–87.
37. Endo M, Lin PP. Surgical margins in the management of extremity soft tissue sarcoma. Chin Clin Oncol. 2018;7(4):37.
38. Hoefkens F, Dehandschutter C, Somville J, Meijnders P, Van Gestel D. Soft tissue sarcoma of the extremities: pending questions on surgery and radiotherapy. Radiat Oncol. 2016;11(1):136.
39. Fujiwara T, Tsuda Y, Le Nail LR, Evans S, Gregory J, Tillman R, Abudu A. The role of radiotherapy in the treatment of superficial soft-tissue sarcomas. Bone Joint J. 2020;102(8):1088–94.
40. Haas RL. Preoperative radiotherapy in soft tissue sarcoma: from general guidelines to personalized medicine. Chin Clin Oncol. 2018;7(4):41.

41. Roeder F. Radiation therapy in adult soft tissue sarcoma—current knowledge and future directions: a review and expert opinion. Cancers. 2020;12(11):3242.
42. Ballo MT, Lee AK. Current results of brachytherapy for soft tissue sarcoma. Curr Opin Oncol. 2003;15(4):313–8.
43. Gronchi A, Maki RG, Jones RL. Treatment of soft tissue sarcoma: a focus on earlier stages. Future Oncol. 2017;13(1s):13–21.
44. Nakamura T, Sudo A. The current status of trabectedin in soft tissue sarcoma. Front Pharmacol. 2022;13:777872.
45. Meyer M, Seetharam M. First-line therapy for metastatic soft tissue sarcoma. Curr Treat Options in Oncol. 2019;20(1):6.
46. Ratan R, Patel SR. Chemotherapy for soft tissue sarcoma. Cancer. 2016;122(19):2952–60. https://doi.org/10.1002/cncr.30191.

Malignant Mesothelioma

25

Jalaluddin Mohammed Zubair, Jahnavi Ramesh Iyer, Meghana Korikani, Seshikala Durisetti, Prapthi Bathini, and Rama Krishna Kancha

25.1 Introduction

25.1.1 Epidemiology and Risk Factors

Mesothelioma is a rare type of cancer that develops from the lining of organs. Worldwide, mesothelioma ranks 32nd in incidence with 30,870 new cases in 2020 [1]. Every year, around 3000 new cases of mesothelioma are reported in the United States. According to the GLOBOCAN 2020, mesothelioma ranks 26th in mortality with a mortality rate of 0.03% (26,278 deaths in the year 2020). As per SEER statistics, the 5-year survival rate is 20%, 16%, and 8% for localized, regional, and metastatic mesothelioma, respectively. Among all cases of mesothelioma, 70–90% are of pleural mesothelioma and the remaining are of peritoneal mesothelioma whereas pericardial and tunica vaginalis are very rare [2]. Eastern Asia has the highest incidence and mortality rates, followed by the Western Europe. The global incidence and mortality rates are significantly higher in males (21,560 cases, cumulative risk 0.05; 18,681 deaths, cumulative risk 0.04) than in females (9310 cases, cumulative risk 0.02; 7597 deaths, cumulative risk 0.02). Most patients diagnosed with mesothelioma are men of >65 years of age. Incidence of mesothelioma is also affected by race: the rate for black Americans is 0.5 per 100,000, which is half than

J. M. Zubair · J. R. Iyer · M. Korikani · R. K. Kancha (✉)
Molecular Medicine and Therapeutics Laboratory, CPMB, Osmania University, Hyderabad, India
e-mail: ramakancha@osmania.ac.in

S. Durisetti
Department of Environmental Sciences, Osmania University, Hyderabad, India

P. Bathini (✉)

Apollo Institute of Medical Sciences and Research, Hyderabad, India

R. K. Kancha (ed.), *Biomedical Aspects of Solid Cancers*,
https://doi.org/10.1007/978-981-97-1802-3_25

that of white Americans (1 per 100,000). Majority of the malignant mesothelioma cases are primarily due to asbestos, often occurring 40 years after the exposure [3]. Exposure to asbestos is reported in 70–80% of people diagnosed with mesothelioma. Zeolites such as erionite, a mineral, are also a cause of malignant mesothelioma [4]. Mesothelioma is also caused due to exposure to high doses of radiation to the chest or abdomen as part of the treatment for Hodgkin lymphoma [5]. Infection with simian virus 40 (SV40) can be a risk factor for developing mesothelioma [6]. Mutations in the *CDK2N, NF2,* and *BAP1* also causes mesothelioma and these mutations could be familial [7]. Tobacco smoking by itself does not increase the risk of mesothelioma, but in combination with asbestos can increase the risk of mesothelioma [8].

25.1.2 Diagnosis

The diagnosis usually involves a combination of imaging studies, biopsy, and markers. X-rays, CT scans, and MRI help identify the tumors in the affected area; they however are not confirmatory. The radiological gold standard for staging of disease is CT scan. Biopsy is usually a confirmatory test. Mesothelioma can be diagnosed by biopsy which include needle aspiration technique in which a fine needle is injected between the ribs to collect the tumor sample and examination of tumor sample is done to confirm mesothelioma [9]. Thoracentesisis, a technique that utilizes both ultrasound and computed tomography (CT) for obtaining tissue for biopsy and draining of excess fluid (effusion), is present in the pleural space [10]. This technique is the safest and accurate for biopsy as it utilizes both ultrasound and computed tomography [11]. Thoracoscopy, a technique for visual examination of lung surfaces and pleural space by passing a tube, is a biopsy technique which provides suction of effusion for diagnosis and examination [12]. High sensitivity and low complication rates are found with thoracoscopy-guided biopsy and CT-guided core biopsies. Biomarkers for mesothelioma include elevated levels of VEGF [13], thioredoxin-1 [14], calretinin [14], fibulin-3 [15], and osteopontin [16].

25.2 Classification

Mesothelioma is classified on the basis of (1) the cell of origin and (2) location of the tumor. (1) Based on type of the cell, mesothelioma is subdivided into 3 types: (a) epithelioid mesothelioma, (b) sarcomatoid mesothelioma, and (c) biphasic mesothelioma (Fig. 25.1) [17]. (a) Epithelioid mesothelioma is caused by mutation in the epithelial cells [18] and accounts for 50–70% of all mesothelioma cases [17]. These mesothelioma cells have square or tubular configuration and are uniform; they divide quickly but remain together with distinguished nuclei [18]. Epithelioid mesothelioma typically is the most responsive to the treatment with best prognosis [19]. (b) *Sarcomatoid mesothelioma:* sarcomatoid cells are spindle shaped, lacks any defining structure and the configuration is irregular, and accounts for 10% of all

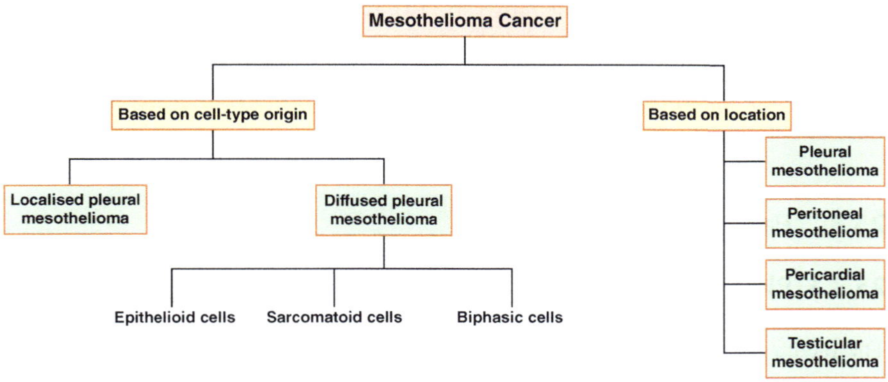

Fig. 25.1 World Health Organization (WHO) classification of mesothelioma

mesothelioma cases [20]. These cells are more aggressive than epithelial cells; they spread more quickly than epithelial cells because they do not tend to stick together as they grow [18]. The treatment response of sarcomatoid cells is less when compared to epithelioid cells [21]. (c) *Biphasic mesothelioma* is considered biphasic when it contains both epithelial and sarcomatoid cells. The biphasic mesothelioma accounts for 10–20% of mesothelioma cases.

(2) Based on the location of tumor, mesothelioma is classified into 4 types: (a) pleural mesothelioma, (b) peritoneal mesothelioma, (c) pericardial mesothelioma, and (d) tunica vaginalis (testicular mesothelioma) [21]. (a) Pleural mesothelioma develops in the pleura, which is the thin lining of tissue that surrounds the lungs [18]. Pleural mesothelioma is the most common type of mesothelioma cancer, accounting for about 75% of cases [18]. Asbestos fiber exposure is the primary cause of pleural mesothelioma [22]. The mechanism of development of tumor in pleural mesothelioma is based on the factors such as asbestos exposure, genetic mutations, SV40, and radiation [23]. When asbestos fibers enter the pleural space of the body, they start damaging the tissue leading to irritability [23]. Intracellular DNA damage and abnormal repair are caused due to the oxygen free radicals released by asbestos fibers [23]. Mesothelial cells release inflammatory cytokines when exposed to asbestos, which also creates a favorable microenvironment for tumor growth [23]. Abnormal cell proliferation and overexpression of proto-oncogenes is seen as a result of phosphorylation of protein kinases due to asbestos fibers [23]. (b) Peritoneal mesothelioma, which accounts for 20% of the cases, is a rare asbestos-related cancer that develops from the abdominal lining, also known as the peritoneum [24]. A much rarer form of peritoneal mesothelioma develops in the omentum, which is a layer of abdominal membrane that covers the stomach and other organs [24]. The primary cause of the peritoneal mesothelioma is asbestos exposure [24]. Patients affected with peritoneal mesothelioma and receiving chemotherapy have a life expectancy of 6–12 months [24]. (c) Pericardial mesothelioma is a rare form of cancer, which accounts for less than 1% of cases, affects the pericardium or the lining of heart [25]. Some benefit was observed in patients after

undergoing surgery or chemotherapy [26]. (d) Testicular mesothelioma is a cancer of tunica vaginalis, which is the membrane lining of the testes [27]. Mesothelioma of tunica vaginalis testes is a rare disease which accounts for <1% of the cases [28]. Inflammation and local trauma may also play a significant role in the pathogenesis [29].

25.3 Pathophysiology

25.3.1 Pleura

The pleura is a membrane structure that surrounds the lungs and is composed of 2 layers: visceral pleura or the inner pleura and parietal pleura or the outer pleura (Fig. 25.2) [30]. Pleural cavity is the space between visceral and parietal pleura and is filled with a small amount of pleural fluid [30]. The visceral pleura covers the lungs and the parietal pleura is located towards the chest wall (Fig. 25.2) [30]. The normal functioning of lungs while breathing is due to the pleural cavity, creating a pressure gradient ensuring proper ventilation during respiration and maintaining lung expansion [30, 31]. The circulation of blood in bronchi supplies visceral pleura with blood and the intercoastal arteries provide blood to parietal pleura [30]. The parietal and visceral pleural surfaces are thin layers of mesothelium, which is derived from embryonic mesoderm [32]. The pleural mesothelium cells are responsible for maintenance of stability of pleural space and also initiates the response to inhaled harmful stimuli such as infections, foreign particles, and irritants [33]. Cytokines and adhesion molecules are produced by pleural mesothelium cells [32].

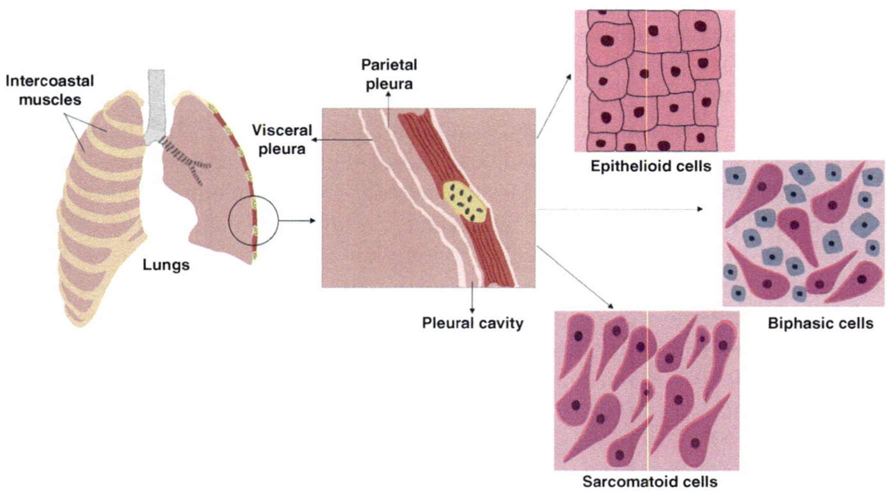

Fig. 25.2 Anatomy of mesothelioma

25.3.2 Peritoneum

The peritoneum is a part of abdominal cavity which covers the abdominal organs that are present in the coelomic cavity of the abdomen [34]. There are 2 types of mesothelium layers in this cavity: (a) the mesothelium layer which covers the internal organs of the abdomen is called as visceral peritoneum and is derived from the splanchnic mesoderm and (b) the layer which lines the abdominal wall called as parietal peritoneum and is derived from the somatic mesoderm [35]. Peritoneum cavity is the space between the visceral and parietal peritoneum, which is filled with fluid rich in leukocytes, macrophages, mast cells, lymphocytes, and granulocytes [36]. The peritoneal mesothelium is mainly composed of epithelial cells that are cuboidal or squamous with round nuclei [35]. These epithelial cells are polygonal in shape and have microvilli at apical surfaces, show cytokeratin expression, have tight junctions, and are also responsible for basement membrane production, which allows selective transport of substances [37]. The mesothelium in the peritoneum is responsible for maintenance of stability, serosal integrity along with induction of tissue repair response, production of anti-friction molecules such as glycosaminoglycans, proteoglycans. and antigen presentation, which allows for the movement of organs during peristalsis and breathing [37]. During inflammation, these cells release cytokines and chemokines such as IL-1BETA, TNF-ALPHA, and IFN-GAMMA for the control of inflammation and tissue repair [38].

25.3.3 Pericardium

The pericardium is a two-membrane layer which covers the heart [39]. The pericardium is made up of 2 layers: the inner serosal pericardium that covers the heart and the outer fibrous pericardium, which is connected to the chest wall [39]. The serosal pericardium is made of 2 layers of mesothelium: (a) the visceral pericardium directly covers the myocardium of the heart and (b) the parietal pericardium which lines the fibrous pericardium on the inner side. It is made up of mesothelial cells supported by fibrous connective tissue [39]. Pericardial space is a cavity present between visceral and parietal pericardium and also contains pericardial fluid that is rich in myocardial interstitial fluid, plasma, and lymph [39]. This pericardial fluid is responsible for maintaining the pressure of the heart during cardiac cycle-dependent change in shape and size of the heart [39]. The cavity between visceral pericardium and myocardium contains epicardial fat, which is rich in coronary arteries, veins, lymphatics, and nerves [39]. In addition to attachment to adventitia of great arteries along with cervical fascia and central tendon, the fibrous pericardium is loosely connected to the esophagus and the remaining diaphragm [39].

25.3.4 Tunica Vaginalis

The entire testis excluding the posterior border is enveloped by tunica vaginalis, which is a mesothelium-lined membrane [40]. The tunica vaginalis contains 2 layers: the visceral layer that covers the testis overall except the posterior and the parietal layer that is attached to the scrotal wall [40]. The transport of spermatozoa towards the rete testis and into the epididymis is facilitated by these layers [40]. During the second and third month of gestation, the tunica vaginalis is derived from peritoneum in the form of processus vaginalis, which later in the ninth month is transformed into tunica vaginalis [40]. Tunica vaginalis is the space between visceral and parietal layer [40]. The free movement of testis in scrotum is facilitated by the tunica vaginalis by the release of lubricant fluid into the tunica vaginalis cavity [40].

25.3.5 Genetics

The mutated genes which are responsible for mesothelioma are *NF2*, *CDKN2A,* and *BAP1* [18]. The loss of *NF2* gene along with combined deletions such as *INK4a* or *ARF* is the cause of mesothelioma [41]. In few mesothelioma cases along with YAP activation, mutations in the *LATS1* and *LATS2* are observed [18]. The down regulation of hippo and mTOR pathways resulting in cell-cell contact inhibition is a result of *LATS1* and *NF2* co-inactivation, which makes the PI3K-AKT-mTOR pathway highly sensitive to inhibitors [42]. p16 and $p14^{ARF}$ are the cell cycle regulators which are encoded by *CDKN2A*; deletion of *CDKN2A* and mutation in *TP53* genes lead to mesothelioma cancer cell growth [18]. *BAP1* along with polycomb repressor complex 2 is responsible for epigenetic regulation of many genes [43]. Deletion of *BAP1* gene makes the PMC2 highly sensitive to PMC inhibitors thereby promoting the tumor growth [44]. Deletion in *BAP1* gene also promotes the sensitivity of mesothelial cells to UV irradiation or ionization [45].

25.4 Treatment

25.4.1 Surgery and Radiotherapy

Patients with clinical stage 1 mesothelioma can undergo surgery. The surgical procedures include *Extrapleural pneumonectomy,* the process in which an entire lung including the visceral and parietal pleura along with diaphragm is removed from the body [46]. The median survival after extrapleural pneumonectomy is 19 months and 5-year survival rate are 15%. For patients with epitheloid histology, negative resection margin and no extrapleural nodal involvement, the median survival was found to be 51 months and 5-year survival rate was 46% [46]. *Lung-sparing cytoreductive surgery:* In this procedure, the parietal pleura of lung is removed along with decortication [46]. The median survival of patients after undergoing this surgery is

15.8 months [46]. *Photodynamic therapy:* A porphyrin-based compound that reacts in the presence of visible light causes direct cellular destruction and initiates a series of apoptotic events. Photodynamic therapy has been approved for the treatment of some malignancies but remains experimental for malignant pleural mesothelioma. *Palliative surgery* is performed to provide relief from shortness of breath because of pleural effusion [46]. A chest tube is permanently fixed in the body and drug is administered through this chest tube [46]. *Radiotherapy* provides temporary reduction in pain and chest wall masses [46]. In intensity modulated radiotherapy, small radiation photon or proton beams are used in a 3D pattern [46]. This procedure is often used after extrapleural pneumonectomy as a precaution against relapse [46]. Radiation does not improve the median survival [46]. External beam radiotherapy (EBRT) is used to kill tumor cells with the help of high-energy X-rays or other types of radiation.

25.4.2 Chemotherapy and Immunotherapy

Cisplatin combined with pemetrexed is used as a first-line treatment. The overall response rate was 41%. The median overall survival (OS) and median progression free survival (PFS) was 52.6 and 24.8 weeks, respectively [47]. Cisplatin plus raltitrexed is also used as a first-line treatment [47]. The overall response rate was 24%. The median overall survival and median progression free survival was 50 and 24 weeks, respectively [47]. A combination of carboplatin and pemetrexed is used as an alternative first-line treatment [48]. The median overall survival (OS) and median progression free survival (PFS) was 12.7 and 6.9 months, respectively; 1-year survival rate was 64% [48]. Gemcitabine with vinorelbine is used as a second-line treatment [49]. The median OS and median PFS was 11.2 and 6 months, respectively [49]. The disease control rate which is a combination of stable disease, partial response, and complete response was 82%. The response rate, which is a sum of partial and complete response was 18% [49]. For unresectable cases of mesothelioma, bevacizumab along with cisplatin—pemetrexed showed significant benefit in a phase III trial and is recommended as a first-line systemic therapy option [50]. Pembrolizumab and nivolumab are checkpoint inhibitors approved for the treatment of mesothelioma for patients who previously received chemotherapy or in whom surgery cannot be performed due to advanced diseases. Nivolumab plus ipilimumab is recommended as a first-line systemic therapy for unresectable malignant mesothelioma [51].

25.5 Conclusion

Malignant mesothelioma, which ranks at 32rd position worldwide in incidence, is a cancer type which affects the lining of internal organs. The main factor contributing to the development of mesothelioma is asbestos exposure, while radiation and viral infections can raise the risk. The majority of cases of mesothelioma are epithelioid, followed by sarcomatoid and biphasic. Upon exposure to asbestos fibers to pleura, a cascade of reactions including tissue damage, attack of reactive oxygen species on DNA, and abnormal repair resulting in uncontrolled proliferation. The purpose of a thoracentesis is to find pleural tumors. Thoracoscopy, a type of biopsy, is further carried out. Other important biomarkers include VEGF, calretinin, osteopontin, etc. Few gene deletions influence the development of malignant mesothelioma. The risk is increased by several-fold when *CDKN2A* deletion and *TP53* mutation are combined. In a number of circumstances, surgeries such as extrapleural pneumonectomy, lung-sparing cytoreductive surgery, photodynamic therapy, and palliative surgery are advised. Chemotherapy and radiation therapy are recommended, just like any other cancer treatment.

References

1. Sung H, Ferlay J, Siegel RL, Laversanne M, Soerjomataram I, Jemal A, Bray F. Global cancer statistics 2020: GLOBOCAN estimates of incidence and mortality worldwide for 36 cancers in 185 countries. CA Cancer J Clin. 2021;71(3):209–49.
2. Hiriart E, Deepe R, Wessels A. Mesothelium and malignant mesothelioma. J Dev Biol. 2019;7(2):7.
3. Kim KC, Vo HP. Localized malignant pleural sarcomatoid mesothelioma misdiagnosed as benign localized fibrous tumor. J Thorac Dis. 2016;8(6):E379.
4. Yang H, Testa JR, Carbone M. Mesothelioma epidemiology, carcinogenesis, and pathogenesis. Curr Treat Options Oncol. 2008;9:147–57.
5. Chirieac LR, Barletta JA, Yeap BY, Richards WG, Tilleman T, Bueno R, Baldini EH, Godleski J, Sugarbaker DJ. Clinicopathologic characteristics of malignant mesotheliomas arising in patients with a history of radiation for Hodgkin and non-Hodgkin lymphoma. J Clin Oncol. 2013;31(36):4544–9.
6. Testa JR, Giordano A. SV40 and cell cycle perturbations in malignant mesothelioma. In: Seminars in cancer biology, vol. 11. Academic Press; 2001. p. 31–8.
7. Singhi AD, Krasinskas AM, Choudry HA, Bartlett DL, Pingpank JF, Zeh HJ, Luvison A, Fuhrer K, Bahary N, Seethala RR, Dacic S. The prognostic significance of BAP1, NF2, and CDKN2A in malignant peritoneal mesothelioma. Mod Pathol. 2016;29(1):14–24.
8. Offermans NS, Vermeulen R, Burdorf A, Goldbohm RA, Kauppinen T, Kromhout H, van den Brandt PA. Occupational asbestos exposure and risk of pleural mesothelioma, lung cancer, and laryngeal cancer in the prospective Netherlands cohort study. J Occup Environ Med. 2014;56(1):6–19.
9. Rezk NA, Aly NY, El-Hadidy TA, Dashti K. CT-guided biopsy versus conventional Abram's needle biopsy in malignant pleural effusion. Egypt J Chest Dis Tuberc. 2015;64(2):405–9.
10. Kohan JM, Poe RH, Israel RH, Kennedy JD, Benazzi RB, Kallay MC, Greenblatt DW. Value of chest ultrasonography versus decubitus roentgenography for thoracentesis. Am Rev Respir Dis. 1986;133(6):1124–6.
11. Rahman NM, Gleeson FV. Image-guided pleural biopsy. Curr Opin Pulm Med. 2008;14(4):331–6.
12. British Thoracic Society Standards of Care Committee. BTS statement on malignant mesothelioma in the UK, 2007. Thorax. 2007;62(Suppl 2):ii1.
13. Demirag F, Ünsal E, Yilmaz A. Prognostic significance of vascular endothelial growth factor, tumor necrosis, and mitotic activity index in malignant pleural mesothelioma. Chest. 2005;128(5):3382–7.

14. Pass HI, Alimi M, Carbone M, Yang H, Goparaju CM. Mesothelioma biomarkers: a review highlighting contributions from the early detection research network. Cancer Epidemiol Biomark Prev. 2020;29(12):2524–40.
15. Pass HI, Levin SM, Harbut MR, Melamed J, Chiriboga L, Donington J, Huflejt M, Carbone M, Chia D, Goodglick L, Goodman GE. Fibulin-3 as a blood and effusion biomarker for pleural mesothelioma. N Engl J Med. 2012;367(15):1417–27.
16. Pass HI, Lott D, Lonardo F, Harbut M, Liu Z, Tang N, Carbone M, Webb C, Wali A. Asbestos exposure, pleural mesothelioma, and serum osteopontin levels. N Engl J Med. 2005;353(15):1564–73.
17. Geltner C, Errhalt P, Baumgartner B, Ambrosch G, Machan B, Eckmayr J, Klikovits T, Hoda MA, Popper H, Klepetko W, Austrian Mesothelioma Interest Group (AMIG). Management of malignant pleural mesothelioma—part 1: epidemiology, diagnosis, and staging: consensus of the Austrian Mesothelioma Interest Group (AMIG). Wien Klin Wochenschr. 2016;128:611–7.
18. Obacz J, Yung H, Shamseddin M, Linnane E, Liu X, Azad AA, Rassl DM, Fairen-Jimenez D, Rintoul RC, Nikolić MZ, Marciniak SJ. Biological basis for novel mesothelioma therapies. Br J Cancer. 2021;125(8):1039–55.
19. Brims FJ, Meniawy TM, Duffus I, de Fonseka D, Segal A, Creaney J, Maskell N, Lake RA, de Klerk N, Nowak AK. A novel clinical prediction model for prognosis in malignant pleural mesothelioma using decision tree analysis. J Thorac Oncol. 2016;11(4):573–82.
20. Marchevsky AM, LeStang N, Hiroshima K, Pelosi G, Attanoos R, Churg A, Chirieac L, Dacic S, Husain A, Khoor A, Klebe S. The differential diagnosis between pleural sarcomatoid mesothelioma and spindle cell/pleomorphic (sarcomatoid) carcinomas of the lung: evidence-based guidelines from the international mesothelioma panel and the MESOPATH National Reference Center. Hum Pathol. 2017;67:160–8.
21. Brcic L, Kern I. Clinical significance of histologic subtyping of malignant pleural mesothelioma. Transl Lung Cancer Res. 2020;9(3):924.
22. Harris EJ, Musk A, de Klerk N, Reid A, Franklin P, Brims FJ. Diagnosis of asbestos-related lung diseases. Expert Rev Respir Med. 2019;13(3):241–9.
23. Bibby AC, Tsim S, Kanellakis N, Ball H, Talbot DC, Blyth KG, Maskell NA, Psallidas I. Malignant pleural mesothelioma: an update on investigation, diagnosis and treatment. Eur Respir Rev. 2016;25(142):472–86.
24. Greenbaum A, Alexander HR. Peritoneal mesothelioma. Transl Lung Cancer Res. 2020;9(Suppl 1):S120.
25. Kahn EI, Rohl A, Barrett EW, Suzuki Y. Primary pericardial mesothelioma following exposure to asbestos. Environ Res. 1980;23(2):270–81.
26. McGehee E, Reisch J, Dowell J, Gerber DE. Treatment and outcomes of primary pericardial mesothelioma: a systematic review.
27. Akin Y, Bassorgun I, Basara I, Yucel S. Malignant mesothelioma of tunica vaginalis: an extremely rare case presenting without risk factors. Singap Med J. 2015;56(3):e53.
28. Nazemi A, Nassiri N, Pearce S, Daneshmand S. Testicular mesothelioma: an analysis of epidemiology, patient outcomes, and prognostic factors. Urology. 2019;126:140–4.
29. Mak CW, Cheng TC, Chuang SS, Wu RH, Chou CK, Chang JM. Malignant mesothelioma of the tunica vaginalis testis. Br J Radiol. 2004;77(921):780–1.
30. Charalampidis C, Youroukou A, Lazaridis G, Baka S, Mpoukovinas I, Karavasilis V, Kioumis I, Pitsiou G, Papaiwannou A, Karavergou A, Tsakiridis K. Pleura space anatomy. J Thorac Dis. 2015;7(Suppl 1):S27.
31. Tschumperlin DJ, Boudreault F, Liu F. Lung mechanobiology. In: Mechanobiology handbook. CRC Press; 2018. p. 407–27.
32. Batra H, Antony VB. Pleural mesothelial cells in pleural and lung diseases. J Thorac Dis. 2015;7(6):964.
33. Owens MW, Grisham MB. Nitric oxide synthesis by rat pleural mesothelial cells: induction by cytokines and lipopolysaccharide. Am J Phys Lung Cell Mol Phys. 1993;265(2):L110–6.

34. Isaza-Restrepo A, Martin-Saavedra JS, Velez-Leal JL, Vargas-Barato F, Riveros-Dueñas R. The peritoneum: beyond the tissue—a review. Front Physiol. 2018;9:738.
35. do Amaral RJ, Arcanjo KD, El-Cheikh MC, de Oliveira FL. The peritoneum: health, disease, and perspectives regarding tissue engineering and cell therapies. Cells Tissues Organs. 2017;204(5–6):211–7.
36. Ray A, Dittel BN. Isolation of mouse peritoneal cavity cells. J Vis Exp. 2010;35:1488.
37. Mutsaers SE, Birnie K, Lansley S, Herrick SE, Lim CB, Prêle CM. Mesothelial cells in tissue repair and fibrosis. Front Pharmacol. 2015;6:113.
38. Visser CE, Tekstra J, Brouwer-Steenbergen JJ, Tuk CW, Boorsma DM, Sampat-Sardjoepersad SC, Meijer S, Krediet RT, Beelen RH. Chemokines produced by mesothelial cells: huGRO-α, IP-10, MCP-1 and RANTES. Clin Exp Immunol. 1998;112(2):270–5.
39. Hoit BD. Anatomy and physiology of the pericardium. Cardiol Clin. 2017;35(4):481–90.
40. Garriga V, Serrano A, Marin A, Medrano S, Roson N, Pruna X. US of the tunica vaginalis testis: anatomic relationships and pathologic conditions. Radiographics. 2009;29(7):2017–32.
41. Jongsma J, van Montfort E, Vooijs M, Zevenhoven J, Krimpenfort P, van der Valk M, van de Vijver M, Berns A. A conditional mouse model for malignant mesothelioma. Cancer Cell. 2008;13(3):261–71.
42. Tranchant R, Quetel L, Tallet A, Meiller C, Renier A, de Koning L, de Reynies A, Le Pimpec-Barthes F, Zucman-Rossi J, Jaurand MC, Jean D. Co-occurring mutations of tumor suppressor genes, LATS2 and NF2, in malignant pleural mesothelioma. Clin Cancer Res. 2017;23(12):3191–202.
43. Carbone M, Yang H, Pass HI, Krausz T, Testa JR, Gaudino G. BAP1 and cancer. Nat Rev Cancer. 2013;13(3):153–9.
44. LaFave LM, Béguelin W, Koche R, Teater M, Spitzer B, Chramiec A, Papalexi E, Keller MD, Hricik T, Konstantinoff K, Micol JB. Loss of BAP1 function leads to EZH2-dependent transformation. Nat Med. 2015;21(11):1344–9.
45. Bononi A, Giorgi C, Patergnani S, Larson D, Verbruggen K, Tanji M, Pellegrini L, Signorato V, Olivetto F, Pastorino S, Nasu M. BAP1 regulates IP3R3-mediated Ca^{2+} flux to mitochondria suppressing cell transformation. Nature. 2017;546(7659):549–53.
46. Mott FE. Mesothelioma: a review. Ochsner J. 2012;12(1):70–9.
47. Cinausero M, Rihawi K, Sperandi F, Melotti B, Ardizzoni A. Chemotherapy treatment in malignant pleural mesothelioma: a difficult history. J Thorac Dis. 2018;10(Suppl 2):S304.
48. Patel SC, Dowell JE. Modern management of malignant pleural mesothelioma. In: Lung cancer: targets and therapy. Taylor & Francis; 2016. p. 63–72.
49. Toyokawa G, Takenoyama M, Hirai F, Toyozawa R, Inamasu E, Kojo M, Morodomi Y, Shiraishi Y, Takenaka T, Yamaguchi M, Shimokawa M. Gemcitabine and vinorelbine as second-line or beyond treatment in patients with malignant pleural mesothelioma pretreated with platinum plus pemetrexed chemotherapy. Int J Clin Oncol. 2014;19:601–6.
50. Zalcman G, Mazieres J, Margery J, Greillier L, Audigier-Valette C, Moro-Sibilot D, Molinier O, Corre R, Monnet I, Gounant V, Rivière F. Bevacizumab for newly diagnosed pleural mesothelioma in the mesothelioma Avastin cisplatin Pemetrexed study (MAPS): a randomised, controlled, open-label, phase 3 trial. Lancet. 2016;387(10026):1405–14.
51. Baas P, Scherpereel A, Nowak AK, Fujimoto N, Peters S, Tsao AS, Mansfield AS, Popat S, Jahan T, Antonia S, Oulkhouir Y. First-line nivolumab plus ipilimumab in unresectable malignant pleural mesothelioma (CheckMate 743): a multicentre, randomised, open-label, phase 3 trial. Lancet. 2021;397(10272):375–86.

Neuroblastoma

26

Ayesha Rahmat Yadwad, Himavarshitha Babbur, Meghana Korikani, Krishna Chaitanya Puligundla, Nageswara Rao Amanchi, and Rama Krishna Kancha

26.1 Introduction

26.1.1 Epidemiology

Neuroblastoma is one of the most common childhood cancers worldwide causing approximately 10% of all pediatric cancer deaths [1–5]. More than 98% of all diagnosed cases are sporadic in nature and the average age at the time of diagnosis is 1–2 years. Over 50% of adolescent patients show metastasis of tumors at the time of diagnosis leading to poor survival [2, 6, 7]. The prognosis depends heavily on the disease stage [8]. In 2014, the overall incidence of pediatric neuroblastoma in USA was 7% making it the third most common type of childhood cancer [7]. The incidence rates of patients up to 19 years old from 2006–2010 were 8.5% for boys and 7.6% for girls, and 5.2%, 9.7%, 6.8% and 5.9% for Hispanic, non-Hispanic (white), non-Hispanic (black) and Asian/Pacific Islander patients, respectively [7]. A population-based study in Netherlands spanning a 25-year period (1990–2014) revealed a 1.6% annual increase in the total incidence of NB since 1990, particularly in patients aged ≥18 months with stage 4 disease along with an improved overall survival from 6 ± 4% (1990–1994) to 43 ± 7% (2010–2014) [9].

A. R. Yadwad · H. Babbur · M. Korikani · R. K. Kancha (✉)
Molecular Medicine and Therapeutics Laboratory, CPMB, Osmania University, Hyderabad, India
e-mail: ramakancha@osmania.ac.in

K. C. Puligundla
Medical Oncology, MNJ Institute of Oncology and Regional Cancer Center, Hyderabad, India

N. R. Amanchi
Department of Zoology, Osmania University, Hyderabad, India

R. K. Kancha (ed.), *Biomedical Aspects of Solid Cancers*,
https://doi.org/10.1007/978-981-97-1802-3_26

26.1.2 Risk Factors

The age, stage of the disease, histopathologic results and various biologic factors contribute to risk stratification of patients with neuroblastoma [10]. The largest meta-analysis in Greece revealed that smoking and alcohol consumption during pregnancy are not significantly associated with increased neuroblastoma risk; however, vitamin intake significantly lowers the risk of the disease [11]. Germline mutations in *ALK*, *TP53*, *NRAS* and *BRCA2* and common polymorphisms in *BARD1* or *LMO1* increase the risk of neuroblastoma [12–14]. Moreover, rearrangements of the TERT locus or inactivating mutations in *ATRX* are associated with high-risk tumors [15–17]. Certain disorders such as neural crest development disorders [12, 18–21], RASopathies and epigenetic syndromes increase the risk of NB.

26.1.3 Diagnosis

Diagnosis of neuroblastoma is primarily based on histological analysis, biochemical testing and imaging [10]. Histological analysis is mainly done through biopsies and bone marrow aspirations [10]. In 1999, the International Neuroblastoma Pathology Committee proposed a modified prognostic classification system based on the morphological features of neuroblastoma which includes the amount of Schwannian stroma, amount of nodules/tumor mass, the degree of differentiation of affected cells and the mitosis-karyorrhexis index (MKI) [10]. On the basis of this system, 2 subgroups are possible: (a) Favorable histological results and (b) Unfavorable histological results. Image-guided percutaneous core needle biopsy (PCNB) is preferred over IB for initial diagnosis and detection of MYCN copy number in pediatric surgical patients due to its low cost with fewer complications that helps to avoid the risks of open surgery [22].

Biochemical tests include complete blood counts to check for anemia and clotting problems (low platelet count), levels of ferritin (chemical released by NB cells) and lactate dehydrogenase (LDH, elevated in NB). Urine tests detect potential tumor markers such as catecholamine metabolites in more than 85% of people with neuroblastoma, with homovanillic acid (HVA) or vanillylmandelic acid (VMA) being the two most commonly detected ones [10, 23]. Molecular tests include identification of mutations in genes such as *ALK* or amplifications in genes such as *MYCN*, which are associated with sporadic cases and to detect germline mutations in *PHOX2B* or *ALK* in familial cases.

Scanning/imaging tests include ultrasound/sonogram, which is the first examination performed when a solid heterogeneous mass, exhibiting approximately 30–90% calcification, is suspected in the child or in the fetus (to facilitate prenatal diagnosis of congenital neuroblastomas) [10, 24]. Computed tomography (CT or CAT) scan and magnetic resonance imaging (MRI) scan are used to detect the tumor and its size. Contrast agents such as the gadolinium may be used for easy detection. This scan is more efficient in detecting tumors around the spinal cord and shows higher sensitivity than CT and MIBG scans, but with low specificity [10].

Meta-iodobenzylguanidine (MIBG) scan in which radioactive iodine linked to MIBG is administered and actively absorbed by neuroblastoma cells in nearly 90% of all cases [10, 25]. It shows high specificity and accuracy, making it the test of choice for the diagnosis of metastatic cases [10]. Positron emission tomography (PET) or PET-CT scan uses radioactive chemicals to detect the tumors. This scan is usually done if the tumor is not responsive to MIBG.

26.2 Classification

Based on various clinical features, molecular factors and disease presentation, patients with NB are classified into 3 basic risk groups: high, intermediate and low-risk groups [8, 26]. There are different systems that are universally used for staging neuroblastoma: (1) The International Neuroblastoma Staging System (INSS) and (2) The International Neuroblastoma Risk Group Staging System (INRGSS) and (3) Modified Curie score and the International Society of Pediatric Oncology Europe Neuroblastoma (SIOPEN) score [10]. For almost 3 decades, INSS was the most commonly used staging system for neuroblastoma [27, 28]. It mainly relies on the extent of surgical resection and the degree of difficulty in resecting the mass [2]; however, it does not have any parameter to stage the disease before surgery. INSS determines the stage after the initiation of treatment based on the amount of tumor resected from the body during surgery [8]. INSS classifies the disease into 5 stages based on the number of tumors remaining after surgery: stages 1, 2, 3, 4 and 4s, with increasing risk of mortality [8]. (2) Since 2004, the INRGSS proposed classification based on image-defined risk factors (IDRFs) at diagnosis, which is being preferred for most research studies and cooperative clinical trials groups [2, 27, 29]. INRGSS determines the stage before treatment based on imaging test results based on CT, MRI and MIBG scans. Based on the extent of metastasis and certain IDRFs, INRGSS classifies neuroblastoma into the following 4 stages (Fig. 26.1): L1 (no metastasis), L2 (little metastasis), M (metastasis to distant body parts) and MS (metastasis in children <18 months) [8]. (3) Another classification is done on the basis of the interpretation of MIBG scans by semiquantitative scoring of skeletal

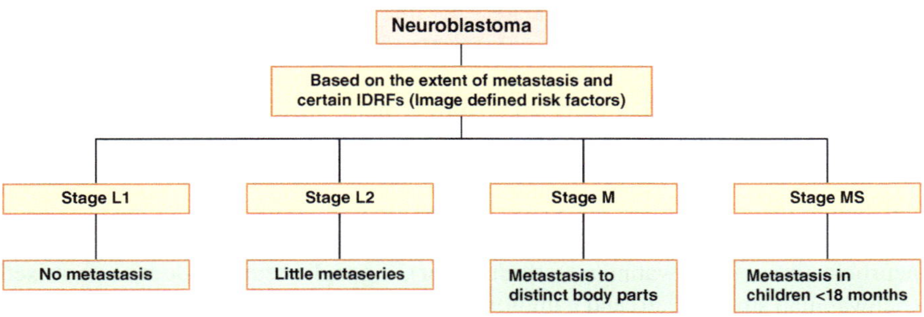

Fig. 26.1 Classification of neuroblastoma based on metastasis and IDRFs

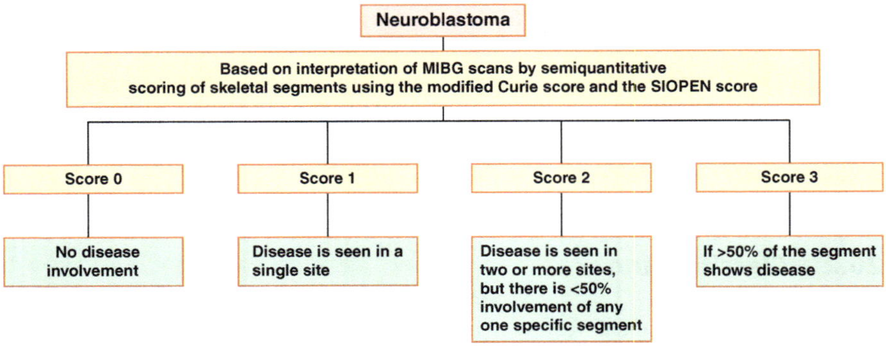

Fig. 26.2 Classification of neuroblastoma based on MIBG (iodine meta-iodobenzylguanidine) scans using the modified Curie score and SIOPEN score

segments using the SIOPEN score (Fig. 26.2) [10]. The body is divided into 9 skeletal segments, with an additional segment for soft-tissue involvement and each segment is assigned a score of 0–3 (maximum score = 30) based on the extent of disease. Score = 0: No disease involvement; Score = 1: Disease is seen in a single site; Score = 2: Disease is seen in two or more sites, but there is <50% involvement of any one specific segment; Score = 3: If >50% of the segment shows disease [10].

26.3 Pathophysiology

Neuroblastoma is a type of cancer that starts in neuroblasts (immature nerve cells) of the sympathetic nervous system. The sympathetic nervous system, which governs the fight-or-flight response is a part of the peripheral nervous system. Neuroblastoma usually affects neuroblasts in the adrenal glands and can develop anywhere in the sympathetic nervous system (Fig. 26.3). It can also advance in the abdomen, nerve tissue of the spinal cord, neck or chest. NB mostly emerges as an abdominal mass in the adrenal gland (most common primary site, 40%) and other abdominal (25%), thoracic (15%), cervical (5%) and pelvic sympathetic ganglia (5%) regions [30, 31]. In about 1/third of all cases, nests of neuroblasts in various stages of differentiation are separated by fine fibrovascular septa and variable amount of Schwannian stroma and rosette formation [32]. The International Neuroblastoma Pathology Classification (INPC), established in 1999 and partly amended in 2003, is often used for distinguishing 'favorable' and 'unfavorable' histology groups and patient stratification and is based on the age-linked morphological changes (cut-offs of 18 and 60 months at diagnosis) caused by 3 major molecular mechanisms: (a) The cross-talk between Schwann cells and neuroblastic cells is essential for tumor maturation, based on which 3 divisions are defined as neuroblastoma (Schwannian stroma-poor), ganglioneuroblastoma-intermixed (Schwannian stroma-rich) and ganglioneuroma (Schwannian stroma-dominant). (b) Based on trkAI/II (high-affinity NGF) expression that is essential for differentiation

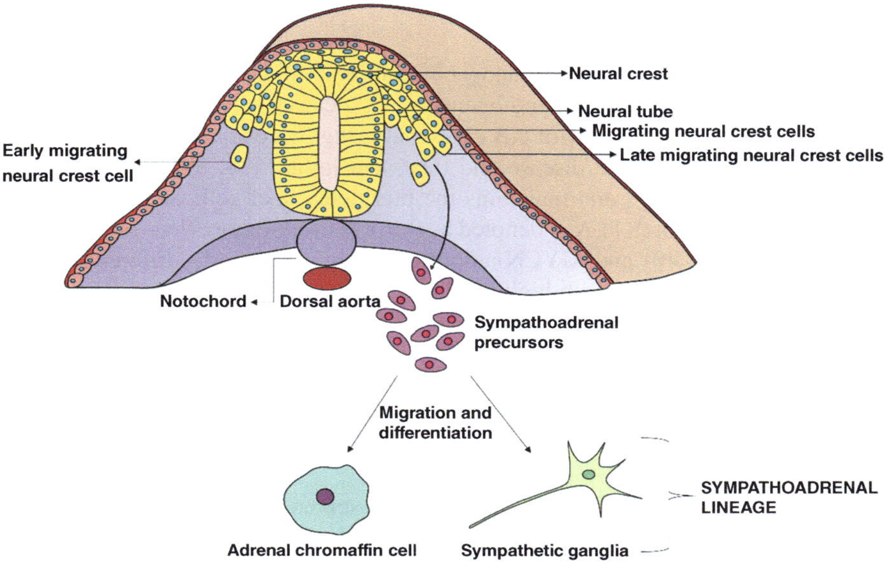

Fig. 26.3 Anatomy and pathophysiology of neuroblastoma. The neural crest cells develop into sympathoadrenal precursors which undergo migration and differentiation, and develop into adrenal chromaffin cell and sympathetic ganglia together constituting sympathoadrenal lineage. Neuroblastoma usually affects neuroblasts of the adrenal gland and can develop anywhere in the sympathetic nervous system

of neuroblasts, 3 subtypes are defined as undifferentiated, poorly differentiated and differentiating. (c) Based on *MYCN* amplification, three classes of mitosis-karyorrhexis index (MKI) are defined as low <100/5000 cells, intermediate 100–200/5000 cells and high >200/5000 cells as it acts as a powerful driving force for preventing neuroblastic differentiation and promotes mitotic and karyorrhectic activities [33].

Tumor-infiltrating lymphocytes (TILs), including T cells and NK cells, are often detected in human neuroblastoma tumors [8]. Invariant natural killer T cells (iNKT), NKT cells and gamma delta (γδ) T cells are often detected in NB tumors [34–37] and B cells are rarely identified [38–40]. $CD3^+$T cells constitute 5% of total cells in the tumor microenvironment (TME) [41–43]. $CD8^+$T cells are more frequently found over $CD4^+$ T cells in the TME, with CD4/CD8 ratios generally ranging between 0.3 and 5 [43–45]. NK cells may be detected in some cases constituting ~30% of total cells in the TME or may be completely absent in other cases [42, 43]. TME consist of immune cells, half of which are myeloid and the other half lymphoid constituting 50% of its total cell components [46]. The lymphoid portion mostly includes $CD4^+$ T helper cells (highest amount), followed by B cells and $CD8^+$ cytotoxic T cells [46]. Infiltration of $CD3^+$ T cells is observed in both primary and relapsed tumors [45].

26.3.1 Genetics

In neuroblastoma, *MYCN* proto-oncogene inhibits immune surveillance and promotes cell proliferation, tumor angiogenesis and metastasis [32]. Amplification of *MYCN* is observed in 20–30% of NB cases and is highly correlated with advanced-stage, clinically aggressive disease and treatment failure [38, 39]. *MYCN* blocks differentiation pathways and maintains the pluripotency of cells and self-renewal [32]. Amplification of *MYCN* is denoted as the presence of more than 10 gene copies of *MYCN* [38, 40] and MYCN-amplified tumors are poorly differentiated or typically undifferentiated with high MKI (mitotic karyorrhectic index), have cells with overexpression of the NMYC protein and prominent nucleoli [32]. Differentiation of neuroblastoma cells is associated with low expression levels of MYCN [47, 48]. *ALK* gene amplification is detected in 2–4% of NB cases, while a gain in copy number of *ALK* was observed in 20–30% of NB cases [49–51]. Gain-of-function mutations in *ALK* are one of the major causes of hereditary diseases in familial NB cases [52, 53].

Diploidy/tetraploidy of cells is commonly observed in advanced-stage tumors and is correlated with amplification of *MYCN* and minimal survival of patients [54]. In tumors without *MYCN* amplification, segmental chromosome aberrations are correlated with a high risk of relapse of NB [55]. Chromosome segmental gain at 1q, 2p or 17q and segmental loss at 1p, 3p, 4p, 11q positions are the most frequently observed and important predictive segmental changes in neuroblastoma [56–58]. Chromatin remodeling proteins cause the alternative lengthening of the telomere, thereby resulting in chronic progression of the disease as well as late recurrence in long-term neuroblastoma survivors [32]. In approximately 11% of NB, mutations are detected in genes encoding chromatin remodeling proteins, such as the AT-rich interactive domain 1A/1B (*ARID1A/1B*; a subunit of the SWI/SNF subfamily of ATP-dependent chromatin remodeling complexes) and are associated with early treatment failure [59]. *ARID1A* is known to act as a tumor suppressor in NB as its knockdown was found to increase the expression and activity of matrix metalloproteinases (MMP-2 and 9), induce E-cadherin downregulation, upregulation of N-cadherin and translocation of β-catenin into the nucleus, thereby enhancing NB cell migration and invasion [60].

Rare mutations at 11p15.4 (*LMO1*), 6p22 (*CASC15-S*), 2q35 (*BARD1*) and a copy number polymorphism at 1q21 are associated with tumor initiation in sporadic cases of high-risk neuroblastoma [5, 61, 62]. Recurrent mutations in *PTPN11*, *TIAM1*, *MYCN* and *TP53* and the RAS-RAF-MAPK pathway genes were observed in neuroblastoma [63]. Some of the aggressive familial neuroblastoma cases arise due to mutations in the *KIF1B* gene and other tumor suppressor genes located in the deleted region of chromosome 1 [64, 65]. Mutations in the *RB* are also observed in familial neuroblastoma patients [66]. Some loci that confer hereditary disposition to NB are present in the region of *GALNT14* gene [66] and an unknown locus at chromosome 16p12–13 [67]. Small nucleolar RNA host gene 7 (*SNHG7*) facilitates NB succession via the miR-653-5p/STAT2 pathway [68].

26.4 Treatment

The standard treatment methods used for NB include surgery, iodine 131-MIBG therapy, radiation therapy, chemotherapy, combination of radiation therapy and high-dose chemotherapy with stem cell transplantation, targeted therapy, and immunotherapy. Treatment options are decided based on several factors such as size of the tumor, location of the tumor, presence or absence of metastasis, risk classification/grade of the tumor, possible side effects, family preferences (for minor patients) and the child's overall health. Low-risk and intermediate-risk neuroblastoma: standard care for patients with low-risk neuroblastoma includes surgery alone or observation without surgery, as most cases show spontaneous regression which is mostly observed in children under 18 months of age [26]. In children with intermediate-risk neuroblastoma, high survival rate can result by outpatient chemotherapy and surgery [26]. The treatment plans are designed to gradually decrease the therapeutic intensity and reduce the associated toxicity in patients with low- and intermediate-risk neuroblastoma [69]. Surgical resection is the only treatment plan in patients with localized and resectable disease and can be combined with chemotherapy for patients showing relapse after resection [69, 70]. The 5-year overall survival rate was 99% for patients with INSS stage 1 and 96% for patients with asymptomatic INSS 2A or 2B tumors, after surgical resection in patients with low-risk neuroblastoma [71]. In infants <6-months old with small adrenal masses, 81% of subjects showed spontaneous regression of tumors and did not require any treatment, while the remaining 19% eventually underwent resection; they showed 3-year event-free survival (EFS) rate of 97% and OS rate of 100% [72]. In children with high-risk neuroblastoma, dose-intensive chemotherapy, surgery, radiation therapy and immunotherapy were used as a means of treatment over an 18-month timespan [26]. For patients with high-risk neuroblastoma, the standard program has 4 main components such as local control, induction chemotherapy, consolidation therapy and maintenance therapy [69].

26.4.1 Induction Therapy

Although the specific regimens may differ for individual patients, the common induction regimen for high-risk neuroblastoma comprises a combination of platinum-containing compounds, anthracyclines, topoisomerase II inhibitors and alkylating agents [69]. In European countries, two different drug combinations are used: (a) cisplatin [C], vincristine [O], carboplatin [J], etoposide [E] and cyclophosphamide [C]—COJEC, which is employed for rapid induction therapy. (b) Vincristine [O], cisplatin [P], etoposide [E], and cyclophosphamide [C]—OPEC, alternated with vincristine [O], carboplatin [J], etoposide [E] and cyclophosphamide [C]—OJEC, which is utilized for standard induction therapy [73]. However, insignificant difference is observed in the overall survival rates in patients undergoing these two induction regimens [74]. *Local control:* Prevention of local recurrence of disease is called as the local control. Local control includes surgical resection usually after 4–6 cycles of induction therapy and external radiation therapy to prevent tumor relapse [69]. *Consolidation therapy:* Myeloablative chemotherapy and autologous stem cell rescue (ASCR) comprise consolidation therapy [69]. Stem cells to be used for ASCR are usually harvested every 2–3 cycles of induction chemotherapy [69]. Due to ease of collection, high yield, low incidence of tumor cell contamination and rapid blood count recovery, peripheral blood is the preferred source of these stem cells [75, 76]. The most routinely used myeloablative program includes 3 days of melphalan with 4 days each of etoposide (CEM) and carboplatin [69]. Combination of busulfan and melphalan (Bu–Mel) causes fewer severe adverse events than carboplatin, etoposide and melphalan (CEM) in children with high-risk neuroblastoma and improved the event-free survival with 3-year EFS rates of 50% and 38%, respectively [77]. Consolidation therapy also makes use of immunotherapy with antibodies targeting the GD2 antigen on neuroblastoma tumor cells [69]. When anti-GD2 immunotherapy is used for consolidation after dose-intensive conventional chemotherapy, myeloablative therapy may not be needed to improve patient outcome [78].

26.4.2 Maintenance Therapy

Maintenance therapy is employed as a last resort when patients with high-risk neuroblastoma still show recurrence after the completion of surgical resection, induction chemotherapy, radiation therapy and myeloablative therapy with ASCR [69]. For the relapse of neuroblastoma, minimal residual disease is an important factor as many patients after achieving complete clinical remission with the above multimodal approach still show recurrence due to residual cancer cells [69]. A synthetic retinoid named as isotretinoin (13-*cis*-retinoic acid) is used to decrease proliferation and induce differentiation of neuroblastoma cells; it is administered to patients showing minimal residual disease even after stem cell rescue or chemotherapy [69]. The 3-year EFS rate was significantly higher in 130 patients receiving isotretinoin compared to 128 that did not receive any further therapy (46 ± 6% vs. 29 ± 5%, $P = 0.027$) [79]. The short-term survival in high-risk patients with both higher EFS (66 ± 5% vs. 46 ± 5% at 2 years, $P = 0.01$) and OS (86 ± 4% vs. 75 ± 5% at 2 years, $P = 0.020$) rates compared to standard therapy after 2 years of follow-up was achieved by performing granulocyte-macrophage colony-stimulating factor (GM-CSF), immunotherapy (anti-GD2 chimeric monoclonal antibody ch14.18 (dinutuximab) and interleukin-2 (IL-2) after standard isotretinoin maintenance therapy [74]. In patients with high-risk neuroblastoma who have received three different treatment regimens (anti-GD2 monoclonal antibody 3F8 alone, 3F8 + intravenous GM-CSF + isotretinoin or 3F8 + subcutaneous GM-CSF + isotretinoin) after first remission indicated that the (3F8 + GM-CSF + CRA) is effective against chemotherapy-resistant neuroblastoma [80]. An irreversible inhibitor of ornithine decarboxylase that is difluoromethylornithine (DFMO) is the rate-limiting enzyme in polyamine synthesis whose gene is a known target of the gene *MYCN* [81]. The maintenance therapy of DFMO for high-risk neuroblastoma patients after completion of standard therapy was associated with improved OS and EFS rates relative to historical controls (5-year OS: 95.1% vs. 81.6%; 5-year EFS: 85.2% vs. 65.6%) [82]. Topoisomerase inhibitors such as topotecan [83] and irinotecan [84, 85] are commonly used for the treatment of relapsed neuroblastoma. Irinotecan is primarily used in combination with the alkylating agent temozolomide, while topotecan is primarily used in combination with cyclophosphamide [69]. Combinations of ifosfamide, carboplatin and etoposide (ICE) are commonly used chemotherapy regimens for children with relapsed neuroblastoma [69]. Nearly 85% of tumors express the norepinephrine transporter on their cell surface, thereby enabling benzylguanidine analogs to bind to this transporter efficiently and selectively target these cells [69]. For the targeted delivery of radiation therapy directly to the active disease site, infusions of 131^{I}-MIBG are used as approximately 90% of neuroblastoma tumors are MIBG-avid [69]. In children with relapsed neuroblastoma, aurora A kinase inhibitor alisertib can be used either alone or in combination with irinotecan and temozolomide [86]. SF1126, a PI-3 kinase inhibitor, exhibited strong antitumor activity in neuroblastoma preclinical models, thereby suggesting PI3K/mTOR/Akt pathway as a therapeutic target in neuroblastoma [87]. Nifurtimox can be used to inhibit neuroblastoma cell growth both in in vitro and in vivo [88].

26.5 Conclusion

Neuroblastoma is a type of cancer that starts in neuroblasts of the sympathetic nervous system and one of the most common types of cancers that arise in childhood worldwide. The stage of disease, age of the patient, histopathologic results and various biologic factors are responsible for the pre-surgical and pre-treatment risk stratification of patients with neuroblastoma. Based on various clinical features, molecular factors and disease presentation including tumor histology, patient age, genomic alterations and localized versus metastatic disease, patients diagnosed with NB can be classified into 3 basic risk-groups: high, intermediate and low-risk groups. Neuroblastoma is diagnosed primarily based on histological assays, biochemical testing and imaging, biopsy and bone marrow aspiration. Treatments associated with neuroblastoma generally include surgery, radiation therapy, consolidation therapy, maintenance therapy and induction therapy. Research on the course of neuroblastoma has long concentrated on the role of oncogene amplification of *MYCN* and the involvement of other genetic changes. The role of tumor microenvironment (TME) is increasingly acknowledged in the development of neuroblastoma; therefore, for improving current and new immunotherapeutic strategies against this pediatric cancer a thorough understanding of the TME of NB is essential.

References

1. Steliarova-Foucher E, Colombet M, Ries LA, Moreno F, Dolya A, Bray F, Hesseling P, Shin HY, Stiller CA, Bouzbid S, Hamdi-Cherif M. International incidence of childhood cancer, 2001–2010: a population-based registry study. Lancet Oncol. 2017;18(6):719–31.
2. Temple WC, Vo KT, Matthay KK, Balliu B, Coleman C, Michlitsch J, Phelps A, Behr S, Zapala MA. Association of image-defined risk factors with clinical features, histopathology, and outcomes in neuroblastoma. Cancer Med. 2021;10(7):2232–41.
3. Brodeur GM. Neuroblastoma: biological insights into a clinical enigma. Nat Rev Cancer. 2003;3(3):203–16.
4. Irwin MS, Park JR. Neuroblastoma: paradigm for precision medicine. Pediatr Clin. 2015;62(1):225–56.
5. Bosse KR, Maris JM. Advances in the translational genomics of neuroblastoma: from improving risk stratification and revealing novel biology to identifying actionable genomic alterations. Cancer. 2016;122(1):20–33.
6. Matthay KK, Maris JM, Schleiermacher G, Nakagawara A, Mackall CL, Diller L, Weiss WA. Neuroblastoma (primer). Nat Rev Dis Primers. 2016;2(1):16078.
7. Ward E, DeSantis C, Robbins A, Kohler B, Jemal A. Childhood and adolescent cancer statistics, 2014. CA Cancer J Clin. 2014;64(2):83–103.
8. Wienke J, Dierselhuis MP, Tytgat GA, Künkele A, Nierkens S, Molenaar JJ. The immune landscape of neuroblastoma: challenges and opportunities for novel therapeutic strategies in pediatric oncology. Eur J Cancer. 2021;144:123–50.
9. Tas ML, Reedijk AM, Karim-Kos HE, Kremer LC, Van de Ven CP, Dierselhuis MP, Van Eijkelenburg NK, van Grotel M, Kraal KC, Peek AM, Coebergh JW. Neuroblastoma between 1990 and 2014 in The Netherlands: increased incidence and improved survival of high-risk neuroblastoma. Eur J Cancer. 2020;124:47–55.
10. Swift CC, Eklund MJ, Kraveka JM, Alazraki AL. Updates in diagnosis, management, and treatment of neuroblastoma. Radiographics. 2018;38(2):566–80.
11. Karalexi MA, Katsimpris A, Panagopoulou P, Bouka P, Schüz J, Ntzani E, Petridou ET, Servitzoglou M, Baka M, Moschovi M, Kourti M. Maternal lifestyle factors and risk of neuroblastoma in the offspring: a meta-analysis including Greek NARECHEM-ST primary data. Cancer Epidemiol. 2022;77:102055.
12. Kamihara J, Bourdeaut F, Foulkes WD, Molenaar JJ, Mossé YP, Nakagawara A, Parareda A, Scollon SR, Schneider KW, Skalet AH, States LJ. Retinoblastoma and neuroblastoma predisposition and surveillance. Clin Cancer Res. 2017;23(13):e98–106.
13. Mossé YP, Laudenslager M, Longo L, Cole KA, Wood A, Attiyeh EF, Laquaglia MJ, Sennett R, Lynch JE, Perri P, Laureys G. Identification of ALK as a major familial neuroblastoma predisposition gene. Nature. 2008;455(7215):930–5.
14. Zhang J, Walsh MF, Wu G, Edmonson MN, Gruber TA, Easton J, Hedges D, Ma X, Zhou X, Yergeau DA, Wilkinson MR. Germline mutations in predisposition genes in pediatric cancer. N Engl J Med. 2015;373(24):2336–46.
15. Ackermann S, Cartolano M, Hero B, Welte A, Kahlert Y, Roderwieser A, Bartenhagen C, Walter E, Gecht J, Kerschke L, Volland R. A mechanistic classification of clinical phenotypes in neuroblastoma. Science. 2018;362(6419):1165–70.
16. Peifer M, Hertwig F, Roels F, Dreidax D, Gartlgruber M, Menon R, Krämer A, Roncaioli JL, Sand F, Heuckmann JM, Ikram F. Telomerase activation by genomic rearrangements in high-risk neuroblastoma. Nature. 2015;526(7575):700–4.
17. Pugh TJ, Morozova O, Attiyeh EF, Asgharzadeh S, Wei JS, Auclair D, Carter SL, Cibulskis K, Hanna M, Kiezun A, Kim J. The genetic landscape of high-risk neuroblastoma. Nat Genet. 2013;45(3):279–84.
18. Moore SW. The contribution of associated congenital anomalies in understanding Hirschsprung's disease. Pediatr Surg Int. 2006;22:305–15.

19. Kratz CP, Franke L, Peters H, Kohlschmidt N, Kazmierczak B, Finckh U, Bier A, Eichhorn B, Blank C, Kraus C, Kohlhase J. Cancer spectrum and frequency among children with Noonan, Costello, and cardio-facio-cutaneous syndromes. Br J Cancer. 2015;112(8):1392–7.
20. Maas SM, Vansenne F, Kadouch DJ, Ibrahim A, Bliek J, Hopman S, Mannens MM, Merks JH, Maher ER, Hennekam RC. Phenotype, cancer risk, and surveillance in Beckwith–Wiedemann syndrome depending on molecular genetic subgroups. Am J Med Genet A. 2016;170(9):2248–60.
21. Mussa A, Molinatto C, Baldassarre G, Riberi E, Russo S, Larizza L, Riccio A, Ferrero GB. Cancer risk in Beckwith–Wiedemann syndrome: a systematic review and meta-analysis outlining a novel (epi) genotype specific histotype targeted screening protocol. J Pediatr. 2016;176:142–9.
22. Overman RE, Kartal TT, Cunningham AJ, Fialkowski EA, Naik-Mathuria BJ, Vasudevan SA, Malek MM, Kalsi R, Le HD, Stafford LC, Lautz TB. Optimization of percutaneous biopsy for diagnosis and pretreatment risk assessment of neuroblastoma. Pediatr Blood Cancer. 2020;67(5):e28153.
23. LaBrosse EH, Com-Nougué C, Zucker JM, Comoy E, Bohuon C, Lemerle J, Schweisguth O. Urinary excretion of 3-methoxy-4-hydroxymandelic acid and 3-methoxy-4-hydroxyphenylacetic acid by 288 patients with neuroblastoma and related neural crest tumors. Cancer Res. 1980;40(6):1995–2001.
24. Dumba M, Jawad N, McHugh K. Neuroblastoma and nephroblastoma: a radiological review. Cancer Imaging. 2015;15:1–4.
25. Vik TA, Pfluger T, Kadota R, Castel V, Tulchinsky M, Farto JA, Heiba S, Serafini A, Tumeh S, Khutoryansky N, Jacobson AF. 123I-mIBG scintigraphy in patients with known or suspected neuroblastoma: results from a prospective multicenter trial. Pediatr Blood Cancer. 2009;52(7):784–90.
26. Brady SW, Liu Y, Ma X, Gout AM, Hagiwara K, Zhou X, Wang J, Macias M, Chen X, Easton J, Mulder HL. Pan-neuroblastoma analysis reveals age-and signature-associated driver alterations. Nat Commun. 2020;11(1):5183.
27. Brisse HJ, McCarville MB, Granata C, Krug KB, Wootton-Gorges SL, Kanegawa K, Giammarile F, Schmidt M, Shulkin BL, Matthay KK, Lewington VJ. Guidelines for imaging and staging of neuroblastic tumors: consensus report from the International Neuroblastoma Risk Group Project. Radiology. 2011;261(1):243–57.
28. Brodeur GM, Pritchard J, Berthold F, Carlsen NL, Castel V, Castelberry RP, De Bernardi B, Evans AE, Favrot M, Hedborg F. Revisions of the international criteria for neuroblastoma diagnosis, staging, and response to treatment. J Clin Oncol. 1993;11(8):1466–77.
29. Monclair T, Brodeur GM, Ambros PF, Brisse HJ, Cecchetto G, Holmes K, Kaneko M, London WB, Matthay KK, Nuchtern JG, Von Schweinitz D. The international neuroblastoma risk group (INRG) staging system: an INRG task force report. J Clin Oncol. 2009;27(2):298.
30. Alexander F. Neuroblastoma. Urol Clin N Am. 2000;27(3):383–92.
31. Schulte JH, Eggert A. Neuroblastoma. Crit Rev Oncog. 2015;20(3–4):245–70.
32. Ahmed AA, Zhang L, Reddivalla N, Hetherington M. Neuroblastoma in children: update on clinicopathologic and genetic prognostic factors. Pediatr Hematol Oncol. 2017;34(3):165–85.
33. Shimada H. International neuroblastoma pathology classification. Pathology. 2012;44(1): S11–2.
34. Karaosmanoglu B, Kocaefe ÇY, Söylemezoğlu F, Anlar B, Varan A, Vargel İ, Ayter S. Heightened CXCR4 and CXCL12 expression in NF1-associated neurofibromas. Childs Nerv Syst. 2018;34:877–82.
35. Ollé Hurtado M, Wolbert J, Fisher J, Flutter B, Stafford S, Barton J, Jain N, Barone G, Majani Y, Anderson J. Tumor infiltrating lymphocytes expanded from pediatric neuroblastoma display heterogeneity of phenotype and function. PLoS One. 2019;14(8):e0216373.
36. Song L, Asgharzadeh S, Salo J, Engell K, Wu HW, Sposto R, Ara T, Silverman AM, DeClerck YA, Seeger RC, Metelitsa LS. Vα24-invariant NKT cells mediate antitumor activity via killing of tumor-associated macrophages. J Clin Invest. 2009;119(6):1524–36.

37. Metelitsa LS, Wu HW, Wang H, Yang Y, Warsi Z, Asgharzadeh S, Groshen S, Wilson SB, Seeger RC. Natural killer T cells infiltrate neuroblastomas expressing the chemokine CCL2. J Exp Med. 2004;199(9):1213–21.
38. Shiloh Y, Shipley J, Brodeur GM, Bruns G, Korf B, Donlon T, Schreck RR, Seeger R, Sakai K, Latt SA. Differential amplification, assembly, and relocation of multiple DNA sequences in human neuroblastomas and neuroblastoma cell lines. Proc Natl Acad Sci. 1985;82(11):3761–5.
39. Bagatell R, Beck-Popovic M, London WB, Zhang Y, Pearson AD, Matthay KK, Monclair T, Ambros PF, Cohn SL. Significance of MYCN amplification in international neuroblastoma staging system stage 1 and 2 neuroblastoma: a report from the International Neuroblastoma Risk Group Database. J Clin Oncol. 2009;27(3):365.
40. Ambros PF, Ambros IM, Brodeur GM, Haber M, Khan J, Nakagawara A, Schleiermacher G, Speleman F, Spitz R, London WB, Cohn SL. International consensus for neuroblastoma molecular diagnostics: report from the International Neuroblastoma Risk Group (INRG) Biology Committee. Br J Cancer. 2009;100(9):1471–82.
41. Slyper M, Porter CB, Ashenberg O, Waldman J, Drokhlyansky E, Wakiro I, Smillie C, Smith-Rosario G, Wu J, Dionne D, Vigneau S. A single-cell and single-nucleus RNA-Seq toolbox for fresh and frozen human tumors. Nat Med. 2020;26(5):792–802.
42. Coughlin CM, Fleming MD, Carroll RG, Pawel BR, Hogarty MD, Shan X, Vance BA, Cohen JN, Jairaj S, Lord EM, Wexler MH. Immunosurveillance and survivin-specific T-cell immunity in children with high-risk neuroblastoma. J Clin Oncol. 2006;24(36):5725–34.
43. Facchetti P, Prigione I, Ghiotto F, Tasso P, Garaventa A, Pistoia V. Functional and molecular characterization of tumour-infiltrating lymphocytes and clones thereof from a major-histocompatibility-complex-negative human tumour: neuroblastoma. Cancer Immunol Immunother. 1996;42:170–8.
44. Carlson LM, De Geer A, Sveinbjørnsson B, Orrego A, Martinsson T, Kogner P, Levitskaya J. The microenvironment of human neuroblastoma supports the activation of tumor-associated T lymphocytes. Onco Targets Ther. 2013;2(3):e23618.
45. Camisaschi C, Renne SL, Beretta V, Rini F, Spagnuolo RD, Tuccitto A, Podda MG, Parmiani G, Rivoltini L, Collini P, Castelli C. Immune landscape and in vivo immunogenicity of NY-ESO-1 tumor antigen in advanced neuroblastoma patients. BMC Cancer. 2018;18(1):1.
46. Zhong X, Zhang Y, Wang L, Zhang H, Liu H, Liu Y. Cellular components in tumor microenvironment of neuroblastoma and the prognostic value. PeerJ. 2019;7:e8017.
47. Huang M, Weiss WA. Neuroblastoma and MYCN. Cold Spring Harb Perspect Med. 2013;3(10):a014415.
48. Westermark UK, Wilhelm M, Frenzel A, Henriksson MA. The MYCN oncogene and differentiation in neuroblastoma. In: Seminars in cancer biology, vol. 21. Academic Press; 2011. p. 256–66.
49. Wang M, Zhou C, Sun Q, Cai R, Li Y, Wang D, Gong L. ALK amplification and protein expression predict inferior prognosis in neuroblastomas. Exp Mol Pathol. 2013;95(2):124–30.
50. Subramaniam MM, Piqueras M, Navarro S, Noguera R. Aberrant copy numbers of ALK gene is a frequent genetic alteration in neuroblastomas. Hum Pathol. 2009;40(11):1638–42.
51. Carén H, Abel F, Kogner P, Martinsson T. High incidence of DNA mutations and gene amplifications of the ALK gene in advanced sporadic neuroblastoma tumours. Biochem J. 2008;416(2):153–9.
52. Bourdeaut F, Ferrand S, Brugières L, Hilbert M, Ribeiro A, Lacroix L, Bénard J, Combaret V, Michon J, Valteau-Couanet D, Isidor B. ALK germline mutations in patients with neuroblastoma: a rare and weakly penetrant syndrome. Eur J Hum Genet. 2012;20(3):291–7.
53. Kwon MJ, Choi YL, Sung KW, Kang SY, Park SM, Choi SY, Kim JS, Suh YL. Oncogenic anaplastic lymphoma kinase (ALK) mutation in neuroblastomas and other pediatric tumors. Pathol Res Pract. 2011;207(10):634–9.
54. George RE, London WB, Cohn SL, Maris JM, Kretschmar C, Diller L, Brodeur GM, Castleberry RP, Look AT. Hyperdiploidy plus nonamplified MYCN confers a favorable prognosis in children 12–18 months old with disseminated neuroblastoma: a pediatric oncology group study. J Clin Oncol. 2005;23(27):6466–73.

55. Schleiermacher G, Michon J, Huon I, d'Enghien CD, Klijanienko J, Brisse H, Ribeiro A, Mosseri V, Rubie H, Munzer C, Thomas C. Chromosomal CGH identifies patients with a higher risk of relapse in neuroblastoma without MYCN amplification. Br J Cancer. 2007;97(2):238–46.
56. Attiyeh EF, London WB, Mossé YP, Wang Q, Winter C, Khazi D, McGrady PW, Seeger RC, Look AT, Shimada H, Brodeur GM. Chromosome 1p and 11q deletions and outcome in neuroblastoma. N Engl J Med. 2005;353(21):2243–53.
57. Spitz R, Hero B, Ernestus K, Berthold F. Deletions in chromosome arms 3p and 11q are new prognostic markers in localized and 4s neuroblastoma. Clin Cancer Res. 2003;9(1):52–8.
58. Caron H, van Sluis P, de Kraker J, Bökkerink J, Egeler M, Laureys G, Slater R, Westerveld A, Voute PA, Versteeg R. Allelic loss of chromosome 1p as a predictor of unfavorable outcome in patients with neuroblastoma. N Engl J Med. 1996;334(4):225–30.
59. Sausen M, Leary RJ, Jones S, Wu J, Reynolds CP, Liu X, Blackford A, Parmigiani G, Diaz LA Jr, Papadopoulos N, Vogelstein B. Integrated genomic analyses identify ARID1A and ARID1B alterations in the childhood cancer neuroblastoma. Nat Genet. 2013;45(1):12–7.
60. Li C, Xu ZL, Zhao Z, An Q, Wang L, Yu Y, Piao DX. ARID1A gene knockdown promotes neuroblastoma migration and invasion. Neoplasma. 2017;64(3):367–76.
61. Oldridge DA, Wood AC, Weichert-Leahey N, Crimmins I, Sussman R, Winter C, McDaniel LD, Diamond M, Hart LS, Zhu S, Durbin AD. Genetic predisposition to neuroblastoma mediated by a LMO1 super-enhancer polymorphism. Nature. 2015;528(7582):418–21.
62. Wang K, Diskin SJ, Zhang H, Attiyeh EF, Winter C, Hou C, Schnepp RW, Diamond M, Bosse K, Mayes PA, Glessner J. Integrative genomics identifies LMO1 as a neuroblastoma oncogene. Nature. 2011;469(7329):216–20.
63. Bagatell R, Cohn SL. Genetic discoveries and treatment advances in neuroblastoma. Curr Opin Pediatr. 2016;28(1):19.
64. Bernards R. Unlikely suspects identified in neuroblastoma conspiracy. Cancer Discov. 2014;4(4):392–3.
65. Ejeskär K, Krona C, Carén H, Zaibak F, Li L, Martinsson T, Ioannou PA. Introduction of in vitro transcribed ENO1 mRNA into neuroblastoma cells induces cell death. BMC Cancer. 2005;5:1–4.
66. De Mariano M, Gallesio R, Chierici M, Furlanello C, Conte M, Garaventa A, Croce M, Ferrini S, Tonini GP, Longo L. Identification of GALNT14 as a novel neuroblastoma predisposition gene. Oncotarget. 2015;6(28):26335.
67. Maris JM, Weiss MJ, Mosse Y, Hii G, Guo C, White PS, Hogarty MD, Mirensky T, Brodeur GM, Rebbeck TR, Urbanek M. Evidence for a hereditary neuroblastoma predisposition locus at chromosome 16p12–13. Cancer Res. 2002;62(22):6651–8.
68. Chi R, Chen X, Liu M, Zhang H, Li F, Fan X, Wang W, Lu H. Role of SNHG7-miR-653-5p-STAT2 feedback loop in regulating neuroblastoma progression. J Cell Physiol. 2019;234(8):13403–12.
69. Whittle SB, Smith V, Doherty E, Zhao S, McCarty S, Zage PE. Overview and recent advances in the treatment of neuroblastoma. Expert Rev Anticancer Ther. 2017;17(4):369–86.
70. De Bernardi B, Mosseri V, Rubie H, Castel V, Foot A, Ladenstein R, Laureys G, Beck-Popovic M, De Lacerda AF, Pearson AD, De Kraker J. Treatment of localised resectable neuroblastoma. Results of the LNESG1 study by the SIOP Europe Neuroblastoma Group. Br J Cancer. 2008;99(7):1027–33.
71. Strother DR, London WB, Schmidt ML, Brodeur GM, Shimada H, Thorner P, Collins MH, Tagge E, Adkins S, Reynolds CP, Murray K. Outcome after surgery alone or with restricted use of chemotherapy for patients with low-risk neuroblastoma: results of Children's Oncology Group study P9641. J Clin Oncol. 2012;30(15):1842.
72. Nuchtern JG, London WB, Barnewolt CE, Naranjo A, McGrady PW, Geiger JD, Diller L, Schmidt ML, Maris JM, Cohn SL, Shamberger RC. A prospective study of expectant observation as primary therapy for neuroblastoma in young infants, a children's oncology group study. Ann Surg. 2012;256(4):573.
73. Pearson AD, Pinkerton CR, Lewis IJ, Imeson J, Ellershaw C, Machin D. High-dose rapid and standard induction chemotherapy for patients aged over 1 year with stage 4 neuroblastoma: a randomised trial. Lancet Oncol. 2008;9(3):247–56.

74. Yu AL, Gilman AL, Ozkaynak MF, London WB, Kreissman SG, Chen HX, Smith M, Anderson B, Villablanca JG, Matthay KK, Shimada H. Anti-GD2 antibody with GM-CSF, interleukin-2, and isotretinoin for neuroblastoma. N Engl J Med. 2010;363(14):1324–34.
75. Grupp SA, Cohn SL, Wall D, Reynolds PC, Hematopoietic Stem Cell Transplant Discipline and the Neuroblastoma Disease Committee, Children's Oncology Group. Collection, storage, and infusion of stem cells in children with high-risk neuroblastoma: saving for a rainy day. Pediatr Blood Cancer. 2006;46(7):719–22.
76. Fish JD, Grupp S. Stem cell transplantation for neuroblastoma. Bone Marrow Transplant. 2008;41(2):159–65.
77. Ladenstein R, Pötschger U, Pearson AD, Brock P, Luksch R, Castel V, Yaniv I, Papadakis V, Laureys G, Malis J, Balwierz W. Busulfan and melphalan versus carboplatin, etoposide, and melphalan as high-dose chemotherapy for high-risk neuroblastoma (HR-NBL1/SIOPEN): an international, randomised, multi-arm, open-label, phase 3 trial. Lancet Oncol. 2017;18(4):500–14.
78. Kushner BH, Ostrovnaya I, Cheung IY, Kuk D, Modak S, Kramer K, Roberts SS, Basu EM, Yataghene K, Cheung NK. Lack of survival advantage with autologous stem-cell transplantation in high-risk neuroblastoma consolidated by anti-GD2 immunotherapy and isotretinoin. Oncotarget. 2016;7(4):4155.
79. Matthay KK, Yanik G, Messina J, Quach A, Huberty J, Cheng SC, Veatch J, Goldsby R, Brophy P, Kersun LS, Hawkins RA. Phase II study on the effect of disease sites, age, and prior therapy on response to iodine-131-metaiodobenzylguanidine therapy in refractory neuroblastoma. J Clin Oncol. 2007;25(9):1054–60.
80. Cheung NK, Cheung IY, Kushner BH, Ostrovnaya I, Chamberlain E, Kramer K, Modak S. Murine anti-GD2 monoclonal antibody 3F8 combined with granulocyte-macrophage colony-stimulating factor and 13-*cis*-retinoic acid in high-risk patients with stage 4 neuroblastoma in first remission. J Clin Oncol. 2012;30(26):3264.
81. Geerts D, Koster J, Albert D, Koomoa DL, Feith DJ, Pegg AE, Volckmann R, Caron H, Versteeg R, Bachmann AS. The polyamine metabolism genes ornithine decarboxylase and antizyme 2 predict aggressive behavior in neuroblastomas with and without MYCN amplification. Int J Cancer. 2010;126(9):2012–24.
82. Lewis EC, Kraveka JM, Ferguson W, Eslin D, Brown VI, Bergendahl G, Roberts W, Wada RK, Oesterheld J, Mitchell D, Foley J. A subset analysis of a phase II trial evaluating the use of DFMO as maintenance therapy for high-risk neuroblastoma. Int J Cancer. 2020;147(11):3152–9.
83. Hawkins DS, Bradfield S, Whitlock JA, Krailo M, Franklin J, Blaney SM, Adamson PC, Reaman G. Topotecan by 21-day continuous infusion in children with relapsed or refractory solid tumors: a Children's Oncology Group study. Pediatr Blood Cancer. 2006;47(6):790–4.
84. Bomgaars LR, Bernstein M, Krailo M, Kadota R, Das S, Chen Z, Adamson PC, Blaney SM. Phase II trial of irinotecan in children with refractory solid tumors: a Children's Oncology Group study. J Clin Oncol. 2007;25(29):4622–7.
85. Blaney S, Berg SL, Pratt C, Weitman S, Sullivan J, Luchtman-Jones L, Bernstein M. A phase I study of irinotecan in pediatric patients: a pediatric oncology group study. Clin Cancer Res. 2001;7(1):32–7.
86. DuBois SG, Marachelian A, Fox E, Kudgus RA, Reid JM, Groshen S, Malvar J, Bagatell R, Wagner L, Maris JM, Hawkins R. Phase I study of the Aurora A kinase inhibitor alisertib in combination with irinotecan and temozolomide for patients with relapsed or refractory neuroblastoma: a NANT (new approaches to neuroblastoma therapy) trial. J Clin Oncol. 2016;34(12):1368.
87. Peirce SK, Findley HW, Prince C, Dasgupta A, Cooper T, Durden DL. The PI-3 kinase-Akt-MDM2-survivin signaling axis in high-risk neuroblastoma: a target for PI-3 kinase inhibitor intervention. Cancer Chemother Pharmacol. 2011;68:325–35.
88. Sholler GL, Brard L, Straub JA, Dorf L, Illyene S, Koto K, Kalkunte S, Bosenberg M, Ashikaga T, Nishi R. Nifurtimox induces apoptosis of neuroblastoma cells in vitro and in vivo. J Pediatr Hematol Oncol. 2009;31(3):187.

GPSR Compliance

The European Union's (EU) General Product Safety Regulation (GPSR) is a set of rules that requires consumer products to be safe and our obligations to ensure this.

If you have any concerns about our products, you can contact us on ProductSafety@springernature.com

In case Publisher is established outside the EU, the EU authorized representative is:

Springer Nature Customer Service Center GmbH
Europaplatz 3
69115 Heidelberg, Germany

Batch number: 10732090

Printed by Printforce, the Netherlands